The Pharmacology Companion

A study guide for students by students

Gary Gallia
MD, PhD Student
Jefferson Medical College
Philadelphia, Pennsylvania

Christine Hann
MD, PhD Student
Jefferson Medical College
Philadelphia, Pennsylvania

William Hewson
Medical Student
Jefferson Medical College
Philadelphia, Pennsylvania

ISBN # 0-9640124-3-X

Notice: the authors have taken care to make certain that the information contained within this book is accurate and up to date. Nonetheless, as the field of medicine is constantly changing, the reader is advised to carefully consult the instructions and information included in the package insert of each drug before treating patients. This book is intended to help with the class, medical pharmacology, and is NOT intended to be a treatment guide.

The authors and publisher disclaim any liability, loss, injury or damage incurred as a consequence, directly or indirectly, of the use or application of this book.

Send all inquiries to:

Alert and Oriented Publishing
616 Church Street, #3
Ann Arbor, MI 48104
1-888-ALERT-44

or

visit our web site at:
www.ALERTandONLINE.com

IV. The Cardiovascular System

V. Antimicrobial Drugs

VI. Cancer Chemotherapy

VII. Endocrine Drugs

VIII. Anti-inflammatory Drugs

Introduction

As was the case for our colleagues and friends who brought you *The Microbiology Companion*, Joel Topf and Sarah Faubel, we were often frustrated with the way in which volumes of medical school facts were presented to us. Our goal in writing *The Pharmacology Companion* was to create an easy, quick reference of all the drugs you will be responsible for in medical pharmacology. Each medically important agent is presented in an easy-to-scan table with all of the important facts. This will save you the frustration of wading through volumes of pharmobabble searching for the pertinent information. The book is laid out in a format which we felt was most useful in studying for medical pharmacology courses and step I of the USMLE. It is our hope that this book will save you time and energy as you study pharmacology.

We tried to provide a framework by categorizing and grouping the therapeutic agents as logically as possible. Additionally, we provided the brand names of the drugs which may or may not be important in your course, but will undoubtedly be important once you start working in the hospital. Different courses may emphasize certain drugs or additional information, so we have provided space for you to add pertinent notes and remarks made by your professors and for new agents which will be introduced after the publication of this edition.

Think of this book as a prearranged notebook. Take it with you everywhere, wherever you'll have even a few minutes to glance at some of the pages. With time, you will find that you can recall the information by visualizing the page.

We are confident that this book will help you throughout your pharmacology course, as well as prepare you for step I of the USMLE. We've worked hard to make this book user friendly, organized and as mistake-free as possible. Please let us know if the book has been useful to you (feel free to let next year's class know too). If you do find any mistakes or have any suggestions on how to make it better we'd like to hear from you. You may reach us at the following email addresses

Gary: galliag@jeflin.tju.edu
Christine: hannc@jeflin.tju.edu
William: hewsonw@jeflin.tju.edu

or you may call our cool publisher, Joel Smith at
1-888-ALERT-44

or contact him at the Alert & Oriented web site:
www.ALERTandONLINE.com

Contributing Author:

Juan Aponte
Medical Student
University of Medicine and Dentistry of New Jersey
Wrote the original draft of the Antimicrobial Drugs

Computer Graphics/Illustrations:

Stacey Broers
staceyb24@aol.com

Acknowledgments:

We would especially like to thank Joel Smith, a JD/MBA student at the University of Michigan, who runs Alert and Oriented Publishing Company. Joel has tirelessly worked with us in every aspect of this publication.

We would like to thank Sarah Faubel, a resident at the University of Colorado and Joel Topf, a resident at Indiana University/Purdue University for their advice, suggestions and review of our material.

We would like to thank Robin Bartlett for contractural advice. We would also like to thank Minturn Wright, Richard Hornstein, Anita Fore and Jayne Skrzysowski.

We would also like to acknowledge the Pharmacology Department of Jefferson Medical College, especially Dr. Anthony Triolo and Dr. Wolfgang Vogel. Others we wish to thank include Dr. Anthony Sorrentino, Rene Guerster, Steve Dunn, Drs. Hann, Mr. and Mrs. Louis Gallia, Dr. and Mrs. James S. Hewson and Dr. Catherine Hu.

Dedication:

We wish to dedicate this book to our families and friends (if they're still talking to us) who endlessly supported and encouraged us during the development of this book.

References:

Hardman JG, Limbird LE, Molinoff, PB, and Ruddon RW (eds). *Goodman & Gilman's The Pharmacological Basis of Therapeutics* (9th ed). New York: Permagon, 1996.

Katzung BG (ed). *Basic and Clinical Pharmacology* (6th ed). Norwalk: Appleton & Lange, 1995.

USPDI. *Drug Information for the Health Care Professional* (16th ed). Taunton: Rand McNally, 1996.

Abbreviations used in the text

ACE	angiotensin converting enzyme
ACh	acetylcholine
ACTH	adrenocorticotropin
ADH	antidiuretic hormone (vasopressin)
ADHD	attention deficit hyperactivity disorder
AIDS	acquired immunodeficiency syndrome
ALL	acute lymphoblastic leukemia
AML	acute myelogenous leukemia
ANS	autonomic nervous system
AV	atrioventricular
AZT	Zidovudine
BCG	Bacillus Calmette-Guerin
BP	blood pressure
cAMP	cyclic adenosine 3',5'-monophosphate
CCNS	cell cycle nonspecific
CCS	cell cycle specific
cGMP	cyclic guanosine monophosphate
CHF	congestive heart failure
CML	chronic myelogenous leukemia
CMV	Cytomegalovirus
CNS	central nervous system
CO	carbon monoxide
CO	cardiac output
CO_2	carbon dioxide
CRH	corticotropin releasing hormone
CSF	cerebral spinal fluid
CT	calcitonin
CV	cardiovascular
DAG	diacylglycerol
DCT	distal convoluted tubule
ddC	Zalcitabine
ddI	Didanosine
DHEA	dehydroepiandrosterone
DHFR	dihydrofolate reductase
DHT	dihydrotestosterone
DIT	diiodotyrosine
DNA	deoxyribonucleic acid
DOC	drug of choice
EBV	Ebstein-Barr virus
FSH	follicle stimulating hormone
G6PD	glucose-6-phosphate dehydrogenase
GABA	gamma-aminobutyric acid
GFR	glomerular filtration rate
GH	growth hormone
GI	gastrointestinal
GnRH	gonadotropin releasing hormone
GU	genitourinary
H_2O	water
hCG	human chorionic gonadotropin
HDL	high density lipoprotein
HIV	human immunodeficiency virus
HR	heart rate
hrs	hours
IA	intra-arterial
IDDM	insulin-dependent diabetes mellitus
IL	interleukin
IM	intramuscular
INH	isoniazid
IP_3	inositol 1,4,5-triphosphate
IT	intrathecal
IV	intravenous
LDL	low density lipoprotein
LH	luteinizing hormone
LSD	lysergic acid diethylamide
MAC	minimum alveolar concentration
MI	myocardial infarction

min	minutes
MIT	monoiodotyrosine
MOA	mechanism of action
MAO	monoamine oxidase
MRSA	methicillin resistant *Staphylococcus aureus*
N_2O	nitrous oxide
NE	norepinephrine
NIDDM	non-insulin-dependent diabetes mellitus
NO	nitric oxide
NO_2	nitrogen dioxide
O_2	oxygen
PABA	para-amino benzoic acid
PCN	penicillin
PCP	phencyclidine
PCT	proximal convoluted tubule
PDA	patent ductus arteriosus
PDE	phosphodiesterase
PG	prostaglandins
PIP_2	phosphatidylinositol 4,5-diphosphate
PNS	peripheral nervous system
PO	by mouth
PR	per rectum
PR	peripheral resistance
PTH	parathyroid hormone
PTU	propylthiouracil
PUD	peptic ulcer disease
PVR	peripheral vascular resistance
RDA	recommended daily allowance
RER	rough endoplasmic reticulum
RNA	ribonucleic acid
SA	sinoatrial
SC	subcutaneous
sec	seconds
SLE	systemic lupus erythematosus
SO2	sulfur dioxide
SSRI	selective serotonin reuptake inhibitors
$t_{1/2}$	half-life
T3	thyroxine
T4	triiodothyronine
TALH	thin ascending loop of Henle
TBG	thyroxine binding globulin
TBPA	thyroxine binding prealbumin
TCA	tricyclic antidepressants
TPO	thyroperoxidase
TRH	thyrotropin releasing hormone
TxA_2	thromboxane
UTI	urinary tract infection
VLDL	very low density lipoprotein
wks	weeks
XO	xanthine oxidase

Introduction

Introduction to Pharmacology

Pharmacology is the study of the relationship between chemical agents and biological systems. It is an extensive field of study which attempts to understand the properties, effects, mechanisms of action, absorption, distribution, metabolism, excretion, as well as the toxic and therapeutic uses, of drugs.

The study of pharmacology is divided into four general areas:

Pharmacokinetics	Describes "what the body does to the drug." This includes the absorption, distribution, metabolism and excretion of drugs.
Pharmacodynamics	Describes "what the drug does to the body." Specifically, it deals with the biochemical and physiological effects of drugs, their characteristics and their mechanisms of action (receptors, agonists, antagonist).
Pharmacotherapeutics	Describes the clinical applications, contraindications and drug interactions useful for the diagnosis, prevention and treatment of disease.
Toxicology	Describes the adverse effects of therapeutic agents on the human body. This field of study also includes the effects of pollutants, poisons and other chemicals on biological systems.

Drugs are chemical agents or substances that affect biological systems.

Drug names	Valium® (diazepam, 7-chloro-1,3-dihydro-1-methyl-5-phenyl-2H-1,4-benzodiazepin-2-one) Valium® → *Brand name*; diazepam → *Generic name*; 7-chloro-1,3-dihydro-1-methyl-5-phenyl-2H-1,4-benzodiazepin-2-one → *Chemical name*
Drug chemistry	Most drugs are compounds of molecular weight between 100 and 1000 Da. Drugs may be solid, liquid or gaseous at room temperature; which state a drug is in often determines the optimal route of administration. Drugs commonly exert their effects by interacting with receptors, which in turn, activate cellular signalling pathways. Drug-receptor bonds may result from covalent, electrostatic or hydrophobic interactions. Rational drug design must take drug chemistry into consideration so that accurate predictions can be made with respect to the molecular structure and the receptors to which a drug binds.
Drug groups	There are thousands of drugs currently available in the US and throughout the world which have been arranged into approximately 70 groups. The members of each group of drugs often have many similar pharmacodynamic and pharmacokinetic properties.

Pharmacokinetics

Pharmacokinetics ("what the body does to the drug") is the study of how drugs move into, through and out of the body including delivery to their target site. Pharmacokinetics encompasses the principles of drug **absorption**, **distribution**, **metabolism** and **excretion**.

Absorption describes the method and rate at which a drug leaves the site of administration and the extent to which this occurs. It depends on the chemical and physical properties of the drug.

Term	Description	Associated Terms and Equations
Routes of administration	**Alimentary canal** routes are among the most common modes of administration. **Parental** (injection) routes usually provide a faster response than alimentary canal routes with accurate dosing to patients who are unconscious or vomiting. **Miscellaneous** routes	1. Oral (PO) 2. Sublingual 3. Buccal 4. Rectal (PR) 5. Intra-arterial (IA) 6. Intravenous (IV) 7. Intrathecal (IT) 8. Intramuscular (IM) 9. Subcutaneous (SC) 11. Respiratory/inhalation 12. Transdermal 13. Topical
Drug solubility	Absorption, distribution and excretion are all affected by drug solubility. Drug solubility is largely determined by charge. Most drugs are weak acids or weak bases and therefore can be ionized. **Lipophilic** drugs are uncharged species which are absorbed easily due to their ability to cross the lipid bilayer of cell membranes and the blood brain barrier. **Hydrophilic** drugs are charged species which are not absorbed easily due to an inability to cross cell membranes and are more readily excreted by the kidney.	The **Henderson-Hasselbalch equation** is used to determine the ionization state of a species at a given pH. $pH = pKa - \log(HA/A^-)$ HA = protonated drug concentration A^- = unprotonated drug concentration

Drug distribution refers to the process by which a drug leaves the systemic circulation and enters the interstitium and tissue cells. It is affected by the blood flow to the target tissue, capillary permeability and plasma protein binding of the drug. Entry of the drug into cells is called drug transport and is described below.

Term	Description	Associated Terms and Equations
Drug transport	Describes the movement of a drug from the site of administration to its target receptor.	There are four general modes of drug transport: 1. **Passive diffusion**: describes the movement of uncharged species down a concentration gradient according to Fick's Law of Diffusion. This is the most common mode of drug transport. 2. **Carrier-mediated (facilitated) diffusion**: describes the movement of drugs down a concentration gradient utilizing carrier proteins. 3. **Active transport**: describes the movement of drugs against a concentration gradient utilizing carrier proteins. This is a energy-consuming process typically in the form of **ATP**. 4. **Endocytosis**: describes the engulfment of drugs via invagination of cell membranes and subsequent release into the cytoplasm. **Fick's Law of Diffusion** measures the passive flux of molecules down a concentration gradient. $\text{Rate} = \frac{(C_1 - C_2) \times PC \times \text{Area}}{\text{Thickness}}$ C_1 = the higher concentration C_2 = the lower concentration PC = permeability coefficient: describes the mobility of a molecule within the medium Area = the area across the diffusion pathway Thickness = the diffusion path

Metabolism is the process by which drugs are chemically altered in the body. This often involves the conversion of lipid-soluble molecules to water-soluble metabolites, the latter of which can be excreted by the kidneys. Metabolism can also convert inactive drugs (prodrugs) to their active form or active drugs to active metabolites. There are two types of reactions: phase I and phase II. Factors affecting drug metabolism include genetics, sex, age, underlying diseases and concurrent use of other drugs.

Term	Description	Associated Terms and Equations
Phase I reactions	These reactions change the structure of the drug resulting in a more hydrophilic species. Most phase I reactions occur in the liver. There are 3 types of phase I reactions: oxidation, reduction and hydrolysis.	1. **Oxidation** (e.g., $C_6H_6 \rightarrow C_6H_5OH$) Usually carried out in the endoplasmic reticulum of hepatocytes by **cytochrome P_{450}** (microsomal mixed function oxidases). Many drugs are able to induce cytochrome P_{450} synthesis, increasing the metabolism of drugs affected by oxidative metabolism. Oxidation is the most common phase I reaction. 2. **Reduction** (e.g., $RNO_2 \rightarrow RNH_2$) This reaction is less common than oxidation and utilizes reductases in the endoplasmic reticulum and/or cytosol. 3. **Hydrolysis** (e.g., $RCO_2R \rightarrow RCO_2H + HOR$) This reaction is also less common than oxidation and utilizes esterases, amidases and related enzymes in hepatocytes and other tissues.
Phase II reactions	These conjugation reactions involve addition of an endogenous substrate to the drug which increases solubility and promotes elimination. These reactions may occur in the liver and other organs.	**Conjugation** reactions may add the following substrates to enhance drug elimination: Glucuronate Acetic acid Glutathione Sulfate
First pass effect	Describes the metabolism of an orally administered drug before it reaches the systemic circulation. The **liver** is the main organ of metabolism, however, other organs such as the kidneys, lung and brain may also contribute to this effect. When a high percentage of a drug is metabolized as it passes through the liver for the first time, less of the drug is available to the systemic circulation, and it is said to have a high "**first pass effect**."	

Elimination is the process by which a drug or metabolite is removed from the body. Elimination generally follows first-order or zero-order kinetics.

Term	Description	Associated Terms and Equations
Routes of elimination	Major routes of elimination include: 1. Kidney: most common route of elimination 2. Biliary tract 3. Intestine 4. Respiration 5. Breast milk 6. Skin	The route of elimination must be considered in patients with decreased organ function. The dose and drug of choice are particularly important in patients with kidney or liver failure.
First-order kinetics	Refers to drug elimination in which a **constant percentage** of substrate is metabolized per unit time. The enzymes are not saturated and the rate of elimination is proportional to the plasma concentration. The plasma drug concentration decreases in an exponential fashion. Most drugs used clinically show this type of elimination and have a characteristic **half-life** of elimination.	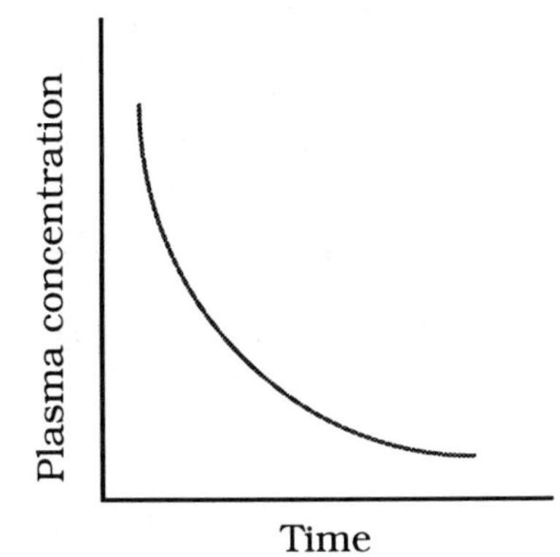
Zero-order kinetics	Refers to drug elimination in which a **constant amount** of drug is metabolized per unit time regardless of the drug concentration. The linear decrease of blood plasma concentration occurs because the enzymes are saturated. The best example of a substance with zero order kinetics is **alcohol**.	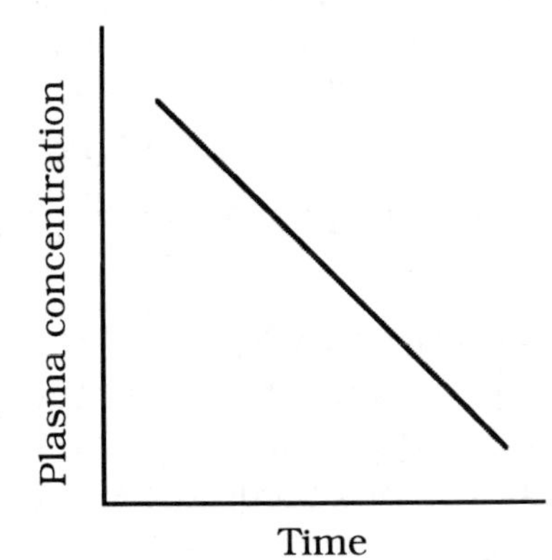

Drug dosing: the following terms and equations are important for learning and understanding drug dosing schedules and the steady state concentrations these schedules are designed to achieve.

Term	Description	Associated Terms and Equations
Bioavailability	The fraction of administered drug which reaches the systemic circulation. By definition bioavailability is 100% with IV administration.	Bioavailability is influenced by: 1. Extent of absorption 2. First pass effect
Half-life ($t_{1/2}$)	The time required to decrease the initial dose of drug by 50% (one half of original value). All drugs are decreased by 96% after 4 half-lives. The $t_{1/2}$ of a drug is important to: 1. Determine the dosing interval necessary to obtain the desired plasma concentration of drug. Generally, the dosing interval is the same as $t_{1/2}$. 2. Predict how long it will take a drug to reach steady-state levels. During multiple dosing or continuous IV infusion it takes approximately 4-5 half-lives to reach steady-state levels. 3. Predict how long it will take a drug concentration to decrease to a lower concentration. 4. Predict the accumulation of a drug in the body for a specific dosing interval.	The $t_{1/2}$ can be calculated using the following equations: $t_{1/2} = 0.693/Ke$ or $= (0.693)Vd/CL$ Ke = elimination rate constant Vd = volume of distribution CL = clearance
Volume of distribution (Vd)	The apparent volume into which a drug distributes and is defined as the ratio of the amount of drug in body tissue to its plasma concentration. The volume of distribution of a drug can be greater than total body volume. Vd is important in estimating the loading dose (D_L).	$Vd = \frac{\text{Total drug in the body}}{\text{Plasma concentration}}$
Clearance (CL)	The measure of the body's ability to eliminate a drug and is defined as the ratio of the rate of elimination of a drug to its plasma concentration. Drug clearance by a single organ is restricted by the blood flow to that organ, therefore hepatic clearance (CL_H) cannot exceed 1.5 L/min and renal clearance (CL_R) cannot exceed 1.2 L/min.	$CL = R/\text{Plasma Concentration}$ or $= Vd \times Ke$ R = rate of elimination Vd = volume of distribution Ke = elimination rate constant

Term	Description	Associated Terms and Equations
Loading dose (D_L)	The volume of distribution multiplied by the desired plasma concentration. A loading dose is sometimes used at the onset of therapy when the therapeutic concentration must be achieved rapidly and the volume of distribution is high. The loading dose is unchanged in patients who have impaired renal or hepatic function.	D_L = Vd x Plasma concentration
Maintenance dose (D_M)	The clearance of a drug multiplied by the desired plasma concentration. The maintenance dose is used to maintain the plasma concentration of a drug within a specific range over extended periods of time. The maintenance dose is decreased in patients who have impaired renal or hepatic function.	D_M = CL x Plasma concentration
Peak and trough concentrations	Describe the maximum and minimum plasma concentrations observed during dosing intervals.	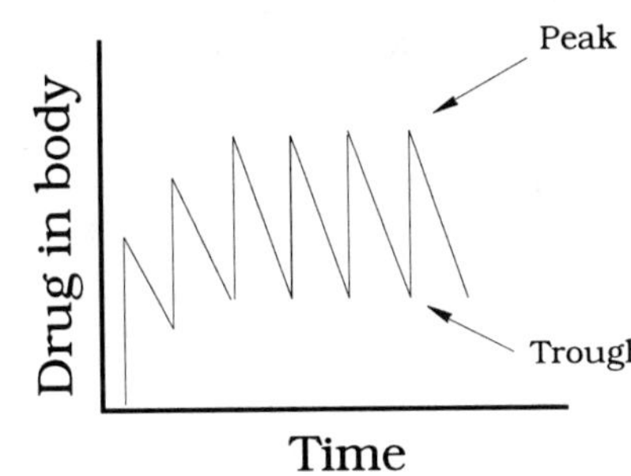
Steady state plasma concentration (Css)	Describes the point at which the rate of drug availability is equal to drug elimination. When the dosing interval is less than four half-lives, the drug accumulates in the body and eventually will reach a plateau. This plateau is referred to as the steady-state plasma concentration (Css) and is the point at which peak and trough levels are identical for each dosing interval. Drugs are commonly administered once every $t_{1/2}$ to achieve Css. During multiple dosing or continuous IV infusion it takes approximately 4-5 half-lives to achieve Css.	When same dose given every half-life: C_{ss} = 1.5 x Dose When same dose given at every second half-life: $C_{ss} = \frac{(1.5 \times Dose)}{2}$

Pharmacodynamics

Pharmacodynamics ("what the drug does to the body") is the study of the biochemical and physiological effects that drugs have on the human body. These are determined by **drug-receptor interactions**, **effector mechanisms** and **dose-response relationships**. These concepts explain the physiologic reactions which occur when a drug is administered as well as the actions of agonists and antagonists at certain receptors. Selected key concepts of drug-receptor interactions, effector mechanisms and dose-response relationships are described below.

Drug + Receptor → Drug-Receptor → Effector → Response

Drug-receptor interactions

Term	Description	Associated Terms and Equations
Receptor	A molecule which interacts with a ligand (drug) to mediate a pharmacologic effect. Receptors can be proteins, carbohydrates, nucleic acids or lipids. The two main functions of receptors are: 1) ligand (drug) **binding** and 2) **activation** of effector mechanisms.	Ligand binding is determined by: • **Affinity** - describes how strongly the drug and the receptor interact. This "attractiveness" depends on the structure of both the drug and receptor. Forces mediating this interaction include Van der Waals, ionic, hydrogen, hydrophobic and covalent bonds. • **Specificity** - refers to the selectivity a receptor has for a drug. This relationship is also dependent on structure and is analogous to the "lock and key" interaction of enzymes and their substrates.
Potency	The **amount** of drug necessary to **elicit a biological effect**. Drugs with greater potency are required in lower concentrations to produce the same effects as drugs with lesser potency. This parameter is determined by the affinity of the receptor for the drug. It is measured along the X-axis.	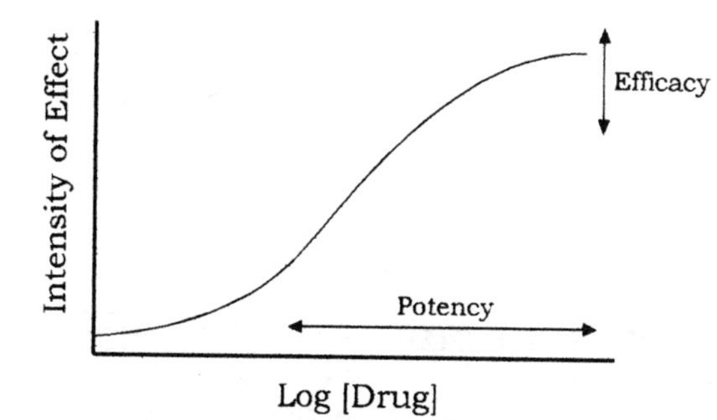
Efficacy	The **ability** of a drug to **produce a biological effect**. Drugs with greater efficacy produce greater biological effects than those with lesser efficacy. This parameter is determined by the ability of the drug-receptor interaction to activate effector mechanisms. It is measured along the Y-axis.	

Term	Description	Associated Terms and Equations
Agonists	Bind to receptors and activate effector mechanisms (elicit biological responses). There are two types of agonists: 1) **Full agonists** are drugs which produce 100% of the maximum biological response and are not dependent upon potency. 2) **Partial agonists** are drugs which produce less than 100% of the maximum biological response no matter how high the concentration. They are also not dependent upon potency.	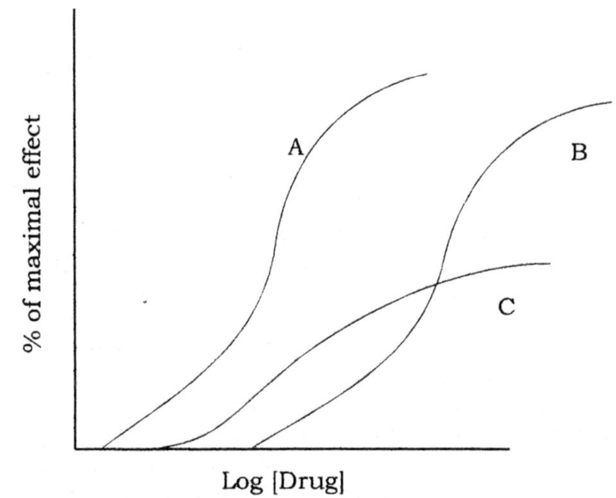 A = Full agonist B = Agonist with full efficacy and lower potency or Competitive antagonist C = Partial agonist or Noncompetitive antagonist
Antagonists	Bind to receptors, but do not activate effector mechanisms (do not produce biological effects). 1) **Competitive antagonists** bind **reversibly** to receptors at the same site as the native drug. They competitively prevent the native drug from binding to the receptor causing a blockade of effects. Graphically, this is observed as a **rightward shift** of the dose-response curve. The effects of competitive antagonists can be overcome by adding higher concentrations of the native drug. Because the same maximum response is attainable, competitive antagonists lower potency but have no effect on efficacy. 2) **Noncompetitive antagonists** bind **irreversibly** to either the same site as the native drug or to an alternative site. Binding to either of these sites block the effects of the native drug. Furthermore, increasing concentrations of the native drug has no effect. Since the interaction is irreversible, bound receptors are no longer available for activation. This lowers the efficacy, but has no effect on potency. Thus, in contrast to competitive inhibition, this interaction results in a **downward shift** of the dose-response curve with no potential for achieving maximum response. 3) **Physiologic antagonists** are drugs which antagonize the biological effects of a drug by binding to a different receptor. 4) **Chemical antagonists** interact with the drug being antagonized to remove it or prevent it from reaching its target.	

Effector mechanisms

Term	Description	Associated Terms and Equations
Effectors	Transduce drug-receptor interactions into cellular effects. There are four types of effector mechanisms that occur within the cell. A given drug works by a single type of effector mechanism. 1. **Intracellular receptors**: some drugs bind receptors within the cytosol or nucleus to form complexes which interact with DNA regulatory elements causing changes in gene expression. Examples include **thyroid** and **steroid hormones**. 2. **Transmembrane receptors**: contain an intracellular domain which possess enzymatic activity. Some drugs bind the extracellular domain of these receptors and activate the intracellular enzymatic activity. An example of this is **insulin** binding to the insulin receptor which stimulates tyrosine kinase activity. 3. **Ligand-gated ion channels**: some drugs bind these receptors and alter the conductance of ions through these channels. Drug binding can either increase or decrease the flow of ions. Examples include **acetylcholine** at nicotinic receptors, **benzodiazepines** at GABA receptors and **calcium channel blockers**. 4. **Receptors coupled to second messenger systems**: some drugs bind receptors which activate second messenger systems involving G-proteins which ultimately produce a cellular response. The main types of second messengers are listed below. Enzymes Activated by Cell Surface Receptors → Second Messenger(s) • Adenylate cyclase -----------> cAMP • Guanylate cyclase ----------> cGMP • Phospholipase C ------------> Inositol triphosphate (IP_3) and Diacylglycerol (DAG)	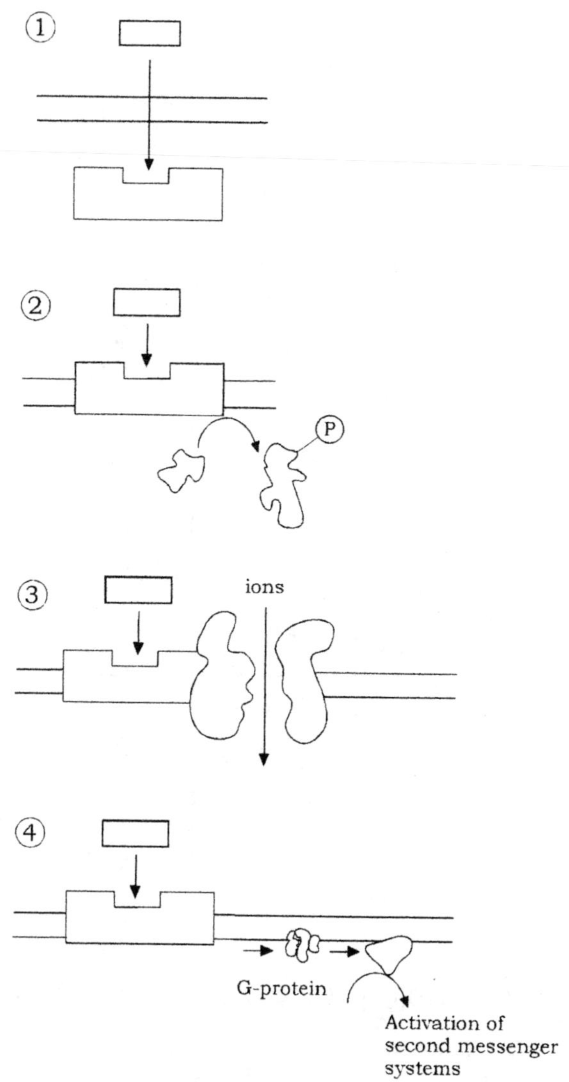

Dose-response relationships

Term	Description	Associated Terms and Equations
Graded dose-response relationships	A dose-response curve graphically plots response vs. drug concentration. This relationship has the following characteristics: drug binding is **dose-dependent** and **saturable** and responses are **graded**. Plotting dose-response data on a linear graph results in a hyperbolic curve. However, when plotted on a semi-log graph, the data produce a sigmoid curve. K_d and EC50 values can be obtained from both types of graphs.	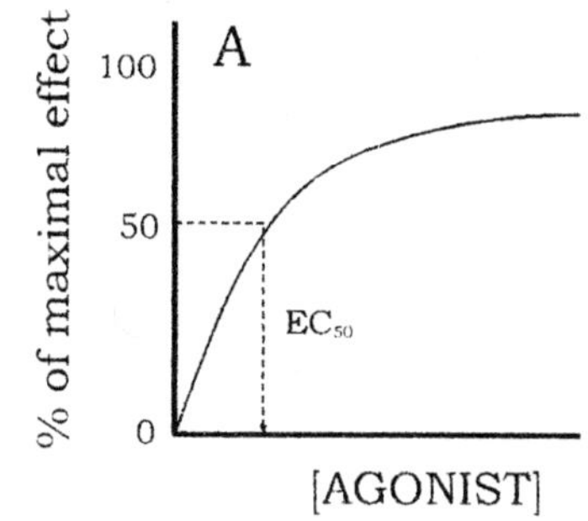
K_d	Is the concentration of drug yielding **50% occupancy of the receptor**. K_d is dependent on the affinity of a drug for its receptor. Drugs with high affinity have a low K_d because only a small amount of drug is required to bind 50% of the receptors. Conversely, drugs with low affinity have a high K_d because a large amount of drug is required to bind 50% of the receptors.	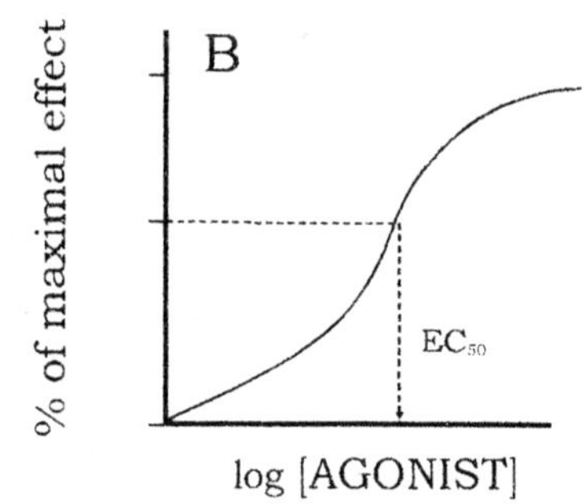
EC50	Is the concentration that produces **50% of the maximum possible response** in graded dose-response curves.	
Quantal dose-response relationships	The quantal dose-response curve graphically plots the percent of the population that responds to a drug vs. the drug dose. **ED50**, the median effective dose, represents the drug dose required to produce an effect in 50% of the population. The **TD50**, the median toxic dose, is the dose required to produce a toxic effect in 50% of the population. The **LD50**, the median lethal dose, is the dose which is lethal to 50% of the population.	

Term	Description	Associated Terms and Equations
Therapeutic window	The difference between the minimum therapeutic concentration and the minimum dose which produces toxicity. This is an important consideration when designing dosing regimens.	
Therapeutic index	The therapeutic index is the ratio of TD50 (or LD50) to ED50. It is an estimate of drug safety and is determined from quantal dose-response curves. Agents with a **high therapeutic index** have a high margin of safety since the therapeutic dose and the lethal dose are far apart. Agents with a **low therapeutic index** have a narrow margin of safety since the therapeutic and lethal dose are close.	$TI = \frac{TD50}{ED50}$

Notes

ANS Drugs

The Autonomic Nervous System

The nervous system is composed of the central nervous system (CNS) and the peripheral nervous system (PNS). The CNS includes the brain and the spinal cord. The PNS is comprised of the peripheral nerves and is divided into somatic and autonomic branches; the somatic nervous system (SNS) is composed of single motor neurons which regulate skeletal muscle through voluntary control. The autonomic nervous system (ANS) is comprised of preganglionic and postganglionic axons separated by ganglia and is responsible for involuntary regulation of smooth muscle, cardiac muscle and glands. It is subdivided into the **sympathetic** and **parasympathetic** systems.

Most organs receive both sympathetic and parasympathetic innervation which mediate antagonistic responses. The parasympathetic nervous system has control over all visceral smooth muscle, glands and skin, while the sympathetic system controls blood vessels. **Sympathetic** outflow is diffuse and activated during times of stress and emergency ("fight or flight") situations. In contrast, **parasympathetic** outflow is discrete, used during times of relaxation, restoration and conservation and is essential for life.

Figure 2.1: Divisions of the nervous system

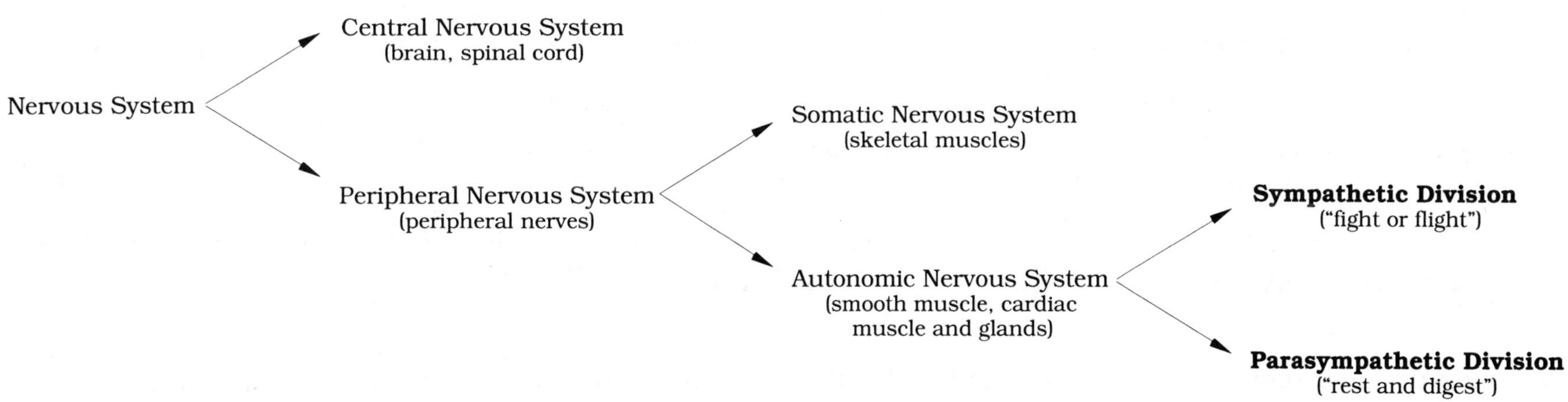

Neurotransmission

The differences in neurotransmission between the sympathetic and parasympathetic branches are summarized below.

	Sympathetic	**Parasympathetic**
Location of neuronal exit from CNS	Thoracic and lumbar nerves (T1-L3)	Cranial (III, VII, IX, X) and sacral (2-4) nerves
Preganglionic axon	Short, myelinated Terminate at ganglia (sympathetic chain)	Long, myelinated Terminate at ganglia within or near target organs
Postganglionic axon	Long, unmyelinated	Short, unmyelinated
Ratio of pre to postganglionic fibers	1:15 (diffuse outflow)	1:1 (discrete outflow)
Synaptic neurotransmitter Between pre and postganglionic neurons At neuroeffector junction	 Acetylcholine Norepinephrine	 Acetylcholine Acetylcholine

Figure 2.2: Schematic of neurotransmission

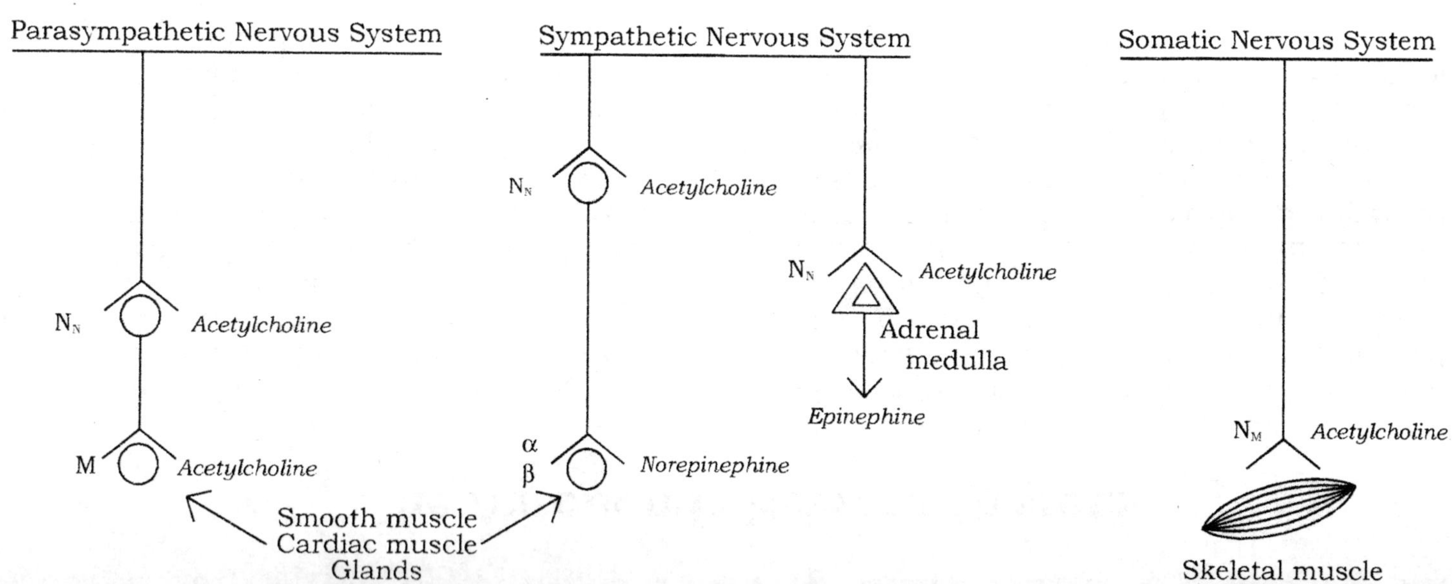

Neurotransmitters and Receptors

Neurotransmitters

Figure 2.3: Summary of the synthesis and degradation of norepinephrine and acetylcholine

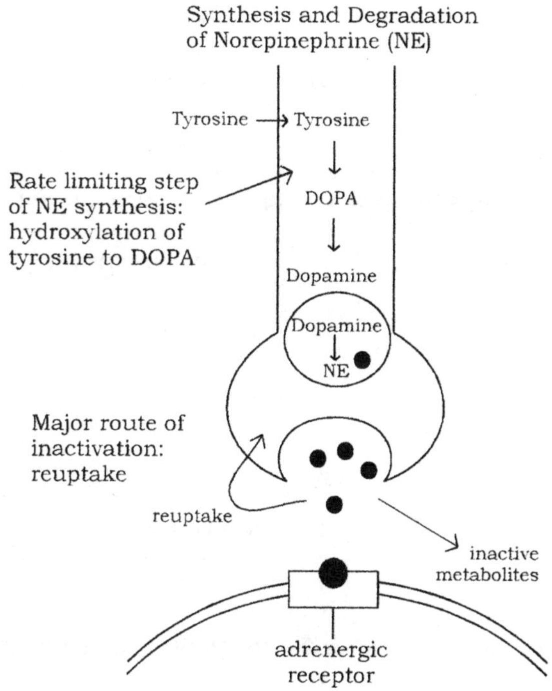

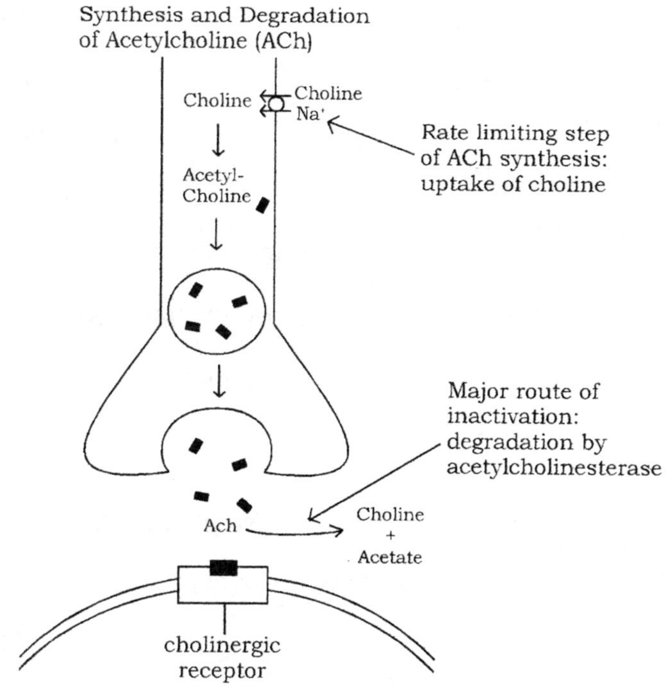

Receptors

There are two types of receptors in the autonomic nervous system: adrenergic and cholinergic. Adrenergic receptors are classified as α, β or dopaminergic (D), each of which can be further subdivided. Cholinergic receptors are classified as muscarinic or nicotinic and also can be further subdivided. Both adrenergic and cholinergic receptors mediate their effects by activating specific intracellular biochemical signalling cascades.

The following pages summarize the subtypes, tissue distribution, effects and intracellular signalling mechanisms of adrenergic and cholinergic receptors.

Adrenergic Receptors

Type	Tissue	Response	G Protein	2nd Messenger
α_1	Radial muscle of the iris	Contraction (mydriasis = pupillary dilation)	G_q	↑ IP_3 and DAG
	Arteriolar smooth muscle	Contraction (↑ peripheral resistance and ↑ blood pressure)		
	GI and GU sphincters	Contraction (retention)		
	Pilomotor smooth muscle	Contraction (piloerection)		
	Seminal vesicle smooth muscle	Contraction (ejaculation)		
	Liver	Glycogenolysis and gluconeogenesis (hyperglycemia)		
α_2	Presynaptic nerve terminals	Inhibits release of norepinephrine (presynaptic inhibition)	G_i	↓ cAMP
	Platelets	Aggregation		
	Pancreatic β cells	Inhibits insulin release (hyperglycemia)		
β_1	Heart	↑ HR, contractility and AV nodal conduction	G_s	↑ cAMP
	Juxtaglomerular cells	Stimulates renin release (↑ blood pressure)		
β_2	Vascular smooth muscle in skeletal muscle	Relaxation (vasodilation)	G_s	↑ cAMP
	Bronchiolar smooth muscle	Relaxation (bronchodilation)		
	GI and urinary bladder smooth muscle	Relaxation (↓ GI and GU motility)		
	Uterine smooth muscle	Relaxation (↓ uterine contraction)		
	Skeletal muscle	Glycogenolysis		
	Liver	Glycogenolysis and gluconeogenesis (hyperglycemia)		
β_3	Adipose tissue	Lipolysis	G_s	↑ cAMP

Dopaminergic

Type	Tissue	Response	G Protein	2nd Messenger
D_1	Smooth muscle of renal, splanchnic, coronary and cerebral arteries	Relaxation (vasodilation)	G_s	↑ cAMP
D_2	Nerve terminals in brain and presynaptic peripheral nerves	Modulation transmitter release	G_i	↓ cAMP, opens K^+ channels and ↓ Ca^{2+} influx

Cholinergic Receptors

Nicotinic

Type	Tissue	Response	Mechanism	Action
N_M	Muscle: neuromuscular junction	Contraction of skeletal muscle	Ion channel	Increased permeability to Na^+ and Ca^{2+} leading to depolarization and excitation.
N_N	Neuronal: autonomic ganglia Adrenal medulla	Depolarization and firing of postganglionic neurons Secretion of catecholamines	Ion channel	Increased permeability to Na^+ and Ca^{2+} leading to depolarization and excitation.

Muscarinic

Type	Tissue	Response	G protein	Mechanism
M_1	Autonomic ganglia	Depolarization (excitatory postsynaptic potential)	G_q	↑ IP_3 and DAG
M_2	Heart	↓ HR, contractility and conduction	G_i	↓ cAMP
M_3	Circular and ciliary muscles of the eye GI smooth muscle Urinary bladder smooth muscle GI and GU sphincters Bronchiolar smooth muscle Secretory glands	Contraction (miosis) and ↓ accommodation Contraction (increase motility and tone) Contraction (micturition) Relaxation Contraction (bronchoconstriction) Increased secretion	G_q	↑ IP_3 and DAG

	Sympathetic		Parasympathetic	
Effector Organs	Receptor	Response	Receptor	Response
Eye				
Radial muscle (iris)	α_1	Contraction (mydriasis)	-	-
Circular muscle (iris)	-	-	M_3	Contraction (miosis)
Ciliary muscle	β_2	Relaxation	M_3	Contraction (accommodation)
Heart				
SA node	β_1	↑ HR	M_2	↓ HR
AV node	β_1	↑ conduction velocity and automaticity	M_2	↓ conduction velocity
Contractility	β_1	↑ force of contraction (atria & ventricles)	M_2	↓ contractility (atria)
Lung				
Bronchial muscle	β_2	Relaxation (bronchodilation)	M_3	Contraction (bronchoconstriction)
Blood Vessels				
Most (except skeletal muscle)	α_1	Constriction	-	-
Skeletal muscle	β_2	Relaxation	-	-
GI (Stomach and Intestine)				
Sphincter	α_1	Constriction (retention)	M_3	Relaxation (defecation)
Motility and tone	α, β_2	Decreases	M_3	Increases motility and tone
GU				
Urinary sphincter	α_1	Constriction	M_3	Relaxation
Bladder wall	β_2	Relaxation (retention)	M_3	Contraction
Uterus, pregnant	α_1; β_2	Contraction; relaxation	-	-
Uterus, non-pregnant	β_2	Relaxation	-	-
Penis, seminal vesicles	α_1	Ejaculation	M	Erection
Secretory glands				
Sweat	α_1	Localized secretion	M	Generalized secretion
Intestinal	α_2	Inhibition	M_3	↑ secretion
Bronchial	-	-	M	↑ secretion
Lacrimal	α	↑ secretion (moderate)	M	Profuse secretion
Metabolism				
Adrenal medulla	N_N	Secretion of catecholamines	-	-
Kidney	β_1	↑ renin release	-	-
Skeletal muscle	β_2	Glycogenolysis, ↑ contractility	-	-
Pancreas (β-cells)	α_2	↓ insulin release	-	-
Fat cells	β_3	Lipolysis	-	-

Note: The parasympathetics control most organs except blood vessels which are regulated by the sympathetic nervous system.

Autonomic Drugs

Adrenergic agonists	Cholinergic agonists	Adrenergic antagonists	Cholinergic antagonists
Catecholamines	**Direct acting**	**Alpha-blockers**	**Antimuscarinics**
Epinephrine	Acetylcholine	Prazosin	Atropine
Norepinephrine	Carbachol	Terazosin	Scopolamine
Isoproterenol	Methacholine	Doxazosin	Propantheline
Dopamine	Bethanechol	Phenoxybenzamine	Methantheline
Dobutamine	Pilocarpine	Phentolamine	Benztropine
	Nicotine	Yohimbine	Cyclopentolate
Non-catecholamines			Pirenzepine
Phenylephrine	**Indirect acting**	**Beta-blockers**	
Tetrahydrozoline	Edrophonium	Metoprolol	**Neuromuscular blocking agents**
Naphazoline	Neostigmine	Atenolol	Tubocurarine
Methoxamine	Physostigmine	Esmolol	Succinylcholine
Clonidine	Pyridostigmine	Acebutolol	Botulinus toxin
Metaproterenol	Isoflurophate	Propranolol	
Albuterol	Echothiophate	Pindolol	**Ganglionic blocking agents**
Terbutaline		Timolol	Nicotine
Ritodrine		Nadolol	Trimethaphan
Tyramine		Butoxamine	Hexamethonium
Amphetamine			
Methamphetamine		**Mixed Antagonist**	
Tricyclic antidepressants		Labetalol	
Cocaine			
Ephedrine			
Phenylpropanolamine			

Adrenergic Agonists (Sympathomimetics)

The adrenergic (sympathomimetic) drugs act on receptors that are stimulated by norepinephrine or epinephrine. These drugs work either **directly** on the receptors or **indirectly** by increasing norepinephrine release from presynaptic terminals or by preventing norepinephrine reuptake.

Catecholamines

Drug	Receptor	Clinical Uses	Side Effects
Epinephrine	Direct: $\alpha_1 = \alpha_2$; $\beta_1 = \beta_2$	Anaphylaxis Cardiac arrest Glaucoma (topical) Adjuvant to local anesthesia	Mydriasis (α_1) Excitation, anxiety, irritability Hypertension (α_1) Hypotension (β_2) Arrhythmias (β_1) Myocardial infarction (β_1)
Norepinephrine	Direct: $\alpha_1 = \alpha_2$; $\beta_1 >> \beta_2$	Hypotension	
Isoproterenol	Direct: $\beta_1 = \beta_2$	CHF	
Dopamine	Direct: $D_1 = D_2 > \beta >> \alpha$	Shock	
Dobutamine	Direct: $\beta_1 > \beta_2$	Shock, CHF	

Non-Catecholamines

Drug	Receptor	Clinical Uses	Side Effects
Phenylephrine	Direct: $\alpha_1 > \alpha_2$	Ocular redness Mydriasis	Excitation, anxiety, irritability Hypertension Constipation Urinary retention
Tetrahydrozoline Naphazoline	Direct: $\alpha_1 > \alpha_2$	Ocular redness	
Methoxamine	Direct: $\alpha_1 > \alpha_2$	Adjuvant to general anesthesia	
Clonidine	Direct: $\alpha_2 > \alpha_1$	Hypertension	
Metaproterenol Albuterol Terbutaline	Direct: $\beta_2 >> \beta_1$	Asthma Labor (terbutaline)	Hypotension Constipation Urinary retention
Ritodrine	Direct: $\beta_2 >> \beta_1$	Premature labor	

Drug	Receptor	Clinical Uses	Side Effects
Tyramine[1]	Indirect		Mydriasis (α_1) Excitation, anxiety, irritability Hypertension (α_1) Hypotension (β_2) Arrhythmias (β_1) Myocardial infarction (β_1) Constipation, urinary retention
Amphetamine Methamphetamine	Indirect	Attention deficit hyperactivity disorder Narcolepsy Weight reduction	
Tricyclic antidepressants	Indirect	Clinical depression	
Cocaine	Indirect	Mucosal anesthetic and vasoconstrictor	
Ephedrine	Mixed: direct on α_1, β_2 and indirect	Hypotension secondary to spinal anesthesia	
Phenylpropanolamine	Mixed: direct on α_1, β_1, β_2 and indirect	Weight reduction	

[1]Tyramine: is found in many foods (cheese, wine, beer) and can cause a hypertensive crisis when ingested while on MAO inhibitors.

Cardiovascular Responses to Selected Catecholamines (low doses)

Norepinephrine possess both α and β activity. When administered in therapeutic doses, however, norepinephrine mainly possess α activity. Thus, only the α responses are listed. At low doses, **epinephrine** primarily exhibits β effects on the vasculature, however, at high doses, α effects prevail.

	Norepinephrine (α)	Epinephrine (α, β)	Isoproterenol (β)
Peripheral vascular resistance	$\uparrow\uparrow\uparrow$	$\downarrow$	$\downarrow\downarrow$
Heart rate	$\downarrow$ (reflex)	$\uparrow$	$\uparrow\uparrow\uparrow$
Cardiac output	–	$\uparrow\uparrow\uparrow$	$\uparrow\uparrow$
Blood pressure	$\uparrow\uparrow$	$\uparrow$	$\downarrow$
Schematic representation: Systolic (s), diastolic (d) and mean blood pressure (arrow)	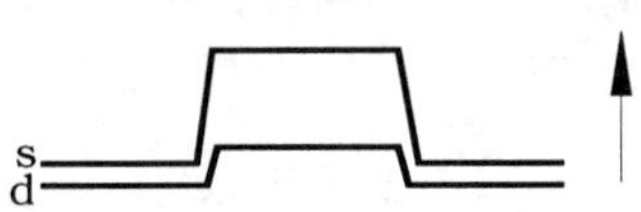	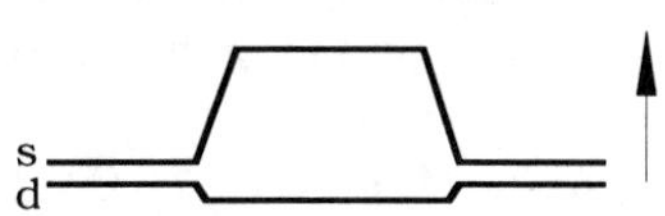	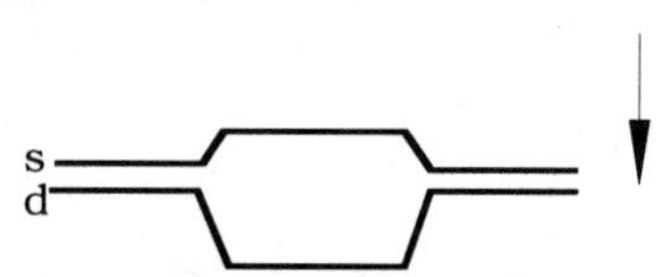

Cholinergic Agonists (Parasympathomimetics)

There are two types of cholinergic agonists: direct and indirect acting. The direct acting cholinergic agonists mimic the effects of acetylcholine by binding to cholinergic receptors. The parasympathetic effect is terminated when these agents are destroyed by acetylcholinesterase. The indirect acting cholinergic agonists work by inhibiting acetylcholinesterase.

Direct Acting Cholinergic Agonists

Drug	Receptor	Duration	Enters CNS	Clinical Uses
Acetylcholine (+)	M, N	seconds	N	None
Carbachol (+)		hrs	N	Glaucoma Pupillary miosis during ophthalmic surgery
Methacholine (+)	M	hrs	N	Asthma: diagnosis and treatment Bronchial airway hyperactivity
Bethanechol (+)		hrs	N	Urinary retention Postoperative GI atony
Pilocarpine		hrs to days	Y	Glaucoma: open angle and closed angle
Nicotine‡	N (low dose) M (high dose)	min to hrs	Y	Nicotine dependence

+ Designates charged molecules which do not cross the blood brain barrier.
‡ Nicotinic escape: at low doses, nicotine stimulates nicotinic receptors. High doses result in the stimulation of muscarinic receptors with no response at nicotinic receptors.

Indirect Acting Cholinergic Agonists (Anticholinesterases)

Anticholinesterases inhibit acetylcholinesterase and cause increased synaptic levels of acetylcholine and prolonged effects at cholinergic receptors. Anticholinesterases cause the stimulation of both **nicotinic** and **muscarinic** receptors with a slight preference for receptors at neuromuscular junctions ($N_M > N_N > M$). These agents can be classified as reversible or irreversible agents.

Drug	Receptor	Reversible	Duration	Enters CNS	Clinical Uses
Edrophonium (+)	M, N	Y	min	N	Myasthenia Gravis (diagnosis) Antidote to non-depolarizing neuromuscular blockade
Neostigmine (+)		Y	hrs	N	Myasthenia Gravis (treatment) Antidote to non-depolarizing neuromuscular blockade Paralytic ileus Postoperative urinary retention
Physostigmine		Y	hrs	Y	Glaucoma (topical) Antidote to anticholinergic poisoning such as atropine
Pyridostigmine (+)		Y	hrs	N	Myasthenia Gravis (treatment) Antidote to non-depolarizing neuromuscular blockade
Isoflurophate (DFP)		N	days	Y	Glaucoma (topical)
Echothiophate (+)		N	days	N	Glaucoma (topical)

Side Effects of Parasympathomimetic Agents

The toxicities of both direct and indirect acting parasympathomimetic agents represent exacerbations of the actions of the parasympathetic branch of the ANS. The most significant side effects are listed below:

Organ	Side Effects
Eye	Miosis (pupillary constriction), loss of accommodation
CNS (if drug crosses BBB)	Excitation, apathy, ataxia and respiratory depression
Lungs	Bronchoconstriction
Heart	Bradycardia
GI and GU	Diarrhea, involuntary micturition
Glands	Sweating, lacrimation, salivation

Notes

Adrenoreceptor-Blocking Agents (Sympatholytics)

Alpha Antagonists

Drug	Receptor Affinities	Clinical Uses	Side Effects
Prazosin Terazosin Doxazosin	Direct: α_1	Hypertension Benign prostatic hypertrophy	Postural hypotension First dose syncope (prazosin)
Phenoxybenzamine	Direct: $\alpha_1 > \alpha_2$	Pheochromocytoma-associated hypertension	Postural hypotension Reflex tachycardia
Phentolamine	Direct: $\alpha_1 = \alpha_2$	Pheochromocytoma-associated hypertension Dermal necrosis following IV norepinephrine	Postural hypotension Reflex tachycardia
Yohimbine	Direct: α_2	No significant uses	

The Effects of α-Blockers on Blood Pressure

Sympathomimetic agent	Agent alone	Pretreatment with α-blocker	Comments
Phenylephrine (α)	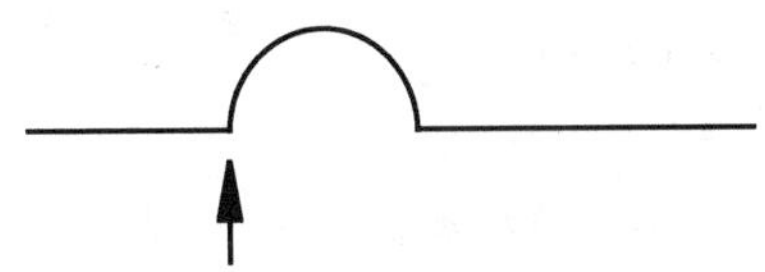	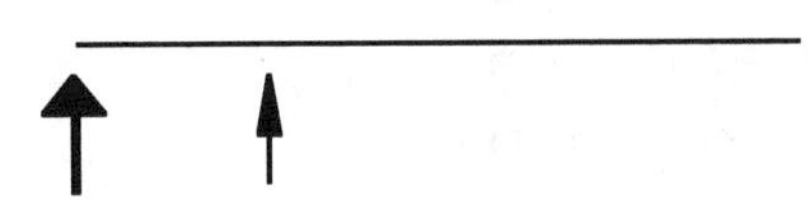	
Epinephrine (α, β)	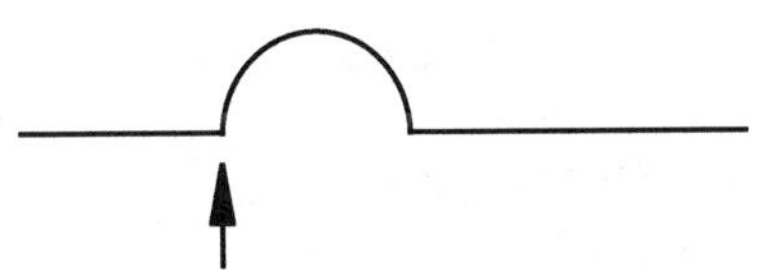	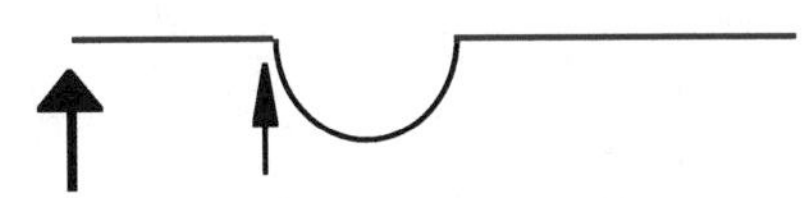	**Epinephrine reversal**: with α receptor blockers, the β effects (vasodilatory) of epinephrine are evident.
Isoproterenol (β)	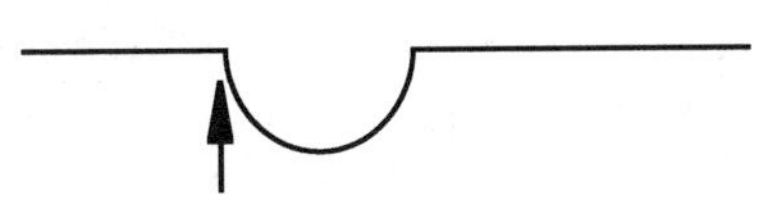	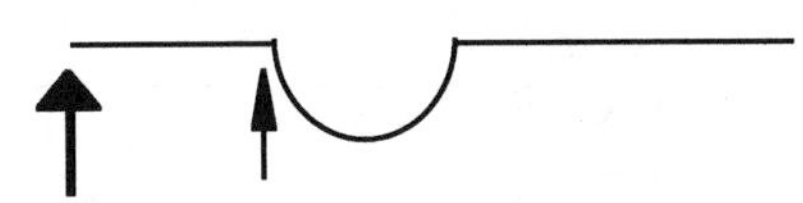	

Beta Antagonists

Drug	Receptor Affinities	Clinical Uses	Side Effects
Metoprolol Atenolol Esmolol	Direct: β_1 Cardioselective	Hypertension Myocardial infarction	Bradycardia CHF CNS effects: sedation, fatigue (metoprolol)
Acebutolol	Direct: β_1 Cardioselective	Hypertension Arrhythmias	
Propranolol	Direct: $\beta_1 = \beta_2$	Hypertension Angina Myocardial infarction Arrhythmia Migraine prophylaxis Hypertrophic cardiomyopathy Pheochromocytoma Stage fright Thyrotoxicosis: adjuvant therapy	Bradycardia CHF Bronchoconstriction CNS effects: sedation, fatigue (propanolol, timolol) May diminish recognition of hypoglycemia
Pindolol Timolol Nadolol	Direct: $\beta_1 = \beta_2$	Hypertension Angina Glaucoma (timolol)	
Butoxamine	Direct: β_2	No significant uses	

Mixed Antagonist

Drug	Receptor Affinities	Clinical Uses	Side Effects
Labetalol	Direct: $\beta_1 = \beta_2 > \alpha_1$	Hypertensive emergencies Hypertension	Postural hypotension Bradycardia Bronchoconstriction Hepatotoxicity

Notable Characteristics of Some Sympatholytics

Lipophilic agents	Intrinsic sympathomimetic*	Notable $t_{1/2}$
Metoprolol Propanolol Timolol	Acebutolol Pindolol Labetalol	Esmolol: short $t_{1/2}$ = 10 min Nadolol: long $t_{1/2}$ = 20 hrs

* These agents exhibit partial agonist activity at β receptors.

The Effects of β-Blockers on Blood Pressure

Sympathomimetic agent	Agent alone	Pretreatment with β-blocker
Phenylephrine (α)	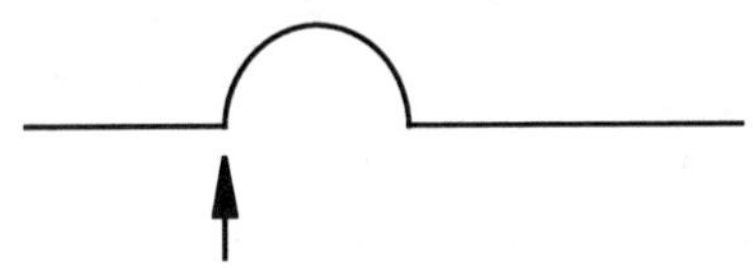	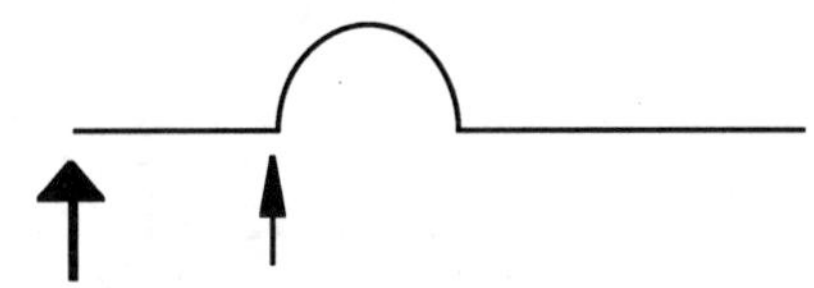
Epinephrine (α, β)	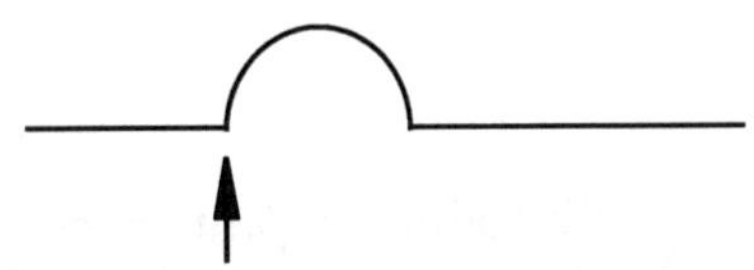	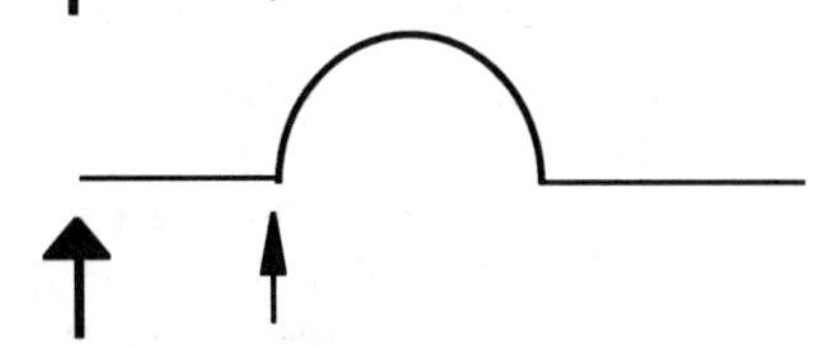
Isoproterenol (β)	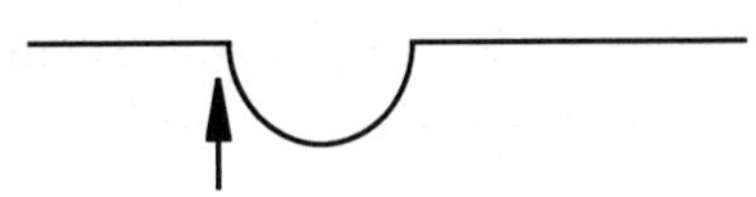	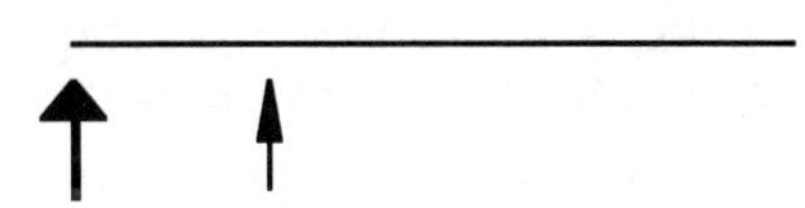

Cholinergic-Blocking Agents (Parasympatholytics)

Antimuscarinic drugs are a class of parasympatholytic agents which competitively block muscarinic receptors. The prototype of this class is **atropine**. Significant properties of other antimuscarinic drugs are noted below.

Drug	Receptor Affinities	Clinical Uses	Side Effects
Atropine A useful mnemonic for remembering atropine's toxicity is: "Dry as a bone" "Red as a beet" "Blind as a bat" "Mad as a hatter"	Nonselective blocker	Antidote for cholinesterase inhibitors, organophosphate pesticides, muscarine (mushroom poisoning), nerve gas Urinary antispasmodic Surgical or dental anesthesia: adjuvant (decreases glandular secretions) Arrhythmic (parenteral) Mydriasis and cycloplegia (ophthalmic)	With increasing doses: **Dry mouth**, **inhibition of sweating** and bronchosecretion, bradycardia Tachycardia, mydriasis, **blurred vision**, **dry skin** Urinary retention, constipation, dry and hot skin, restlessness, headache **Overdose** → Rapid pulse → Dry, red and hot skin → Blurred vision → Delirium and hallucinations → Convulsions and coma Treatment of overdose: **physostigmine** and **PAM** (pralidoxime)

Other antimuscarinics

Drug	Receptor Affinities	Clinical Uses
Scopolamine	Nonselective blocker	Motion sickness GI and urinary spasms Dysmenorrhea Anesthesia: adjuvant
Propantheline (+) Methantheline (+) Benztropine Cyclopentolate	Nonselective blocker	
Pirenzepine	Selective M_1 blocker	

+ Designates charged molecules which do not cross the blood brain barrier.

Neuromuscular Blocking Agents

Neuromuscular blocking agents represent a class of parasympatholytic agents which block cholinergic transmission at neuromuscular junctions (N_M receptors). There are 3 classes of neuromuscular blocking agents which are differentiated by their mechanism of blockade and duration of action.

Drug	Mechanism of Blockade	Duration	Notes
Tubocurarine (+) Pancuronium Vecuronium Atracurium	**Non-depolarizing** agents which competitively block N_M receptors at the motor endplate. This blockade results in muscle weakness followed by paralysis. Small, rapidly moving muscles are affected first. The activity of these drugs is antagonized by anticholinesterases.	30 to 60 min	**Tubocurarine** can cause **histamine release** resulting in bronchospasm, skin wheals and, in conjunction with sympathetic ganglionic blockade, **hypotension**.
Succinylcholine (+)	A **depolarizing**, **desensitizing** agent which competes with acetylcholine to activate N_M receptors at the motor endplate. Due to its high affinity for cholinergic receptors and resistance to cholinesterases, it produces a more prolonged depolarization than acetylcholine. This results in fasciculations and subsequently paralysis. Not antagonized by anticholinesterases. Hydrolyzed by pseudocholinesterase. Patients with "atypical cholinesterases" exhibit a prolonged duration of action.	5 to 10 min	May cause **malignant hyperthermia** (see below) which is treated with **dantrolene** and cooling. Can cause **histamine release** resulting in bronchospasm, skin wheals and, in conjunction with sympathetic ganglionic blockade, **hypotension**.
Botulinus toxin	**Inhibits** the **release** of acetylcholine.	weeks to months	Extremely potent toxin produced from *Clostridium botulinus.*

+ Designates charged molecules which do not cross the blood brain barrier.

Malignant hyperthermia is an autosomal dominant disorder which is a major cause of anesthesia related deaths. It is caused by fluorinated hydrocarbons and depolarizing muscle relaxants such as succinylcholine. Malignant hyperthermia results from an excessive release of Ca^{2+} from the sarcoplasmic reticulum and clinically presents as hyperthermia, metabolic acidosis, tachycardia and accelerated muscle contractions. **Treatment** includes rapid cooling, 100% O_2, control of the acidosis and IV administration of **dantrolene** which blocks the release of Ca^{2+} from the sarcoplasmic reticulum.

Ganglionic Blocking Agents

Neurotransmission at autonomic ganglia involves acetylcholine and, in general, nicotinic receptors. Ganglionic blockers inhibit neurotransmission in both the sympathetic and parasympathetic branches of the ANS. Significant properties of ganglionic blockers are listed below.

Drug	Notes
Nicotine	At low doses causes stimulation of nicotinic receptors. High doses result in no response (nicotinic escape) at nicotinic receptors and stimulation of muscarinic receptors. Clinical use: transdermal patch for tobacco withdrawal.
Trimethaphan	The only ganglionic blocker clinically used (hypertensive crisis).
Hexamethonium	

CNS Drugs

Page	Topic

Anxiolytic and Hypnotic Agents

Anxiolytic and hypnotic agents are drugs which produce dose-dependent CNS depressant effects ranging from anxiety reduction to sleep induction and coma (Figure 3.1). Although these agents have overlapping activities, they can be generally classified as anxiolytics or hypnotics based on their major clinical use. **Anxiolytics** are used to **reduce anxiety** and include benzodiazepines, meprobamate and buspirone. Flumazenil is a benzodiazepine antagonist which is used to reverse benzodiazepine induced sedation. **Hypnotic drugs** are used to induce **drowsiness** and include benzodiazepines, barbiturates, zolpidem and chloral hydrate.

Anxiolytics	Benzodiazepine Antagonist	Hypnotics
Benzodiazepines Meprobamate Buspirone	Flumazenil	Benzodiazepines Barbiturates Zolpidem Chloral hydrate

Two well-known anxiolytic and hypnotic drug classes are barbiturates and benzodiazepines. One of the most distinguishing features between these classes is their therapeutic index.

Barbiturates were once considered the prototypic anxiolytic and hypnotic agent. However, their major drawback is that they exhibit a **low therapeutic index** (small margin of safety). As depicted on the right, the drug doses required for therapeutic effects are close to those which can cause medullary depression and coma.

Benzodiazepines, on the other hand, possess a **high therapeutic index** (higher margin of safety), and have replaced barbiturates for many uses, especially anxiolytic indications.

Figure 3.1: Comparison of dose-response relationships of benzodiazepines and barbiturates

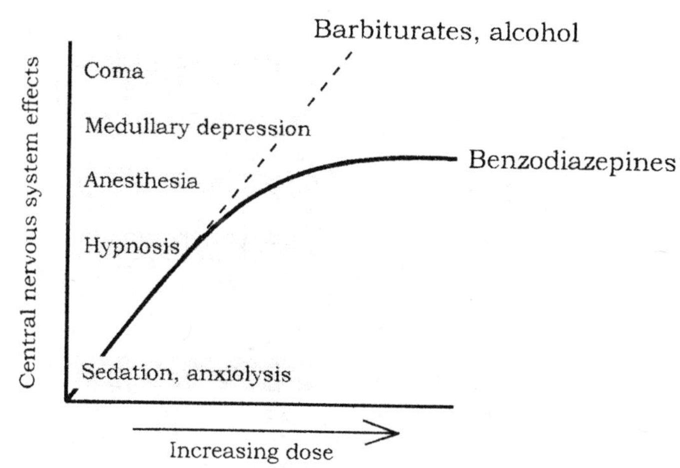

Benzodiazepines and **barbiturates** act at different sites of the **$GABA_A$ receptor** to enhance GABA binding (Figure 3.2). Activation of GABA receptors inhibits neurotransmission by increasing chloride conductance and causing membrane hyperpolarization. The inhibition of neurotransmission is responsible for the CNS depressant effects of these drugs

Flumazenil is an antagonist at the benzodiazepine binding site of the $GABA_A$ receptor.

Zolpidem is an agonist at the ω1-subtype of $GABA_A$ receptors.

Figure 3.2: The $GABA_A$ receptor

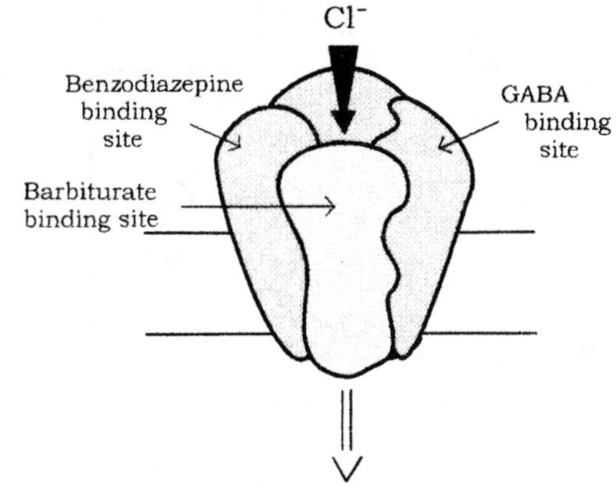

Anxiolytics

Drug	MOA & Pharmacokinetics	Clinical Uses	Side Effects
Benzodiazepines *Long Acting (1-3 days)* Chlordiazepoxide (Librium®) Diazepam (Valium®) Flurazepam (Dalmane®) *Intermediate Acting (10-20 hrs)* Alprazolam (Xanax®) Lorazepam (Ativan®) Temazepam (Restoril®) *Short Acting (2-8 hrs)* Clonazepam (Klonopin®) Oxazepam (Serax®) Midazolam (Versed®) Triazolam (Halcion®)	Bind to the α subunit of the $GABA_A$ receptor causing allosteric changes which enhance GABA binding to the β1 subunit. This results in an **increased frequency** of **chloride channel opening** leading to membrane hyperpolarization and a decrease in neuronal excitability. Most benzodiazepines have active metabolites some of which have long half-lives, particularly flurazepam and diazepam. Given PO, IM, IV	**Anxiety**: *diazepam* **Panic disorders**: *alprazolam* **Insomnia**: *flurazepam, triazolam, temazepam* Antegrade amnesia: *lorazepam* Muscle spasms: *diazepam* Alcohol withdrawal: *diazepam, lorazepam, oxazepam, chlordiazepoxide* Status epilepticus: *diazepam* Absence and myoclonic seizures: *clonazepam* Reduction of ketamine induced hallucinations and unpleasant dreams: *midazolam*	Drowsiness Decreased cognitive function Ataxia Respiratory depression Dizziness Convulsions (rare) Rebound insomnia (withdrawal symptom)

Drug	MOA & Pharmacokinetics	Clinical Uses	Side Effects
Meprobamate (Miltown®)	A carbamate whose MOA is unknown. Given PO	Anxiety	Ataxia, drowsiness Respiratory depression, confusion Hypotension, shock, cardiac failure Withdrawal syndrome: anxiety, insomnia, tremors
Buspirone (BuSpar®)	**Partial serotonin agonist** at $5HT_{1A}$ receptors. Differences from benzodiazepines: • No drug dependence • No withdrawal symptoms • No cross tolerance with other sedatives • No anticonvulsant actions • No muscle relaxant properties • Less sedation Slow onset (weeks) Given PO	Anxiety: especially generalized anxiety disorders.	Dizziness Headache Nausea Restlessness

Benzodiazepine Antagonist

Drug	MOA & Pharmacokinetics	Clinical Uses	Side Effects
Flumazenil (Romazicon®)	**Competitive antagonist** of benzodiazepines at the $GABA_A$ receptor in the CNS. It will NOT reverse benzodiazepine-induced respiratory depression. Duration of action: 1 hr. Note: the duration of action of flumazenil is much shorter than those of benzodiazepines. Thus repeat doses may be necessary. Given IV	Reversal of benzodiazepine-induced sedation following anesthesia. Zolpidem overdose: reversal of sedative and respiratory depressant effects. Suspected **acute benzodiazepine overdose** (if administered to a chronic benzodiazepine user, seizures will result).	Few effects in benzodiazepine-free individuals; effects are mainly due to reversal of benzodiazepine activity. Agitation Dizziness, headache, nausea Visual disturbances Seizures in benzodiazepine-dependent individuals

Hypnotics

Drug	MOA & Pharmacokinetics	Clinical Uses	Side Effects
Barbiturates *Long Acting (3-5 days)* Phenobarbital (Luminal®) *Short Acting (10-50 hrs)* Pentobarbital (Nembutal®) Secobarbital (Seconal®) Amobarbital (Amytal®) *Ultra-short Acting (3-10 hrs)* Thiopental (Pentothal®) Methohexital (Brevital®)	Binds the $GABA_A$ receptor causing allosteric changes which enhance GABA binding resulting in **prolonged duration** of **chloride channel opening**. This causes membrane hyperpolarization and a decrease in neuronal excitability. These drugs vary in their lipid solubilities. Drugs which possess high lipophilicity (**thiopental**) enter the CNS quickly and have a rapid onset of action. CNS effects of **thiopental** are attenuated by **redistribution** from the brain to other tissues. Given PO, IV	Status epilepticus: *phenobarbital* Partial and generalized tonic-clonic seizures: *phenobarbital* Anesthetic adjuvant: often *thiopental* Narco-analysis (truth serum): *amobarbital*	Clumsiness, dizziness, drowsiness Chronic toxicity: confusion, irritability, poor judgement Withdrawal symptoms: anxiety, nausea, hypotension, convulsions and hallucinations Induction of the P_{450} system ◆ Contraindication: Acute intermittent porphyria
Zolpidem (Ambien®)	**Agonist** at ω-1 subtype of $GABA_A$ receptors enhancing GABA binding. Differences from benzodiazepines: • Less drug dependence • No anticonvulsant actions • No muscle relaxant properties Given PO	Insomnia	Rare but include ataxia, confusion and mental depression
Chloral Hydrate (Noctec®)	Reduced by the liver to the active metabolite **trichloroethanol**. Given PO	Hypnotic Sedation in children	GI irritation: nausea, vomiting Unpleasant taste

Antidepressant Drugs

Affective disorders are a group of psychiatric illnesses characterized by extreme alterations in mood. Depression is the most common affective disorder. Common symptoms of depression include feelings of hopelessness, decreased energy, loss of appetite, insomnia and low self-esteem. The most common form of depression is reactive (secondary) depression which results from an unhappy occurrence and usually does not require therapy. Endogenous depression does not arise from a specific causative event and may benefit from pharmacological intervention. Four classes of drugs are used clinically in the treatment of depression.

Monoamine Oxidase (MOA) Inhibitors	Tricyclic Antidepressants (TCA)	Selective Serotonin Reuptake Inhibitors (SSRI)	Second Generation Antidepressants
<u>Hydrazine</u> Isocarboxazid Phenelzine <u>Non-hydrazines</u> Tranylcypromine	Imipramine Desipramine Amitriptyline Nortriptyline Clomipramine	Fluoxetine Sertraline Paroxetine	Trazodone Bupropion

The Catecholamine Indoleamine Hypothesis of Depression

The biogenic amine theory of depression postulates that depression is due to a **deficiency of monoamines** such as **norepinephrine** and **serotonin** at functionally important receptor sites within the brain (conversely, mania might be associated with an excess of these amines). Agents effective in treating depression increase the concentration of these neurotransmitters within the synaptic cleft. The sites of action of the major classes of antidepressants are shown below:

Figure 3.3: Site of action of antidepressants

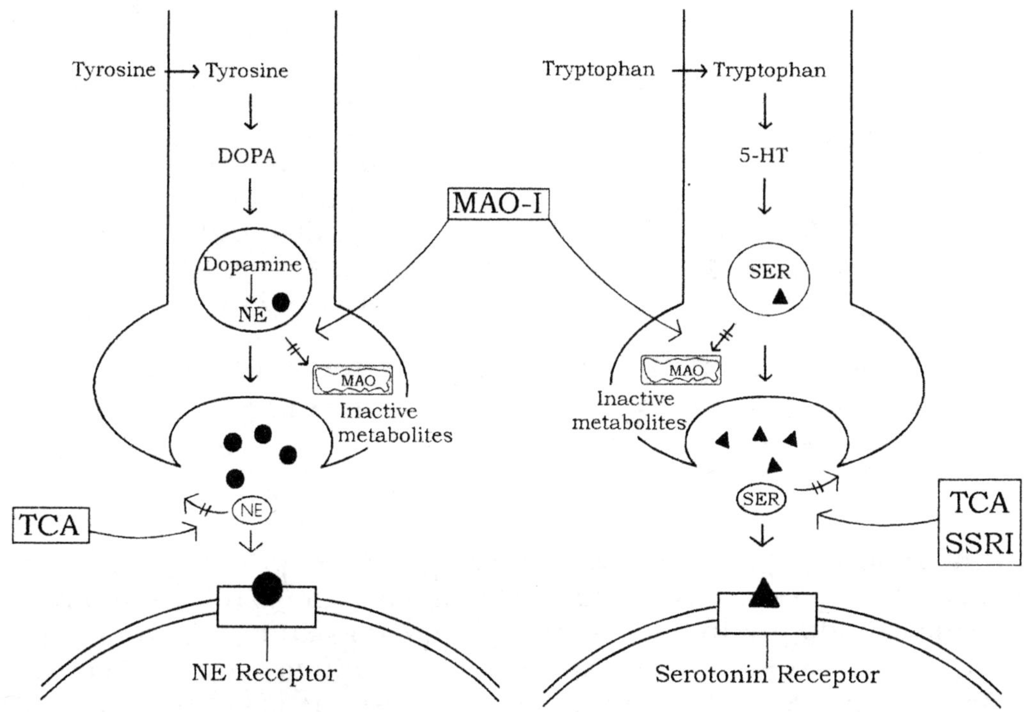

Monoamine Oxidase (MAO) Inhibitors

Monoamine oxidase (MAO) is a mitochondrial enzyme that metabolizes catecholamines (norepinephrine, dopamine and serotonin). There are two types of MAOs: **MAO-A** which is selective for serotonin, norepinephrine and tyramine and **MAO-B** which is selective for dopamine. **MAO inhibitors** may reversibly or irreversibly inactivate MAO resulting in an accumulation of the neurotransmitters in the presynaptic neuron and the synaptic cleft. The major MAO inhibitors are isocarboxazid, phenelzine and tranylcypromine.

The clinical use of MAO inhibitors is limited mainly because of their side effects. The tricyclic antidepressants (TCA) are more efficacious and less toxic. Additionally, the stimulating effect of MAO inhibitors, makes them poor for treating severely depressed patients who have suicidal tendencies.

Drug	MOA & Pharmacokinetics	Clinical Uses	Side Effects
Isocarboxazid (Marplan®) Phenelzine (Nardil®) Tranylcypromine (Parnate®) Note: Isocarboxazid and phenelzine are hydrazine derivatives. Tranylcypromine is a non-hydrazine derivative.	Inhibit the activity of intraneuronal MAO which increases the release of **norepinephrine** and/or **serotonin** from the presynaptic neuron. Phenelzine and isocarboxazid are **irreversible** MAO inhibitors. Tranylcypromine is a **reversible** MAO inhibitor. Phenelzine and tranylcypromine have mild amphetamine-like stimulating activity. A therapeutic response is not observed for 2-3 weeks even though MAO is inhibited after several days of treatment. Given PO	**Depression**: indicated for patients resistant to TCA therapy or who are highly anxious.	**Orthostatic hypotension** **Hypertensive crisis**: characterized by headache, nausea, tachycardia, hypertension, cardiac arrhythmias and possibly stroke. MAO metabolizes **tyramine** which is found in such foods as cheese and wine. With MAO activity inhibited, tyramine acts as an indirect sympathomimetic releasing norepinephrine causing a hypertensive crisis. Patients are therefore instructed to avoid foods containing tyramine. Impotence Weight gain CNS stimulation: agitation, seizures Drug Interactions: **Alcohol** and other **CNS depressants** may increase CNS depressant effects. **TCA** and **SSRI** may produce a potentially lethal hyperserotonergic state (**serotonin syndrome**) characterized by mental status changes, myoclonus and restlessness.

Tricyclic Antidepressants (TCA)

Tricyclic antidepressant (TCA) drugs are more efficacious and less toxic than MAO inhibitors. These drugs inhibit the reuptake of **norepinephrine** (NE) and **serotonin** (5-HT) and increase the levels of these neurotransmitters in the synaptic space. This action is thought to account for the antidepressant effects of these drugs. The antidepressant effects of these drugs, however, are not seen for several weeks. Thus, inhibition of norepinephrine and serotonin reuptake is not the sole effect responsible for the antidepressant effects of this class of drugs. Down-regulation of receptors may contribute to TCA's antidepressant activity.

Drugs in this class can also block cholinergic receptors, histamine receptors and α_1 and α_2-adrenergic receptors. These actions account for most of the observed side effects.

Drug	MOA & Pharmacokinetics	Clinical Uses	Side Effects
Imipramine (Tofranil®) Desipramine (Norpramin®) Amitriptyline (Elavil®) Nortriptyline (Aventyl®) Clomipramine (Anafranil®)	Block the active uptake of norepinephrine and serotonin at the cell membrane of presynaptic neurons causing desensitization of postsynaptic adrenergic and serotonergic receptors. A therapeutic response is not observed for 2-3 weeks even though the uptake mechanism is inhibited acutely. Imipramine is converted to **desipramine**. Amitriptyline is converted to **nortriptyline**. Given PO	**Depression** **Enuresis** in childhood: *imipramine* **Obsessive-compulsive disorder**: *clomipramine* Neurogenic pain	**Orthostatic hypotension**, tachycardia: due to α_1-adrenergic blockade Excessive **sedation**: due to H_1 blockade **Anticholinergic effects**: dry mouth, urinary retention, blurred vision, constipation, tachycardia, sweating (most severe with amitriptyline) Arrhythmias Drug Interactions: **Alcohol** and other **CNS depressants** may increased CNS depression. TCA may reverse the antihypertensive effects of **guanethidine**. Serotonin syndrome with **MAO inhibitors**. **Overdose**: characterized by severe anticholinergic effects, convulsions, coma, respiratory depression, even death. Treatment includes gastric lavage, activated charcoal, $NaHCO_3$, lidocaine, diazepam and/or physostigmine.

Selective Serotonin Reuptake Inhibitors (SSRI)

SSRI selectively inhibit the reuptake of serotonin (5-HT). These drugs have a more benign side effect profile than TCA. Like the other antidepressants, the beneficial effects of SSRI are not observed for several weeks after initiation of treatment.

Drug	MOA & Pharmacokinetics	Clinical Uses	Side Effects
Fluoxetine (Prozac®)	Selectively inhibits serotonin reuptake. A **pro-drug** which is converted to its active metabolite, **norfluoxetine**. Highly protein bound Half-life of **active metabolite** is **7-15 days**. Given PO	**Depression**: DOC **Obsessive compulsive disorder**	Nervousness, restlessness, irritability Sleep disturbances (insomnia) Nausea, diarrhea Drug Interactions: **Alcohol** and other **CNS depressants** may increase CNS depressant effects. **Highly protein bound medications** may lead to elevated plasma levels of either drug. Serotonin syndrome with **MAO inhibitors**.
Sertraline (Zoloft®)	Selectively inhibits serotonin reuptake. Highly protein bound The half-life is short (1 day). Thus, the time required to attain steady-state is quicker (1 wk) than with fluoxetine (4-5 wks). When switching from sertraline to another antidepressant, the time required for drug wash out will be less than with fluoxetine. Given PO	**Depression**	Decreased appetite, anorexia and diarrhea Dizziness, tremors Sexual dysfunction (inhibit ejaculation) Drug Interactions: **Highly protein bound medications** may lead to elevated plasma levels of either drug. Serotonin syndrome with **MAO inhibitors**
Paroxetine (Paxil®)	Selectively inhibits serotonin reuptake. More selective and potent than other SSRI. Highly protein bound Given PO	**Depression**	Dizziness, drowsiness Tremors Drug Interaction: Serotonin syndrome with **MAO inhibitors**

Second Generation Antidepressants

Drug	MOA & Pharmacokinetics	Clinical Uses	Side Effects
Trazodone (Desyrel®)	**Selectively inhibits serotonin reuptake**. Highly protein bound Given PO	**Depression**	Dizziness, drowsiness Nausea Confusion, tremors Drug Interactions: **Alcohol** and other **CNS depressants** may increase CNS depressant effects. May increase hypotension when given concurrently with **antihypertensives**.
Bupropion (Wellbutrin®)	Not clearly established, but at high doses, it weakly blocks dopamine reuptake (does not correlate with antidepressant activity). Antidepressant effects are thought to be mediated via noradrenergic pathways. Given PO	Depression	CNS stimulation Tachycardia Headache Anticholinergic effects

Neuroleptic Drugs (Antipsychotics) and Lithium

Neuroleptic drugs are used primarily to treat severe forms of mental illness such as **schizophrenia**, **manic states** and **acute-manic depression**. This class of agents in known by several aliases: antischizophrenic drugs, antipsychotic drugs and major tranquilizers (minor tranquilizers are anxiolytic agents such as benzodiazepines). Major tranquilizers are selective depressants of the CNS which control emotions without affecting intellectual functions.

Neuroleptic drugs can be divided into four major classes based on their structure. The general mechanism of action of most of these agents is to **decrease dopamine activity**.

Phenothiazines	Thioxanthene	Butyrophenone	Atypical	Antimanic
Chlorpromazine Fluphenazine Trifluoperazine Thioridazine	Thiothixene	Haloperidol	Clozapine Risperidone	Lithium

Proposed Biochemical Mechanism for Schizophrenia

The **Dopamine Hypothesis** proposes that increased activity of dopaminergic transmission through mesolimbic and/or mesocortical pathways leads to schizophrenia. The hypothesis was originally developed from observations that drugs with dopamine-releasing properties (amphetamines) can induce a psychosis indistinguishable from acute paranoid schizophrenia. This hypothesis was further supported by the observations that most antipsychotic agents antagonize CNS dopamine receptors and that dopamine receptor density is increased in the brains of schizophrenic patients.

Antipsychotic drugs exert their neuroleptic effects by antagonizing dopamine receptors. However, the various side effects of these drugs result from their activity at other receptors including **muscarinic**, α-**adrenergic**, **serotonergic** and **histaminic receptors**. Listed below is a summary of the relative activities of selected antipsychotic drugs at various receptors:

Drug	Dopamine receptor	Antihistaminic (H_1)	Antiserotinergic (5-HT)	Antiadrenergic (α_1)	Anticholinergic
Chlorpromazine	D_2	+++	+	+++	++
Fluphenazine	D_2	+	+	+	++++
Trifluoperazine	D_2	+	+	+	+++
Thioridazine	D_2	+++	+	+++	+
Thiothixene	D_2	+	+	++	+++
Haloperidol	D_2	+	-	+	++++
Clozapine	D_2, D_4	+++	++	+++	-
Risperidone	D_2	++	+++	+++	++

Extrapyramidal side effects are some of the most significant consequences of antipsychotic medication. These occur secondary to the blockade of dopamine in the CNS which can disturb the dopamine:acetylcholine balance. Acute manifestations include parkinsonism (rigidity, tremor), akathisia (inability to remain in a seated posture) and acute dystonic reactions. Long term effects include tardive dyskinesia (choreoathetoid movements and lip smacking). **Anticholinergic** agents, such as **benztropine** and **diphenhydramine**, are useful in the treatment of acute extrapyramidal side effects, however, they are ineffective in ameliorating the long term sequelae.

Phenothiazine Derivatives

Drug	MOA & Pharmacokinetics	Clinical Uses	Side Effects
Chlorpromazine (Thorazine®)	**Antipsychotic**: blocks postsynaptic dopaminergic receptors (D_2) in the brain. Also blocks α-adrenergic receptors. Antiemetic: blocks dopamine receptors in the medullary chemoreceptor trigger zone and blocks of the vagus nerve in the GI tract.	**Schizophrenia** and other psychotic disorders **Emesis** Intractable hiccups Tetanus: adjunct treatment Acute intermittent porphyria	**Antiemetic effects** (strong) **Hypotensive effects** (strong) **Sedative properties** (strong) Anticholinergic (moderate to strong) Extrapyramidal (weak to moderate)
Fluphenazine (Permitil®, Prolixin®)	**Antipsychotic**: blocks postsynaptic dopaminergic receptors (D_2) in the brain. Also blocks α-adrenergic receptors.	**Schizophrenia** and other psychotic disorders	**Extrapyramidal effects** (strong) Antiemetic (weak) Hypotensive (weak) Sedative (weak) Anticholinergic (weak)
Trifluoperazine (Stelazine®, Suprazine®)	Same MOA as fluphenazine.	**Schizophrenia** and other psychotic disorders Anxiety	**Antiemetic effects** (strong) **Extrapyramidal effects** (strong) Hypotensive (weak) Sedative (weak) Anticholinergic (weak)
Thioridazine (Mellaril®)	Same MOA as fluphenazine.	**Schizophrenia** and other psychotic disorders	**Pigmentary retinopathy** Hypotensive (moderate to strong) Anticholinergic (moderate) Sedative (moderate) Antiemetic effects (weak) Extrapyramidal effects (weak) Ventricular arrhythmias/sudden death (rare)

Thioxanthene Derivative

Drug	MOA & Pharmacokinetics	Clinical Uses	Side Effects
Thiothixene (Navane®)	Blocks postsynaptic dopaminergic receptors (D_2) in the brain. Also blocks α-adrenergic receptors.	Schizophrenia and other psychotic disorders	Extrapyramidal effects Anticholinergic effects Hypotension

Butyrophenone

Drug	Mechanism of Action	Clinical Uses	Side Effects
Haloperidol (Haldol®)	Competitive blocker of postsynaptic dopamine (D_2) receptors in the CNS. Exhibits the highest affinity for D_2 receptors of antipsychotics. Also blocks α-adrenergic receptors.	**Psychotic disorders** including schizophrenia, manic states and drug-induced psychosis **Gilles de la Tourette's Syndrome** Huntington's disease	**Extrapyramidal effects** (strong) Anticholinergic effects Allergic reactions Orthostatic hypotension Drug Interactions: **Alcohol** and other **CNS depressants** may result in increased CNS and respiratory depression and increased hypotensive effects.

Atypical Antipsychotics

Drug	Mechanism of Action	Clinical Uses	Side Effects
Clozapine (Clozaril®)	Less affinity for blocking D_2 than chlorpromazine. Greater affinity for blocking D_4 than chlorpromazine. Antagonist at α_1-adrenergic, serotonin (5-HT_2), histamine H_1 and cholinergic receptors.	**Schizophrenia**: used in severely ill schizophrenics who are refractory to other neuroleptic agents.	**Agranulocytosis**: can lead to aplastic anemia. **Convulsions**: due to decreased seizure threshold **Sedation**: due to antihistaminic action **Cardiovascular effects: hypotension**, tachycardia Anticholinergic effects Sialorrhea: this is a poorly understood side effect because one would expect a dry mouth with anti-cholinergic effects. Benign Hyperthermia Syndrome (fever)
Risperidone (Risperdal®)	Antagonist at 5-HT_2 (high affinity) and D_2 (weak affinity) receptors. Also blocks α-adrenergic receptors (moderate affinity).	**Schizophrenia** and other psychotic disorders	**Hypotension** Extrapyramidal effects (limited with low doses)

Antimanic Agent

Drug	MOA & Pharmacokinetics	Clinical Uses	Side Effects
Lithium Carbonate (Eskalith®)	The mechanism is unclear but involves the inhibition of inositol phosphate recycling. This results in a decrease in the level of phosphatidylinositol bisphosphate (PIP_2) which leads to a depletion of IP_3 and DAG. The therapeutic blood level of lithium ions is 0.9 to 1.1 mEq/L. Levels must be checked regularly. Given PO Renal excretion	**Bipolar disorder** **Mania**	CNS effects: nausea, vomiting, diarrhea, tremors, ataxia, convulsion, coma, death Nephrogenic diabetes insipidus Leukocytosis Thyroid enlargement (but thyroid function usually remains unchanged). Teratogenic Drug Interactions: Concurrent use with **thiazide diuretics** may enhance lithium toxicity by decreasing its excretion.

Antiepileptic Drugs

Epilepsy is a common neurologic disorder affecting approximately 1% of the population. It comprises a heterogenous group of chronic syndromes characterized by recurrent seizures which result from excessive and disorderly discharges from cerebral neurons. The origin of these electrical discharges determines the symptoms that are produced during a seizure. Epilepsy can be classified as **idiopathic epilepsy** (70%) or **neurologic epilepsy**. Some causes of neurologic epilepsy include brain infections, ischemic injury, head trauma, mass lesions, metabolic disorders, drug or alcohol overdose and trauma at birth.

Term	Definition
Aura	The premonitory symptom of an impending seizure that is recognized by the patient.
Ictal period	The time during which the seizure occurs.
Status epilepticus	Seizure activity ≥ 30 minutes in duration regardless of seizure type. This syndrome is rare, but it is life-threatening when the repeating seizures are of the tonic-clonic variety.
Postictal period	The period of recovery from seizures. Postictal symptoms range from none to headache, confusion and profound exhaustion which depend on the intensity and duration of the ictal period.

Drugs Used to Treat Seizure Disorders

Grand mal and partial seizures	Absence seizures	Myoclonic seizures	Status epilepticus
Phenytoin Carbamazepine Primidone Phenobarbital	Ethosuximide Valproic acid Clonazepam	Valproic acid Clonazepam	Diazepam Phenytoin Phenobarbital

Classification of Seizure Types

Seizures have been classified as either partial or generalized. **Partial seizures** (focal seizures) begin in a limited region of the brain and either remain localized or spread to adjacent regions of the cortex. There are three types of partial seizures: simple partial, complex partial and partial seizures secondarily generalized. **Generalized seizures** begin in both hemispheres without local onset. Generalized seizures are characterized by a loss of consciousness and are either convulsive (tonic-clonic seizures) or nonconvulsive (myoclonic, atonic and absence seizures).

	Seizure type	Description
Partial Seizures	Simple partial seizures (focal seizures)	No loss of consciousness. May present with motor, somatosensory, special sensory or autonomic symptoms.
	Complex partial seizures (temporal or psychomotor seizures)	Consciousness is impaired. May begin as a simple partial seizure which progresses to impairment of consciousness or the impairment of consciousness may be present at the onset. These seizures may originate in limbic structures within the temporal lobe such as the hippocampus or amygdala.
	Partial seizures secondarily generalized (Jacksonian epilepsy)	Either simple partial or complex partial seizures which spread elsewhere to involve the entire brain, producing a generalized tonic-clonic seizure. Clinically seizures begin in one limb and then progress to include the rest of the body.
Generalized Seizures	Tonic-clonic seizures (grand mal seizures)	Tonic phase is associated with sustained cerebral discharge. The patient becomes stiff with stretched out arms and legs, ventilation is arrested as the respiratory muscles become fixed and the jaw is tightly closed. After the tonic phase the person enters the clonic phase, which consists of alternating relaxation and contraction of skeletal muscles. These seizures usually last 2-3 minutes.
	Absence seizures (petit mal seizures)	Non-convulsive seizures that usually begin in childhood and may persist into adulthood. Characterized by a sudden brief loss of consciousness; however, postural tone is preserved. The attacks are usually brief (5 and 30 seconds) and may occur up to one hundred times a day.
	Tonic seizures	Involve tonic contractions of certain muscle groups without progression to a clonic phase. Ocular phenomena are common (fixation of the eyes, eyelid retraction, nystagmus and mydriasis). Usually brief (10 seconds).
	Clonic seizures	Characterized by repetitive clonic jerks (lack a tonic component). Usually occurs in early childhood.
	Myoclonic seizures	Characterized by single or multiple sudden, brief contractions which may be generalized or confined to individual muscles or groups of muscles.
	Atonic seizures (drop attacks)	Sudden loss of postural tone.

Drugs for Partial and Generalized Tonic-Clonic Seizures

Drug	MOA & Pharmacokinetics	Clinical Uses	Side Effects
Phenytoin (Dilantin®)	Binds to and prolongs the inactivated state of **Na^+ channels** (prevents high frequency firing of action potentials). Metabolized by hepatic cytochrome P_{450} to inactive metabolites. At elevated serum levels, phenytoin saturates the cytochrome system and exhibits **zero-order kinetics**.	**Generalized tonic-clonic seizures** **Partial seizures** **Status epilepticus**: prophylaxis only Arrhythmias	**Gingival hyperplasia** CNS toxicity: nystagmus, diplopia and ataxia Hirsutism Induction of cytochrome P_{450} enzymes which can lead to increased metabolism and clearance of other drugs. Hypersensitivity reactions: SLE, Stevens-Johnson syndrome Peripheral neuropathy: diminished deep tendon reflexes in extremities occurs with long term use. Sedation occurs at higher levels. Megaloblastic anemia due to alteration in folate metabolism. Teratogenic: fetal hydantoin syndrome which is characterized by abnormal growth and development.
Carbamazepine (Tegretol®)	Anticonvulsant mechanism is similar to phenytoin. Metabolized by the liver to an **active metabolite** (carbamazepine-10, 11-epoxide) which also exhibits antiepileptic activity. Antineuralgic activity may involve interaction with $GABA_B$ receptors.	**Generalized tonic-clonic seizures** **Partial seizures**: DOC **Trigeminal neuralgia**: DOC	**CNS toxicity**: diplopia, nystagmus, and ataxia Induction of cytochrome P_{450} enzymes: can lead to increased metabolism and clearance of other drugs. Blood dyscrasias: rare

Drug	MOA & Pharmacokinetics	Clinical Uses	Side Effects
Primidone (Mysoline®)	Primidone has an antiepileptic action similar to phenytoin. Metabolized to active metabolites phenobarbital and phenyl-ethylmalonamide (PEMA). The phenobarbital metabolite generated enhances GABA-mediated inhibition of neuronal activity and reduces glutamate-mediated excitation.	Generalized tonic-clonic seizures Partial seizures	CNS toxicity: sedation, dizziness, ataxia, diplopia and nystagmus Nausea and vomiting Hypersensitivity reactions: SLE, Stevens-Johnson syndrome (rare) Blood dyscrasias (rare)
Phenobarbital (Barbita®, Luminal®)	A long acting barbiturate which binds the $GABA_A$ receptor causing allosteric changes which enhance GABA binding resulting in prolonged periods of chloride channel opening. This causes membrane hyper-polarization and a ↓ in neuronal excitability. Also blocks the excitatory responses in CNS synapses induced by glutamic acid.	**Generalized tonic-clonic seizures** **Partial seizures** **Status epilepticus** Sedative-hypnotic	**Sedation** CNS and respiratory depression Induction of cytochrome P_{450} enzymes which can lead to increased metabolism and clearance of other drugs. Tolerance, dependence Exfoliative dermatitis and Stevens-Johnson syndrome (rare)

Drugs Used to Treat Absence Seizures

Drug	MOA & Pharmacokinetics	Clinical Uses	Side Effects
Ethosuximide (Zarontin®)	**Inhibits Ca^{2+} influx** through low threshold T-type channels in thalamic neurons. Metabolized to an active metabolite N-desmethylmethsuximide.	**Absence seizures**: DOC	GI disturbances: nausea, vomiting CNS effects: lethargy, sedation, dizziness Hypersensitivity reactions and blood dyscrasias (rare)
Valproic Acid (Depakene®)	Inhibits high-frequency repetitive firing of neurons by **inhibiting Na^+ influx** through specific voltage-gated ion channels (similar to phenytoin). Inhibits Ca^{2+} influx through low threshold T-type channels. May have an effect on GABA metabolism. Blood level is poorly correlated with anticonvulsant activity, thus plasma concentration is not useful in determining dose.	Absence seizures Mixed seizures: generalized tonic-clonic concomitant with absence seizures. Myoclonic seizures Generalized tonic-clonic seizures	GI disturbances: nausea, vomiting Hepatotoxicity: may be due to toxic metabolite. CNS effects: sedation, ataxia, tremor Teratogenic: neural tube defects and digital abnormalities Drug Interactions: Inhibits metabolism of phenobarbital, phenytoin and carbamazepine.
Benzodiazepines Diazepam (Valium®) Clonazepam (Klonopin®)	Bind the $GABA_A$ receptor causing allosteric changes which enhance GABA binding. This results in an increased frequency of chloride channel opening leading to membrane hyperpolarization and a decrease in neuronal excitability. Also enhances glycine binding in the spinal cord.	**Status epilepticus**: *diazepam* is DOC Absence seizures: *clonazepam* Myoclonic seizures: *clonazepam*	Drowsiness and lethargy Respiratory and cardiovascular depression

Notes

Drugs Used to Treat Movement Disorders

The two major movement disorders are **Parkinson's** and **Huntington's diseases**.

Parkinson's disease

Parkinson's disease is a common disease of the elderly. It presents as a range of motor disorders including resting tremors, muscular rigidity, bradykinesia, expressionless countenance and emotional disturbances. Most cases of Parkinson's disease are idiopathic, however, some cases may involve previous viral encephalitis or exposure to particular compounds such as MPTP, an impurity found in some heroin preparations. Parkinson's disease is a neurodegenerative disorder which results from the loss of dopamine producing cells in the basal ganglia. The basal ganglia, composed of the substantia nigra and corpus striatum, is the region of the brain responsible for motor control. Dopamine is an inhibitory neurotransmitter which acts on the neostriatum in a tonic manner to maintain motion. Loss of these dopaminergic neurons is the underlying cause of the decreased motor activity which characterizes Parkinson's disease. Pharmacologic therapy attempts to increase dopaminergic activity in the CNS.

Figure 3.4: Schematic of pathophysiology of Parkinson's and Huntington's diseases

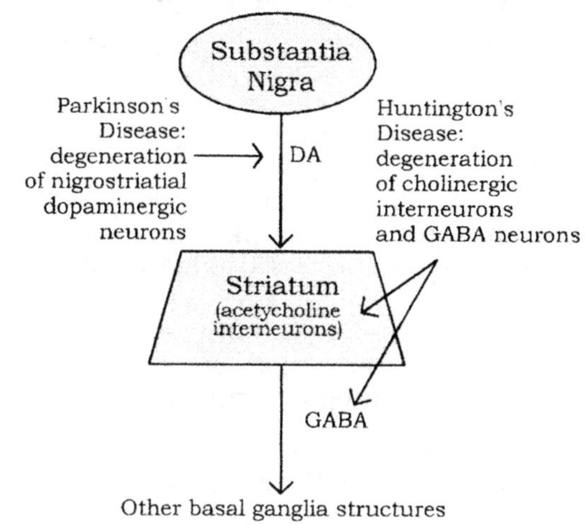

Huntington's disease

Chorea and **dementia** are characteristic of this **autosomal dominant** disorder. A relative increase of dopamine, or decrease of acetylcholine or GABA, in the basal ganglia seem to be the underlying causes of this motor disorder. Drugs used to treat Huntington's disease either impair the action of dopamine or increase the amounts of acetylcholine or GABA.

Drugs for Parkinson's Disease	Drugs for Huntington's Disease
Levodopa Carbidopa Selegiline Bromocriptine Pergolide Benztropine Amantadine	Haloperidol Phenothiazines Reserpine Tetrabenazine

Drugs for Parkinson's Disease

Treatment for Parkinson's disease focuses on ameliorating the clinical manifestations. Therefore, therapy is targeted towards increasing dopamine activity or reducing the effect of cholinergic stimulation. Dopamine itself can not be given because it does not cross the blood brain barrier.

Drug	MOA & Pharmacokinetics	Clinical Uses	Side Effects
Levodopa (L-dopa) (Dopar®, Larodopa®)	L-dopa is rapidly **converted to dopamine** by **dopa decarboxylase** in the periphery and nervous system. 95% is decarboxylated in the periphery, therefore, some α– and β–adrenergic effects are seen. L-dopa **crosses the blood brain barrier**. Metabolized to dihydroxyphenylacetic acid (DOPAC) and homovanillic acid (HVA). Given PO	**Parkinson's disease**: idiopathic, postencephalitic and carbon monoxide or manganese induced. Tolerance develops over time, therefore, patients should be taken off medication periodically (drug holidays).	**GI disturbances**: anorexia, nausea, vomiting **Dyskinesia**: choreoathetosis, chorea, ballismus, myoclonus, tics or tremors **Cardiovascular effects**: tachycardia, orthostatic hypotension, arrhythmias CNS effects: hallucinations, delusions, agitation, confusion
Levodopa plus Carbidopa (Sinemet®)	**Carbidopa** increases cerebral concentrations of dopamine by **inhibiting peripheral dopa decarboxylase**. Carbidopa **does not cross the blood brain barrier**. Sinemet is a mixture of L-dopa and carbidopa (either 10:1 or 4:1).		Drug Interactions: Pyridoxine enhances peripheral metabolism of L-dopa. Phenothiazines, reserpine and butyrophenones antagonize L-dopa effects. MAO inhibitors should be discontinued prior to treatment (risk of hypertensive crisis).
Selegiline (Eldepryl®, Deprenyl®)	Increases dopamine concentrations by **selectively inhibiting MAO-B** (more selective for metabolizing dopamine than norepinephrine or serotonin). The use of selegiline enhances the actions of L-dopa, allowing for decreased dosage.	**Parkinson's disease**: idiopathic. Used as an adjuvant with L-dopa or L-dopa/carbidopa.	**Dyskinesias**: may enhance L-dopa induced dyskinesia Mood alterations

Drug	MOA & Pharmacokinetics	Clinical Uses	Side Effects
Bromocriptine (Parlodel®)	Ergot alkaloid which acts as a strong agonist at D_2 receptors and a partial antagonist at D_1 receptors. Growth hormone stimulant	**Parkinson's disease**: idiopathic and postencephalitic. Used as an adjuvant with L-dopa/carbidopa. **Hyperprolactinemia**: DOC Acromegaly	Hypotension CNS effects: confusion, hallucinations, dyskinesias Retroperitoneal fibrosis (rare) Erythromyalgia (rare)
Pergolide (Permax®)	A dopamine agonist at D_1 and D_2 receptors. More potent than bromocriptine.	**Parkinson's disease**: idiopathic and postencephalitic. Used as an adjuvant with L-dopa or L-dopa/carbidopa.	**CNS effects**: confusion, hallucinations, dyskinesias **Urinary tract infections** Hypotension Retroperitoneal fibrosis (rare) Erythromyalgia (rare)
Benztropine (Cogentin®)	Alkaloid which is thought to act as an antimuscarinic agent in the CNS, specifically the corpus striatum. Crosses the blood brain barrier. Helps to balance the dopaminergic-cholinergic ratio in the basal ganglia.	**Parkinson's disease**: idiopathic, postencephalitic or drug (antipsychotic) induced.	Anticholinergic effects: glaucoma, dry mouth, constipation, urinary retention, blurred vision, sedation CNS effects: amnesia, delirium, hallucinations ◆ Contraindication: Narrow angle glaucoma
Amantadine (Symmetrel®)	An antiviral agent which **increases synthesis, release** and **delays reuptake of dopamine** in the nigra striatum. Prevents the uncoating of influenza virus. Given PO	**Parkinson's disease**: idiopathic, postencephalitic or drug (antipsychotic) induced. **Influenza A** prophylaxis and treatment	Infrequent but include: Anticholinergic effects CNS effects: restlessness, agitation, confusion Livedo reticularis, a bluish discoloration of the legs and hands, is seen with long-term use.

Drugs Used to Treat Huntington's Disease

The drugs used to treat Huntington's disease are listed below. Huntington's disease is not listed as an indication in U.S. product labelling for these agents. Furthermore, tetrabenazine is not currently available in the U.S.

Dopamine receptor blocking agents	Dopamine depleting agents
Haloperidol Phenothiazines	Reserpine Tetrabenazine

Anesthetic Drugs

Anesthesia is defined as the loss of feeling or sensation. There are two types of anesthesia: general and local. General anesthetics act within the CNS and/or ANS to produce a loss of consciousness, amnesia, analgesia, skeletal muscle relaxation and loss of reflexes. Local anesthetics block nerve conduction in the periphery causing only a focal loss of sensation.

General Anesthetics

All general anesthetics are **CNS depressants**. There are two types of general anesthetics: inhalation agents and intravenous agents. Inhalation agents are further subdivided into volatile liquids and gases; intravenous agents are further subdivided into barbiturates, benzodiazepines, opioids, dissociative agents and others.

Inhalation Agents	
Volatile liquids	Gas
Halothane Enflurane Isoflurane Desflurane	Nitrous oxide (N_2O)

Intravenous Agents					
Barbiturates	Benzodiazepines	Opioids	Neuroleptic-Opioid	Dissociative	Others
Thiopental	Midazolam Diazepam Lorazepam	Morphine Fentanyl	Fentanyl plus Droperidol	Ketamine	Propofol

Gases and Vapors

Inhalation anesthesia is produced by the inhalation of certain gases (nitrous oxide) and vaporized liquid halogens (halothane, desflurane, enflurane and isoflurane). A measure of potency of these compounds is the **minimum alveolar concentration (MAC)**. The MAC is defined as the steady state alveolar concentration necessary for 50% of the population not to react to a surgical stimulus. The lower the MAC, the more potent the anesthetic. The MAC is related to the lipid solubility of the agent; as lipid solubility increases, the MAC decreases (see below).

Since these compounds are administered either as a gas or a vapor, the concentration in the body is reflected by the **partial pressure** of the agent in the blood. There are several factors which influence the uptake of an inhaled agent and affect the onset of anesthesia. The faster the uptake the earlier the onset of anesthesia.

Factor	Effect on Uptake	Explanation
Inspired Gas Concentration	**↑ concentration = ↑ uptake**	Increases in the inspired gas concentration of an inhaled agent increases the alveolar concentration and subsequently the blood partial pressure. This results in quicker onset of anesthesia. Thus, a concentration higher than the maintenance dose is used to induce anesthesia.
Alveolar Ventilation	**↑ ventilation = ↑ uptake**	An increase in pulmonary ventilation results in a higher alveolar and blood concentration leading to a faster onset of anesthesia. This is more pronounced with agents with high solubility. Mechanical hyperventilation can be employed to hasten the induction of anesthesia with agents that normally have a slow onset.
Solubility	**↑ solubility = ↓ uptake**	There is an inverse relationship between the solubility of an anesthetic agent and the rate of rise of its partial pressure in the blood. Molecules which dissolve in the blood do not contribute to the pressure of the gas in the blood. Thus the partial pressure of agents with low solubility increases faster than those with high solubility. Solubility is measured by the blood-gas partition coefficient (PC) which is a comparison between the affinity of an agent for blood compared to air.
Cardiac Output	**↑ cardiac output = ↓ uptake**	As cardiac output increases, pulmonary output also increases; this results in a slower rise in the gas partial pressure (slower uptake of anesthetic) and a reduction in the speed of onset of anesthesia.

<table>
<tr><th rowspan="2">Drug</th><th rowspan="2">Metabolism</th><th rowspan="2">PC</th><th rowspan="2">MAC</th><th colspan="5">Cardiovascular Effects</th><th rowspan="2">Respiratory Effects</th><th rowspan="2">Toxicity</th></tr>
<tr><th>HR</th><th>BP</th><th>CO</th><th>PR</th><th>Myo</th></tr>
<tr><td>Halothane</td><td>20%; the rest is eliminated unchanged in exhaled air</td><td>2.3</td><td>0.75%</td><td>↓</td><td>↓</td><td>↓</td><td>↓</td><td>+++</td><td rowspan="4">Decrease tidal volume and minute ventilation (↑CO_2) resulting in an increased respiratory rate.

Decrease hypoxic and hypercarbic ventilatory response ('respiratory depression').

Inhibit hypoxic pulmonary vasoconstriction.

Decrease bronchial smooth muscle tone.

Decrease pulmonary vascular resistance.</td><td rowspan="4">Malignant hyperthermia: potentially fatal disorder observed as hyperthermia, metabolic acidosis, tachycardia and accelerated muscle contraction. Treated with dantrolene.

Hepatic necrosis (with halothane): halothane hepatitis occurs in 1/10,000 administrations usually with repeat administrations over a short period of time. It is unlikely to occur in children and thus halothane is the DOC for inhalational anesthesia in children.

Renal failure (with enflurane): free fluoride is released which can cause renal failure in patients with pre-existing renal disease.</td></tr>
<tr><td>Enflurane</td><td>Less than for halothane</td><td>1.8</td><td>1.6%</td><td>↑</td><td>↓</td><td>↓</td><td>↓</td><td>+</td></tr>
<tr><td>Isoflurane</td><td>Minimal</td><td>1.4</td><td>1.2%</td><td>↑</td><td>↓</td><td></td><td>↓↓</td><td>+</td></tr>
<tr><td>Desflurane</td><td>Minimal</td><td>.4</td><td>6%</td><td>↑</td><td>↓</td><td></td><td>↓</td><td>+</td></tr>
<tr><td>Nitrous oxide (N_2O)</td><td>Not metabolized; termination of action is by exhalation.</td><td>.5</td><td>> 100%</td><td colspan="5">↑

Note: This agent cannot be used alone for general anesthesia. It is often combined with other anesthetics to provide complete anesthesia.</td><td>Very little effect</td><td>Irreversibly inactivates methionine synthase (a vitamin B_{12}-dependent enzyme) which can cause bone marrow depression (megaloblastic anemia) with prolonged administration.

High concentration may cause neuropathy.

◆ Contraindication: Patients with closed air cavities (pneumothorax)</td></tr>
</table>

PC = blood-gas partition coefficient; MAC = minimal alveolar concentration; HR = heart rate; BP = blood pressure; CO = cardiac output; PR = peripheral resistance; Myo = sensitization of the myocardium to catecholamines.

Intravenous Anesthetic Agents

Various classes of drugs are used as intravenous anesthetics: barbiturates, benzodiazepines, opioids, a dissociative anesthetic and propofol. Because several of these compounds have been discussed in other chapters, this section will focus on the anesthetic property of these agents.

Barbiturate

Drug	General Notes & Physiological Effects	Clinical Uses	Side Effects
Thiopental (Pentothal®)	An ultrashort acting barbiturate which binds the $GABA_A$ receptor causing allosteric changes which enhance GABA binding resulting in **prolonged duration** of **chloride channel opening**. This causes membrane hyperpolarization and a decrease in neuronal excitability. Unconsciousness occurs in about 15 seconds after IV administration. Thiopental is metabolized in the liver but the anesthetic effects are terminated by **redistribution** to other organs in the body. **Respiratory depression**: decreases response to CO_2 or hypoxia. Cerebral blood flow and intracranial pressure are markedly reduced. Thiopental and other barbiturates are **poor analgesics** and could even increase sensitivity to pain if inadequate doses are administered.	**Induction of anesthesia** with subsequent administration of other agents for maintenance. Used alone for short procedures associated with little pain.	Cough, laryngospasm and bronchospasm There is no effective agent to antagonize barbiturates in overdose. ◆ Contraindication: Variegate porphyria (South African) or acute intermittent porphyria. Thiopental and other barbiturates may precipitate CNS and PNS demyelination resulting in weakness, paralysis, even death.

Benzodiazepines

Drug	General Notes & Physiological Effects	Clinical Uses	Side Effects
Midazolam (Versed®) Diazepam (Valium®) Lorazepam (Ativan®)	Bind the $GABA_A$ receptor causing allosteric changes which enhance GABA binding. This results in an **increased frequency** of **chloride channel opening** leading to membrane hyperpolarization and a decrease in neuronal excitability. Slower onset than barbiturates (several minutes) after IV administration. Midazolam is the preferred benzodiazepine for induction and maintenance of anesthesia due to its shorter onset of action, its greater potency, and its more rapid elimination when compared to diazepam. When used alone, benzodiazepines cause moderate circulatory and respiratory depression. Given PO, IM, IV	**Preanesthetic medication** **Anesthesia**: sole agent for procedures that do not require analgesia (ie. endoscopy, cardioversion, cardiac catheterization, radiographic diagnostic procedures). Since benzodiazepines are not analgesic and cannot alone produce a state of surgical anesthesia, a combination of drugs is necessary to achieve surgical anesthesia. Diagnostic procedures in patients with cardiac pathology (due to the minor cardiovascular effects). Antegrade amnesia: *lorazepam* Muscle spasms: *diazepam* Alcohol withdrawal: *diazepam, lorazepam* Status epilepticus: *diazepam* Reduction of ketamine induced hallucinations and unpleasant dreams: *midazolam.*	Drowsiness Decreased cognitive function When given in conjunction with opioids, severe cardiovascular and respiratory depression may occur. CNS depression caused by benzodiazepine is antagonized by **flumazenil**.

Opioids and Neuroleptic-Opioid Combination

Drug	General Notes & Physiological Effects	Clinical Uses	Side Effects
Fentanyl (Sublimaze®) Morphine	Large doses of opioid analgesics are required to produce general anesthesia. These agents cause respiratory system depression while the cardiovascular system remains relatively preserved. Fentanyl has replaced morphine due to its higher potency and a decreased incidence of respiratory depression.	General anesthesia in conjunction with skeletal muscle relaxants and N_2O or other inhalational anesthetics Surgery in cardiac patients	Nausea and vomiting IV opioids may increase chest wall rigidity which may impair ventilation. Postoperative respiratory depression antagonized by **naloxone**.
Droperidol plus Fentanyl (Innovar® is a combination of droperidol and fentanyl).	When a neuroleptic drug is combined with a narcotic, a state of **neurolept analgesia** is produced; most often produced by combining droperidol with fentanyl. If anesthesia is required, neurolept analgesia can be converted to **neurolept anesthesia** by the administration of 65% N_2O in O_2. Induction of the above states is slow. Since fentanyl has such a short analgesic duration of action (30-60 minutes) compared to the effect of droperidol, supplementary doses of fentanyl are usually administered. Respiratory depression is severe and outlasts the analgesic effect. Cardiovascular effects are mild. Droperidol possesses mild α-adrenergic blocking activity and can produce hypotension. Fentanyl possesses parasympathetic activity and can produce bradycardia.	Analgesia: during minor surgical procedures, the changing of burn dressings and diagnostic procedures such as endoscopy and radiographic procedures General anesthesia: in combination with N_20	Nausea and vomiting Confusion and mental depression Respiratory depression during recovery is antagonized by **naloxone**. Neuroleptic malignant syndrome (droperidol-induced) Extrapyramidal symptoms (due to droperidol) can be controlled with atropine. ◆ Contraindication: Patients with Parkinson's disease

Dissociative anesthetic and propofol

Drug	General Notes & Physiological Effects	Clinical Uses	Side Effects
Ketamine (Ketalar®)	Structurally similar to PCP (the original dissociative anesthetic). Blocks **NMDA** receptors. Patients experience **dissociation anesthesia** in which they have a feeling of dissociation from their environment and experience sedation, immobility, amnesia and marked analgesia. Not a respiratory depressant **Cardiovascular stimulant**: ↑HR, CO and BP Cerebral blood flow and intracranial pressure are increased. Given IV, IM	Trauma and emergency surgical procedures (because of its cardiostimulatory properties). Radiological procedures in children	**Hallucinations** and unpleasant dreams frequently occur during recovery and are more common in adults than children. These adverse psychological experiences can be reduced by preoperative administration of a **benzodiazepine**, especially midazolam. ◆ Contraindication: Not to be used in patients with head trauma because of increased intracranial pressure.
Propofol (Diprivan®)	Produces anesthesia as rapidly as thiopental, but recovery is more rapid. Does not have the hangover effect after anesthesia that barbiturates have. Decreases arterial pressure due to peripheral vasodilation. Respiration is severely depressed: tidal volume, minute volume and the responses to CO_2 and hypoxia are reduced. Cerebral blood flow and intracranial pressure are reduced. Given IV	Induction and maintenance of general anesthesia Sedation during regional anesthesia or intensive care	Severe hypotension Pain at the site of injection Apnea

Local Anesthetics

Local anesthetics affect nerve **conductance**. These drugs cause a loss of sensation without loss of consciousness. Local anesthetics are administered topically or injected into areas where anesthesia is needed. There are two classes of local anesthetics: esters and amides.

Esters	Amides
Cocaine Benzocaine Procaine Tetracaine	Lidocaine Mepivacaine Bupivacaine Prilocaine

Characteristics of nerve fibers most sensitive to local anesthetics:
• Small diameter • Myelinated fibers • Rapidly firing nerves • Peripheral fibers in a nerve bundle • Pain fibers (C- and $A\partial$) > Sensory fibers ($A\beta$) > Motor neurons ($A\alpha$)

Drug	MOA & Pharmacokinetics	Clinical Uses	Side Effects
Esters: Cocaine Benzocaine Procaine Tetracaine *Amides:* Lidocaine Mepivacaine Bupivacaine Prilocaine	Block nerve transmission by inhibiting **Na^+ channels**. Local anesthetics are **weak bases** which exist in protonated or unprotonated forms. Only the protonated form is pharmacologically active, but only the unprotonated form can penetrate nerve sheaths. Areas of inflammation tend to have a lower pH resulting in a predominance of the protonated form. Consequently, there is little tissue penetration and poor anesthesia. **Esters** are **more rapidly metabolized** by blood/tissue esterases and have shorter half-lives. **Amides** are metabolized by **hepatic microsomal enzymes** (amidases) and have longer half-lives.	Surface anesthesia Nerve block anesthesia Spinal anesthesia Epidural anesthesia Arrhythmias: lidocaine	**CNS effects**: • Lightheadedness • Restlessness • Sensory disturbances • Euphoria • Convulsions, coma and death at high doses **Cardiovascular effects** (more pronounced with bupivacaine): • Hypotension • Myocardial depression • **Cocaine** is the exception: causing **vasoconstriction** and **hypertension** Allergic reactions: mostly with **esters** due to the formation of the metabolite **p-amino benzoic acid** (PABA) Methemoglobinemia: prilocaine

Figure 3.5: The mechanism of local anesthetics

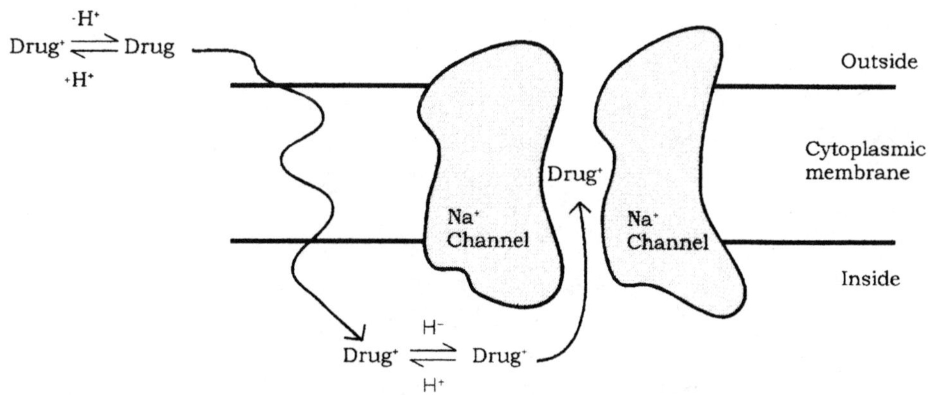

Notes

Opioid Agonists and Antagonists

Opioid agonists, also known as **narcotic analgesics**, stimulate opioid receptors to produce morphine-like effects, most importantly analgesia. Also included in this section are opioid receptor antagonists and drugs with mixed agonist-antagonist activities.

Opioid Agonists		
Severe pain	Mild to moderate pain	Special uses
Morphine Meperidine Methadone Fentanyl Hydromorphone Heroin	Hydrocodone Oxycodone Codeine Propoxyphene	Diphenoxylate Loperamide

Opioid Receptor	
Antagonists	Agonist-Antagonists
Naloxone Naltrexone	Pentazocine Nalbuphine

Endogenous Opioids and Receptors

Endogenous opioids include β-endorphin, enkephalins and dynorphins which impart their effects via several classes of opioid receptors. There are four known opioid receptors, μ, κ, δ and σ. These receptors are differentially distributed throughout the nervous system including the spinal cord, brainstem, thalamus, limbic system and cortex. The pharmacological significance of δ receptors is unclear.

Figure. 3.6: Opioid receptors

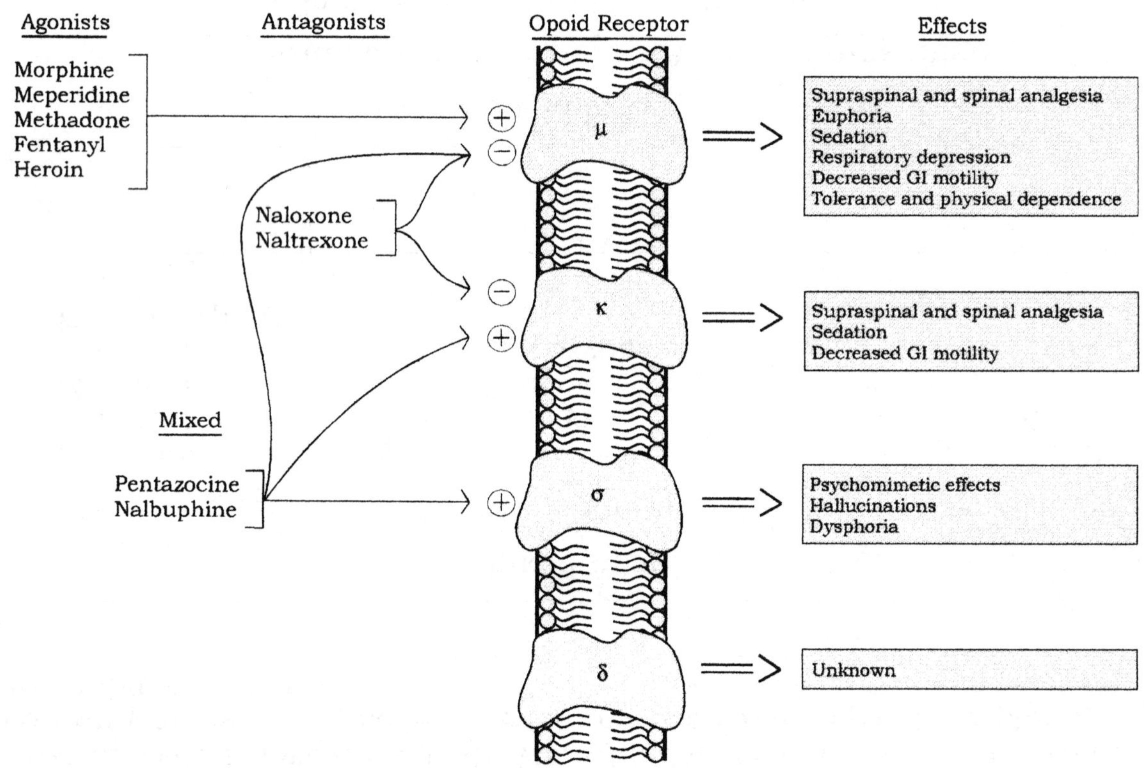

Effects of Morphine

The following table summarizes the acute effects of opioids. Two noteworthy chronic effects of opioids are **tolerance** and **dependence**. Tolerance develops to all of these effects except miosis and constipation. Dependence may occur with the more potent opioids. Physical dependence is observed upon discontinuance as a **withdrawal syndrome** including chills, diarrhea, myalgia, anxiety and hostility.

Effect	Notes
1. **Analgesia**	occurs primarily by the stimulation of μ receptors which suppresses the peripheral nociceptive pathway and the pain processing cortex.
2. **Respiratory depression**	occurs by the stimulation of μ receptors. Opioids decrease the sensitivity of chemoreceptors to carbon dioxide in the medullary respiratory center. This is the major cause of death in overdose.
3. **Sedation and euphoria**	occur by the stimulation of μ receptors at sub-analgesic doses.
4. **Miosis**	is characteristic of opioid exposure. Tolerance does NOT develop.
5. **Constipation**	is caused by decreased intestinal motility. Tolerance does NOT develop.
6. **Antitussive effects**	are due to the depression of the medullary cough center which occurs at sub-analgesic doses.
7. **Emetic effects**	are due to stimulation of the chemoreceptor trigger zone (CTZ) and emetic center. Opioids initially stimulate the CTZ and cause nausea, however, chronic use of opioids suppresses the medullary emetic center and imparts an antiemetic effect.
8. **Convulsant effects**	are seen in a portion of the population. Additionally, metabolites of codeine and meperidine exhibit convulsant activity.
9. **Cardiovascular effects**	include **postural hypotension** from administration of a large IV dose of morphine.
10. **Smooth muscle effects**	include an increase in circular muscle tone, resulting in biliary, ureteral and bronchial spasms.
11. **Histamine release**	results in urticaria, vasodilation and bronchoconstriction.

Opioid Agonists

Severe Pain

Drug	MOA & Pharmacokinetics	Clinical Uses	Side Effects
Morphine (Roxanol®, MS Contin®) Schedule II drug	Naturally occurring opioid agonist at μ receptors. Has an **active** metabolite, **morphine 6-glucuronide**. Duration = 5 hrs Given PO, IM, SC, or IV	**Analgesia: DOC** for **acute myocardial infarction**, also for chronic pain **Acute pulmonary edema** due to left ventricular failure: adjunct therapy. Antitussive	Constipation Histamine release Convulsions: due to the formation of normorphine, an inactive metabolite
Meperidine (Demerol®) Schedule II drug	Synthetic opioid agonist at μ receptors. Metabolized to **normeperidine** which is both active and toxic. Potency is 1/10 that of morphine. Causes **mydriasis** (not miosis) due to an atropine like effect. Duration: 2-3 hrs Given PO, parenterally	**Analgesia**: moderate to severe pain. Also used for **obstetrical analgesia** because it has less respiratory effects on the fetus than other opioids.	Constipation Histamine release ◆ Contraindication: Use of MAO inhibitors 14-21 days prior to meperidine administration.
Methadone (Dolophine®) Schedule II drug	A synthetic opioid agonist at μ receptors. Potency is equivalent to morphine. Duration = 6 hrs Given PO	Analgesia: moderate to severe pain **Narcotic addiction**: **methadone detoxification** cures a narcotic addiction by the administration of a gradually decreasing dose (to control withdrawal symptoms); **methadone maintenance** is a constant dose given as a substitute for illicit narcotics. Antitussive	Constipation Drug Interactions: Phenytoin and rifampin increase the metabolism of methadone and exacerbate withdrawal symptoms in dependent individuals.

Drug	MOA & Pharmacokinetics	Clinical Uses	Side Effects
Fentanyl (Sublimaze®, Duragesic®) Schedule II drug	A synthetic opioid agonist at μ receptors. Potency is 80x that of morphine. Duration = 1 hr (parenteral) = days (transdermal patch) Given parenterally or **transdermally**	**Analgesia**: for chronic and post-operative pain Anesthesia: used in combination with droperidol as a supplement to general anesthesia.	**Apnea** **CNS depression** **Hypoventilation** ◆ Contraindications: Patients with diarrhea or respiratory depression. Drug Interactions: Can enhance CNS depression when used in combination with alcohol, CNS depressants or naltrexone.
Hydromorphone (Dilaudid®) Schedule II drug	An opioid agonist at μ receptors. Potency is 7x that of morphine. Duration: 4-5 hrs	**Analgesia**: moderate to severe pain Antitussive	
Heroin Schedule I drug	A semisynthetic opioid agonist which is metabolized to 6-acetyl morphine and, subsequently, to morphine. Both of these metabolites are active. Both heroin and 6-acetylmorphine are more lipophilic than morphine.	Not used therapeutically in the U.S.	

Mild to Moderate Pain

Drug	MOA & Pharmacokinetics	Clinical Uses	Side Effects
Hydrocodone (Dihydrocodeinone) (Hydocan®) Schedule III drug	An opioid agonist at μ receptors. Duration = 4 hrs	Analgesia: mild to moderate pain Antitussive	Histamine release
Oxycodone (Roxicodone®, Supeudol®) Percodan® contains oxycodone and aspirin. Percocet® contains oxycodone and acetaminophen. Schedule II drug	An opioid agonist at μ receptors. Potency is 2/3 that of morphine. Duration = 4 hrs Given PO	Analgesia: mild to moderate pain	
Codeine Schedule II drug	A naturally occurring opioid agonist with low affinity at μ receptors. 10% is demethylated to morphine. Potency is 1/8 that of morphine. Given PO	Analgesia: mild to moderate pain at high doses. This effect is mediated through the formation of morphine. **Antitussive**: at low doses due to codeine itself.	Constipation
Propoxyphene (Darvon®) Schedule IV drug	A synthetic opioid agonist at μ receptors. Potency is 1/6 that of morphine.	Analgesia	Convulsions Hepatotoxicity

Special Use Opioid Agonists and Dextromethorphan

Drug	MOA & Pharmacokinetics	Clinical Uses	Side Effects
Diphenoxylate HCl Lomotil® is diphenoxylate and atropine Motofen® is diphenoxin and atropine	A meperidine analog which acts at opioid receptors in the enteric nervous system to increase intestinal motility. Diphenoxylate is metabolized to **diphenoxin**, which exhibits equivalent activity. Duration = 4 hrs Given PO	**Diarrhea** at low doses. It is only available in preparations containing atropine to discourage abuse. Analgesia only at high dose	Anticholinergic effects: dry mouth, blurred vision due to the presence of atropine.
Loperamide (Imodium®, Imodium-AD®)	A meperidine analog which acts at opioid receptors in the enteric nervous system to decrease intestinal motility. Given PO	**Antidiarrheal**	Abdominal cramps
Dextromethorphan (Benylin DM®, Delsym®) Non-narcotic antitussive	A synthetic derivative of morphine which acts directly on the medullary cough center to suppress the cough reflex. Does not have any activity at opioid receptors. Duration = 6 hrs Given PO	**Antitussive**	Drug Interactions: CNS depressants can potentiate depressant effects. MAO inhibitors may cause an adrenergic crisis.

Opioid Antagonists

Drug	MOA & Pharmacokinetics	Clinical Uses	Side Effects
Naloxone (Narcan®)	Antagonist at opioid receptors with high binding specificity. Given IV, IM	**Opioid toxicity**: diagnosis and treatment **Respiratory depression**: post-operative and opioid induced.	Tachycardia Arrhythmias
Naltrexone (Trexan®)	Antagonist at opioid receptors. Given PO	Maintaining an **opioid-free state** in former opioid addicts: adjuvant therapy. Chronic alcoholism	Hepatotoxicity Drug Interaction: Opioid medication ◆ Contraindications: Patients with liver failure or hepatitis Opioid dependency

Opioid Agonist-Antagonists

Drug	MOA & Pharmacokinetics	Clinical Uses	Side Effects
Pentazocine (Talwin®)	**Agonist** at κ and σ receptors. **Antagonist** at μ receptors. Potency is 1/15 that of morphine. Duration = 3 hrs Given PO, IV, IM, SC	Analgesia	Subjective/psychotomimetic effects due to stimulation of σ receptors. Respiratory depression: exhibits a "**ceiling effect**" where the degree of respiratory depression reaches a plateau despite increasing drug level.
Nalbuphine (Nubain®)	**Agonist** at κ receptors **Weak agonist** at σ receptors **Antagonist** at μ receptors. Potency is equivalent to morphine. Duration = 3-6 hrs Given IV	Analgesia Anesthesia adjuvant	Histamine release Subjective/psychotomimetic effects due to stimulation of σ receptors (rare). Exhibits a "**ceiling effect**" for respiratory depression.

Alcohols and Disulfiram

Alcohol is a CNS depressant whose effects and abuse potential are well documented. The following section describes its metabolism and clinical uses.

Ethanol is metabolized to acetaldehyde by either of the following systems:

1. **alcohol dehydrogenase:** a cytosolic, NAD-dependent enzyme which metabolizes low to moderate doses (up to 7-10 gm/hr) of ethyl alcohol. This reaction has **zero order kinetics** due to the limited cellular supply of NAD.
2. **microsomal ethanol-oxidizing system (MEOS)** is a NADPH-dependent liver microsomal mixed-function oxidase system whose activity is induced by chronic exposure to ethanol (potential mechanism of tolerance).

Acetaldehyde is rapidly converted to acetic acid by acetaldehyde dehydrogenase. **Disulfiram** is an inhibitor of acetaldehyde dehydrogenase and is used in therapy for alcohol abuse. Other inhibitors of acetaldehyde dehydrogenase include metronidazole, oral hypoglycemics and some cephalosporin antibiotics.

Figure 3.7: The metabolic pathway of ethanol

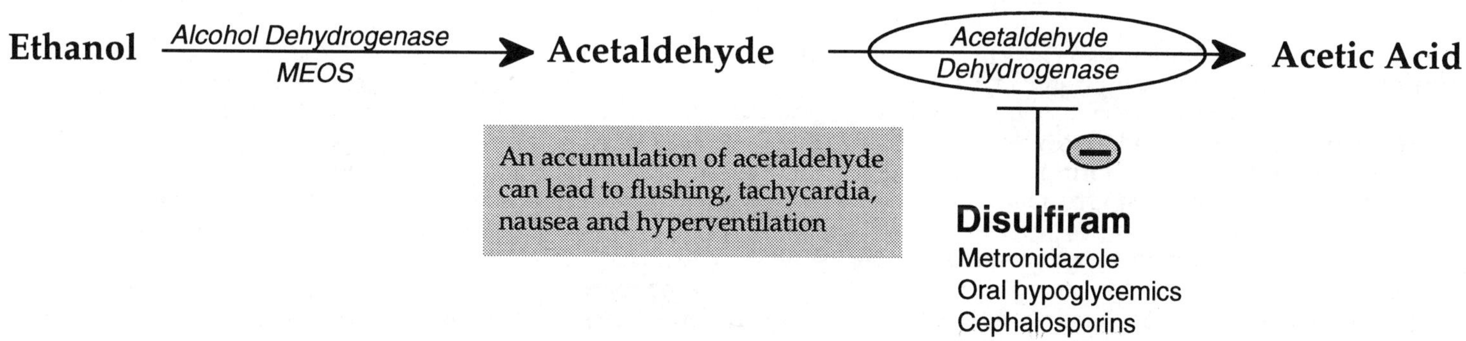

Alcohols

Drug	MOA & Pharmacokinetics	Clinical Uses	Effects
Ethanol (Ethyl alcohol)	A CNS depressant which works through GABA receptors to enhance GABA mediated synaptic neurotransmission. Preferred substrate for alcohol dehydrogenase and, therefore, inhibits the metabolism of other alcohols. This is the rationale for its use in the treatment of methanol and ethylene glycol overdose. Rapidly absorbed from the stomach, small intestine and colon.	**Methanol overdose** **Ethylene glycol overdose**	**Acute** effects include disinhibition, sedation, euphoria, slurred speech, reduced visual acuity, dizziness, ataxia, decreased myocardial contractility and vasodilation. **Chronic** effects include: • Tolerance and dependence • ↓ liver function, fatty liver, hepatitis and cirrhosis • GI irritation, inflammation and bleeding • ↑ risk of hypertension and myocardial infarction • ↑ incidence of cancer • Wernicke-Korsakoff syndrome: ophthalmoplegia, ataxia, confusion, amnesia and confabulation A withdrawal syndrome is observed upon discontinuation of chronic alcohol use. It is initially characterized by tremor, insomnia and headache; later, delirium tremens and convulsions may appear. Teratogenic: fetal alcohol syndrome Drug Interactions: Additive sedation, ataxia and depression with other sedative-hypnotic drugs
Methanol (Wood alcohol, Methyl alcohol)	Found in industrial solvents, varnishes and paint removers. Metabolized by alcohol dehydrogenase to **formaldehyde** which is responsible for toxicities.	None	**Retinal damage** (blindness), metabolic acidosis, shortness of breath and death. Treatment of exposure: **ethanol**

Disulfiram

Drug	MOA & Pharmacokinetics	Clinical Uses	Effects
Disulfiram (Antabuse®)	An **aldehyde dehydrogenase inhibitor** which causes the accumulation of acetaldehyde when ethanol is consumed.	**Alcoholism**: used as adjunctive therapy	An accumulation of acetaldehyde can cause flushing, nausea, hypotension and tachycardia.

Drugs of Abuse

Drug abuse refers to the use of illicit drugs as well as misuse of legal drugs. Implicit in this definition is that this behavior can ultimately harm the user and/or society. Drugs of abuse include street drugs, such as LSD and marijuana and clinically used drugs such as sedative-hypnotics, opioid analgesics and CNS stimulants. All of these drugs are able to cause euphoria which is most likely a factor in their frequent abuse.

Drugs which possess abuse potential are listed below. Hypnotic drugs, alcohol and opioid analgesics have been described in previous sections, therefore, only stimulants, hallucinogens and "others" will be discussed in this section.

Sedative-Hypnotics	Opioid Analgesics	Stimulants	Hallucinogens	Others
Ethanol Barbiturates Benzodiazepines	Heroin Morphine Meperidine Fentanyl	Caffeine Theophylline Nicotine Amphetamines Methylphenidate Cocaine	LSD Mescaline Phencyclidine	Marijuana Inhalants

The following definitions may aid in the understanding of this section:

Tolerance	Refers to an altered physiological state in which the user experiences a **decreased response to a drug**. Factors which may contribute to tolerance include pharmacokinetic (↑ drug metabolism), pharmacodynamic (↓ receptors), and behavioral compensation. Cross tolerance among substances is based on similar pharmacologic properties.
Physical dependence	Is revealed as a **withdrawal** (or abstinence) syndrome when drug use is discontinued. Symptoms are usually opposite to those caused by the drug and can be life-threatening. Drugs with severe withdrawal syndromes include **alcohol** and **barbiturates**. Cross dependence is observed among drugs with similar pharmacologic effects such as ethanol and diazepam.
Addiction	Is distinct from physical dependence and usually described as **compulsive** drug abuse despite significant substance related problems. Addicted persons also exhibit a high tendency to relapse after cessation.

CNS Stimulants

Drug	MOA & Pharmacokinetics	Effects
Caffeine	Blocks adenosine (purinergic) receptors.	Vasoconstriction (low dose), vasodilation (high dose), tachycardia, smooth muscle relaxation, inhibition of mast cell secretion **Clinical Uses**: fatigue, drowsiness, analgesia adjuvant, adjuvant with ergotamine to treat migraine and cluster headaches, apnea in prematurity, USMLE Step 1. **Withdrawal** includes fatigue and sedation. Nausea and headache at higher doses.
Nicotine	Agonist at CNS and PNS nicotinic receptors. Initially stimulates then blocks these receptors.	CNS stimulation, increased heart rate, respiratory rate and blood pressure followed by CNS depression, decreased heart rate, respiratory rate and blood pressure Psychological dependence. **Clinical uses**: transdermal patch for tobacco withdrawal **Withdrawal**: includes irritability, impatience, hostility, anxiety, restlessness, decreased heart rate and weight gain.
Amphetamines: Dextroamphetamine (Dexedrine®) Methamphetamine (Methedrine®, "speed") Methylphenidate (Ritalin®)	Stimulates presynaptic dopamine release.	Euphoria, increased attention, insomnia, decreased appetite, increased motor activity, increased respiration, increased initiative, self-confidence **Clinical uses**: Methylphenidate: attention deficit hyperactivity disorder (ADHD), narcolepsy Dextroamphetamine: attention deficit hyperactivity disorder (ADHD), narcolepsy, obesity **Overdose**: confusion, anxiety, aggressiveness, delusions, headache, hallucinations, palpitations, cardiac arrhythmias and circulatory collapse.

Drug	MOA & Pharmacokinetics	Effects
Cocaine	Blocks the dopamine transporter (↑ dopaminergic stimulation) and prevents norepinephrine and serotonin reuptake. Cocaine is a salt and is snorted. **"Free base"** is free alkaloid cocaine and is the pure uncharged form. **"Crack"** is cocaine salt combined with bicarbonate to form an uncharged species. Both free base and crack are more volatile and can be smoked. Additionally, free base and crack are absorbed rapidly and have an intense onset.	Clinical uses: **local anesthesia** and vasoconstriction to control bleeding in ENT procedures. Effects include arousal, euphoria, increased heart rate and blood pressure, and increased body temperature. Sense of well-being and increased alertness. **Overdose**: excitation, psychosis such as formication ("cocaine bugs"), convulsions, respiratory depression and coma.

Hallucinogens

Drug	MOA & Pharmacokinetics	Effects
LSD (Lysergic acid diethylamide)	Interacts with 5-HT receptors. Other related hallucinogens include **psilocybin** and **mescaline**.	**CNS effects**: arousal, excitation, hallucinations, disturbed perception (time and space), labile mood and panic. "Bad trips" are usually marked by severe anxiety. **Peripheral effects**: mydriasis, hypertension, tachycardia, flushing, increase in body temperature and tremors. Very few drug-related fatalities (wide margin of safety).
Phencyclidine (PCP, "Angel dust")	A **dissociative anesthetic** which blocks NMDA (glutamate) receptors.	**CNS effects**: distortion of time, space and body image, impaired judgment, hostile and reckless behavior and hallucinations, Can cause a **schizophrenia-like psychosis** several weeks in duration. **Peripheral effects**: increased blood pressure and heart rate, limb numbness, hypersalivation, sweating, muscular rigidity and ataxia. Overdose may include extreme hypertension and seizures. Can be fatal.

Other Drugs of Abuse

Drug	MOA & Pharmacokinetics	Effects
Marijuana Schedule I Drug	The active component is ∂-**9THC**, derived from the flowering tops of hemp plants, which acts on its own receptors. "Hashish" is a partially purified form which is more potent. **Dronabinol**, a pharmaceutical preparation of ∂-9THC, is used in AIDS-related anorexia and as an antiemetic agent in chemotherapy. Wide margin of safety. There have been very few drug-related fatalities.	**CNS effects**: euphoria, sedation, decreased psychomotor activity. Altered judgement and time sense. At high doses: delusions, hallucinations and depersonalization. **Peripheral effects**: increased heart rate and blood pressure, hunger, **reddening of conjunctiva**, dry mouth and bronchodilation. Decreased intraocular pressure may occur at high doses.

Inhalants

Drug	Examples	Notes and Effects
Anesthetics	Nitrous oxide, chloroform, diethyl ether	Produce euphoria, analgesia and loss of consciousness. Chronic use may result in peripheral neuropathy. Chloroform can cause liver damage.
Industrial solvents	Gasoline, kerosene, paint thinner, glues	Active components include benzene, hexane, methylketone, toluene and trichloroethylene. Euphoria, disinhibition. Toxicities: hepatic, renal, pulmonary, bone marrow and neuronal damage.
Organic nitrates	Amyl nitrite, isobutyl nitrite, organic nitrates	Euphoria, disinhibition, dizziness, tachycardia, and hypotension.

Cardiovascular Drugs

Antihypertensive Drugs

Hypertension is defined as a systolic blood pressure (BP) ≥ 140 mm Hg and/or diastolic BP ≥ 90 mm Hg. It represents one of the most common and important cardiovascular diseases in the United States, afflicting 20% of the adult population. Hypertension is a major cause of stroke, coronary artery disease, myocardial infarction, congestive heart failure, atherosclerosis, renal insufficiency and dissecting aortic aneurysms. Major risk factors for the development of hypertension include smoking, obesity, diabetes, race and family history. There are two types of hypertension, idiopathic and secondary.

Classification	Description
Idiopathic (essential or primary) hypertension	Represents the vast majority (90%) of patients with hypertension. It is a disorder of unknown etiology characterized by hypertension in the absence of other pathologic processes. Current evidence suggests that genetic inheritance in the principal cause of idiopathic hypertension. Essential hypertension usually appears between the ages of 15 - 40 years old.
Secondary hypertension	Represents a small percentage of patients (10%) with hypertension and is a disorder caused by one of several known pathological processes. Causes include: renal artery disease, primary aldosteronism (Conn's syndrome), pheochromocytoma, renal parenchymal disease, glomerulonephritis, toxemia of pregnancy, CNS disorders and estrogen use.

Hypertension is categorized in stages described below (values listed are for adults 18 years and older).

Status	Systolic BP (mmHg)	Diastolic BP (mmHg)	Risk of Morbidity
Normal	< 140	< 90	None
Hypertension			
Stage 1 (mild)	140 - 159	90 - 99	Long-term
Stage 2 (moderate)	160 - 179	100 - 109	~ 50% in 5 years
Stage 3 (severe)	180 - 209	110 - 119	~ 40% in 2 years
Stage 4 (very severe)	> 210	> 120	High, emergency

Antihypertensive drugs include a wide range of substances used to control hypertension. All antihypertensive drugs work by inhibiting cardiac output, decreasing peripheral vascular resistance (PVR) or both. Antihypertensive drugs can be classified according to their mechanism of action or the site at which they work. Examples of each class of drugs and their antihypertensive effects are listed below; they are discussed in more detail in the pages that follow.

Class	Major Antihypertensive Effect	Drugs
Diuretics	Initially decrease blood volume and thus cardiac output. Eventually, cardiac output returns to normal but is accompanied by a decrease in PVR.	Hydrochlorothiazide Furosemide Spironolactone
Peripheral Sympatholytics	Decrease PVR and/or cardiac output.	Reserpine Guanethidine α_1-adrenergic blockers β-adrenergic blockers
Central Sympatholytics	Decrease PVR by inhibiting sympathetic outflow centrally.	Methyldopa Clonidine
Direct Vasodilators	Decrease PVR by directly vasodilating arterioles.	Hydralazine Minoxidil
ACE Inhibitors	Decrease PVR by reducing the level of the vasoconstrictor angiotensin II. Decrease blood volume by reducing the secretion of aldosterone.	Captopril Enalapril Lisinopril
Angiotensin II Receptor Antagonist	Decreases PVR by blocking the vasoconstricting activity of angiotensin II. Decreases blood volume by reducing the secretion of aldosterone.	Losartan
Calcium Channel Blockers	Decrease PVR by arteriolar vasodilation and/or decreases HR.	Nifedipine Diltiazem Verapamil
Drugs used to treat Hypertensive Emergencies	Decrease PVR by vasodilating arterioles and/or veins.	Sodium nitroprusside Diazoxide Trimethaphan Labetalol

Diuretics

Loop Diuretics

Drug	MOA & Pharmacokinetics	Clinical Uses	Side Effects
Furosemide (Lasix®) Note: loop diuretics are the most efficacious diuretics available and are thus called "high ceiling diuretics." The name lasix comes from "lasts six" hours.	**Sulfonamide** derivative which inhibits the **Na^+- K^+- $2Cl^-$ symporter** in the luminal membrane of the **thick ascending limb of the loop of Henle** (TALH) by interfering with the Cl^- binding site of this symporter. Delivery of these electrolytes to distal regions of the nephron results in secretion of K^+ and H^+ (hypokalemic alkalosis). A decrease in the TALH membrane potential inhibits the reabsorption of Ca^{2+} and Mg^{2+}. Antihypertensive effect results from an initial decrease in blood volume and thus cardiac output. Eventually, cardiac output returns to normal but is accompanied by a decrease in peripheral resistance which maintains the hypotensive effects. Very short $t_{1/2}$ Given PO, IV	**Edema**: associated with CHF, liver and renal disease (including nephrotic syndrome) **Pulmonary edema** **Hypertension**: usually reserved for patients refractory to other diuretics. **Hypercalcemia**: due to the stimulation of tubular Ca^{2+} secretion	Hypokalemic metabolic alkalosis Hyponatremia Hypochloremia Hypomagnesemia Hyperuricemia leading to gouty attacks Hypercalciuria: leading to kidney stone formation Orthostatic hypotension (hypovolemia) Ototoxicity occurs especially with ethacrynic acid and the concurrent use of other ototoxic drugs Allergic reactions occur with the sulfonamide derivatives: furosemide, bumetanide, torsemide
Bumetanide (Bumex®)	Sulfonamide derivative with activity similar to furosemide, but is 10 to 40 times more potent.		
Torsemide (Demadex®)	A newer sulfonamide derivative with activity similar to furosemide, but has a longer $t_{1/2}$ (due to an active metabolite).		
Ethacrynic acid (Edecrin®)	**Non-**sulfonamide derivative which possesses activity and potency similar to furosemide. Useful in patients allergic to sulfa drugs.		

Thiazide Diuretics

Drug	MOA & Pharmacokinetics	Clinical Uses	Side Effects
Hydrochlorothiazide (HydroDIURIL®) Chlorthalidone (Hygroton®) Indapamide (Lozol®) Metolazone (Mykrox®) Note: Thiazide diuretics have a synergistic effect when combined with loop diuretics.	Sulfonamide derivatives which inhibit the **Na^+-Cl^- symporter** on the luminal side of the epithelial cells in the early **distal convoluted tubules** (DCT) resulting in decreased reabsorption of NaCl. This decrease in Na^+ reabsorption promotes Na^+-Ca^{2+} exchange which leads to hypercalcemia and H_2O excretion. Delivery of Na^+ to distal regions of the nephron results in secretion of K^+ and H^+ (hypokalemic alkalosis). These agents are only moderately efficacious since most of the filtered load is reabsorbed before reaching the DCT. Possess a mild antidiuretic effect resulting from Na^+ and H_2O depletion which leads to increased reabsorption of the glomerular filtrate in the PCT. Antihypertensive effect results from an initial decrease in blood volume and thus cardiac output. Eventually, cardiac output returns to normal but is accompanied by a decrease in peripheral resistance which maintains the hypotensive effects. Indapamide possesses the strongest vasodilatory effects of the thiazide diuretics. Given PO	**Hypertension** (mild to severe) in black and elderly patients with low plasma renin and increased plasma volume. **Edema** associated with **CHF**, hepatic disease, renal disease and corticosteroid therapy. Nephrogenic diabetes insipidus: thiazide diuretics decrease urine volume due to volume contraction which leads to increased proximal tubular reabsorption. Calcium nephrolithiasis	Hypokalemic metabolic alkalosis Hyponatremia Hypochloremia Hypomagnesemia Hypercalcemia Hyperuricemia leading to gouty attacks Hyperglycemia: ↓ insulin release Hyperlipidemia: ↑ cholesterol and triglycerides Orthostatic hypotension Allergic reactions Photosensitivity Drug Interactions: May increase the toxicity of lithium by decreasing its renal clearance. May enhance digitalis toxicity associated with hypokalemia.

Potassium Sparing Diuretics

These drugs are rarely used alone and are often combined with thiazide or loop diuretics to offset urinary K^+ loss.

Drug	MOA & Pharmacokinetics	Clinical Uses	Side Effects
Spironolactone (Aldactone®)	**Aldosterone antagonist** at mineralocorticoid receptors in the late distal tubule and collecting ducts leading to decreased synthesis of Na^+ channels and Na^+/K^+-ATPase. This activity causes an increase in Na^+ clearance and a decrease in K^+ and H^+ excretion in the distal nephron. Antihypertensive effect results from an initial decrease in blood volume and thus cardiac output. Eventually, cardiac output returns to normal but is accompanied by a decrease in peripheral resistance which maintains the hypotensive effects. Antiandrogenic effect is due to both antagonism at androgen receptors and inhibition of steroid biosynthesis. Given PO	**Edematous states** including those associated with secondary hyperaldosteronism such as cardiac failure, hepatic cirrhosis, ascites and nephrotic syndrome. **Hypertension** (mild to severe) especially useful when combined with thiazide and loop diuretics. **Primary hyperaldosteronism** (Conn's syndrome) Hirsutism	**Hyperkalemia** Metabolic acidosis Endocrine effects: impotence, gynecomastia and menstrual irregularities CNS effects: drowsiness, lethargy, ataxia, confusion and headache GI effects: diarrhea, gastritis, gastric bleeding and peptic ulcers ◆Contraindication: Conditions predisposing to hyperkalemia especially renal insufficiency
Amiloride (Midamor®) Triamterene (Dyrenium®)	Block Na^+ channels in the late distal convoluted tubule and collecting ducts. This activity causes an increase in Na^+ clearance and a decrease in K^+ and H^+ excretion in the distal nephron. Given PO	**Edematous states** including those associated with secondary hyperaldosteronism such as cardiac failure, hepatic cirrhosis, ascites and nephrotic syndrome. **Hypertension** (mild to severe) especially useful when combined with thiazide and loop diuretics.	**Hyperkalemia** Metabolic acidosis Headache GI effects: nausea, vomiting, diarrhea Megaloblastic anemia: triamterene ◆Contraindication: Conditions predisposing to hyperkalemia especially renal insufficiency

Peripheral Sympatholytics

This group of drugs includes reserpine, guanethidine, α-adrenergic blockers and β-adrenergic blockers.

Drug	MOA & Pharmacokinetics	Clinical Uses	Side Effects
Reserpine (Serpasil®) An alkaloid extracted from the roots of the plant *Rauwolfia serpentina*.	**Irreversibly** binds to storage vesicles in adrenergic neurons causing reduced uptake and storage of norepinephrine, dopamine and serotonin both centrally and peripherally. Decreases cardiac output and PVR; these antihypertensive effects are thought to be due to both central and peripheral activities. Side effects are mainly due to reserpine's effect on the CNS. The major compensatory responses are salt and H_2O retention. $t_{1/2}$ = 4.5 hrs. Duration of action = 1-6 weeks due to its irreversible binding to storage vesicles of biogenic amines. Given PO	Hypertension (mild to moderate): often combined with a diuretic. Huntington's disease	**Sedation** **Inability to concentrate** **Dizziness** Loss of appetite Nasal congestion Dryness of mouth Nausea and vomiting ↑ gastric acid secretion Extrapyramidal effects Depression: insidious in onset, may even lead to suicide.
Guanethidine (Ismelin®)	Enters neuron by norepinephrine reuptake transporter and slowly displaces norepinephrine in the synaptic vesicles. ("substitute neurotransmitter"). This blocks the release of norepinephrine normally produced by nerve stimulation. Depletion of catecholamines leads to vasodilation. Does **not** enter the CNS (unlike reserpine). The major compensatory responses are salt and H_2O retention. Given PO	Hypertension (severe): given to patients who cannot tolerate other antihypertensive medications. Frequently combined with a thiazide diuretic.	**Orthostatic hypotension** **Impotence** Diarrhea Bradycardia Weakness Peripheral edema ◆ Contraindication: Patients with pheochromocytoma due to potential for norepinephrine release.

α-Adrenergic Blockers

Drug	MOA & Pharmacokinetics	Clinical Uses	Side Effects
Doxazosin (Cardura®) Prazosin (Minipress®) Terazosin (Hytrin®)	Potent selective α_1-adrenergic receptor antagonists at arterioles and veins causing a decrease in PVR and venous return to the heart. Decrease cardiac preload and afterload with minimal effects on cardiac output and heart rate. Relax smooth muscle in the bladder neck and prostate by blocking α_1-adrenergic receptors. This results in a reduction of urethral resistance, pressure and symptoms of urinary obstruction. ↓ plasma lipid and LDL and ↑ HDL. Duration of action: 4-6 hours (prazosin); ≥18 hrs (terazosin). Given PO	**Hypertension** (mild to moderate): often given with a diuretic to compensate for salt and H_20 retention. **Benign prostatic hyperplasia** by decreasing urinary obstruction.	**First-Dose Phenomenon**: orthostatic hypotension, syncope and dizziness occur within 30-90 minutes of administration of initial dose. These effects are more pronounced with high initial dose and/or salt and water depletion. Tolerance develops with repeated dosage. Dizziness Headache Palpitations Lassitude

β-Adrenergic Blockers

Drug	MOA & Pharmacokinetics	Clinical Uses	Side Effects
Propranolol (Inderal®) Note: timolol, another non-selective β-blocker, is also used to treat hypertension.	Nonselective β_1 and β_2-adrenergic receptor antagonist. Antianginal effect is due to negative inotropic and chronotropic effects which decrease myocardial oxygen demand. Antiarrhythmic effects (Class II): these agents decrease phase 4 (resting potential) depolarization leading to ↓ rate of firing of sinus and ectopic pacemakers and ↓ AV node conduction. Antihypertensive effects may include reduced cardiac output, ↓ sympathetic outflow to peripheral vasculature (↓PVR) and inhibition of renin release by the kidney. Crosses the blood brain barrier. Given PO	**Hypertension** (mild to moderate) especially in young patients with high plasma renin and rapid pulse. Often given in combination with a thiazide diuretic. **Angina**: stable **Arrhythmias** (supraventricular arrhythmia, ventricular tachycardia, digitalis-induced tachyarrhythmia) Myocardial infarction: reduces myocardial ischemia by decreasing myocardial oxygen demand. Hypertrophic cardiomyopathy Pheochromocytoma (adjuvant) Hyperthyroidism Migraine prophylaxis Panic symptoms such as stage fright	Impotence CNS effects: drowsiness, insomnia, fatigue Bronchoconstriction Abrupt withdrawal may result in arrhythmias, heart failure or angina. Hypoglycemia due to a ↓ glucagon secretion and glycogenolysis (use with caution in patients with labile diabetes) Masks hypoglycemia-induced tachycardia Lipidemia due to ↑ plasma triglycerides and ↓ HDL Claudication of peripheral vessels

Drug	MOA & Pharmacokinetics	Clinical Uses	Side Effects
Metoprolol (Lopressor®) Note: atenolol, another β_1-selective blocker, is also used to treat hypertension.	Selective β_1-adrenergic receptor antagonist (cardioselective). Antianginal effect is due to negative inotropic and chronotropic effects which decrease myocardial oxygen demand. Antiarrhythmic effects (Class II): these agents decrease phase 4 depolarization leading to ↓ rate of firing of sinus and ectopic pacemakers and ↓ AV node conduction. Antihypertensive effects are due to reduced cardiac output, ↓ sympathetic outflow to peripheral vasculature (↓PVR) and inhibition of renin release by the kidney.	**Hypertension** in patients with asthma or diabetes. **Angina**: stable Arrhythmias Myocardial infarction: used to reduce myocardial ischemia by decreasing myocardial oxygen demand.	Bradycardia CNS effects: sedation, fatigue Bronchospasm, hypoglycemia, peripheral vasoconstriction and hyperlipidemia, but less than non-selective β-blockers. Congestive heart failure may occur due to the reduction of cardiac output.

Central Sympatholytics

Methyldopa and clonidine stimulate presynaptic α_2-**adrenergic receptors**. Unlike true agonists, however, these agents inhibit the release of norepinephrine from presynaptic nerve terminals and thus impart sympatholytic effects. Interestingly, both drugs cause minimal postural hypotension.

Drug	MOA & Pharmacokinetics	Clinical Uses	Side Effects
Methyldopa (Aldomet®)	**Prodrug** converted in the brain to its active metabolite methyl-norepinephrine which activates α_2-adrenergic receptors to inhibit sympathetic outflow. Antihypertensive effect is mediated by a decrease in **peripheral vascular resistance** (major effect) and a decrease in cardiac output. Renal blood flow is maintained. Duration of action ~ 24 hrs Given PO, IV	**Hypertension** (moderate to severe): often used in combination with a thiazide diuretic. Useful in treating hypertension complicated by renal disease.	Edema Drowsiness Dry mouth and nasal mucosa Headache Reduced libido Development of a **(+) Coombs test** which may progress to hemolytic anemia. Hepatotoxicity
Clonidine (Catapres®)	Stimulates α_2-adrenergic receptors in the CNS inhibiting sympathetic outflow. Antihypertensive effect is mediated primarily by decreasing **peripheral vascular resistance** and secondarily by decreasing cardiac output. Renal blood flow is maintained. Duration of action <8 hrs Given PO, IV, transdermal patch	**Hypertension** (mild to moderate): often used in combination with a thiazide diuretic. Useful in treating hypertension complicated by renal disease.	Dry mouth and nasal mucosa Drowsiness Itching and redness of skin may occur with the patch Dizziness Constipation Reduced libido Rebound hypertension: more likely to occur after abrupt withdrawal

Direct Vasodilators

Drug	MOA & Pharmacokinetics	Clinical Uses	Side Effects
Hydralazine (Apresoline®)	Direct vasodilator of **arteriolar** smooth muscle resulting in a significant ↓PVR. This action elicits a compensatory sympathetic response including ↑ HR and stroke volume (↑ cardiac output) and fluid retention. Because of the sympathetic responses, hydralazine is often combined with a diuretic and/or a β-blocker. Increases renal blood flow. Given PO, IV, IM	**Hypertension** (moderate to severe): used in combination with a diuretic to decrease sodium retention and a β-blocker to prevent reflex tachycardia. Congestive heart failure	Headache Nausea Diarrhea Cardiovascular effects: hypotension, palpitations, tachycardia and angina pectoris **Lupus-like syndrome**: especially in slow acetylators Edema ◆ Contraindications: Dissecting aortic aneurysm Coronary artery disease
Minoxidil (Loniten®) Note: also available as a topical formulation (Rogaine®) which is used to treat alopecia androgenetica (male pattern baldness).	**Prodrug** metabolized to minoxidil N-O sulfate which is an **arteriolar** smooth muscle vasodilator. Minoxidil sulfate increases K^+ efflux by opening K^+ channels causing hyperpolarization and relaxation of smooth muscle. The vasodilatory activity results in a ↓PVR. This action elicits a compensatory sympathetic response including ↑ HR and stroke volume (↑ cardiac output) and fluid retention. Because of these sympathetic responses, minoxidil is often combined with a diuretic and/or a β-blocker. More potent than hydralazine. Given PO	**Hypertension**: used in patients with symptomatic or organ damaging hypertension refractory to other antihypertensive medications. Used in combination with a diuretic to decrease sodium retention and a β-blocker to prevent reflex tachycardia.	Edema Reflex tachycardia Flushing Hypertrichosis (increased hair growth)

ACE (Angiotensin Converting Enzyme) Inhibitors

Drug	MOA & Pharmacokinetics	Clinical Uses	Side Effects
Captopril (Capoten®)	Reversibly inhibits angiotensin converting enzyme (ACE, kininase II) preventing the conversion of angiotensin I into the vasoconstrictor **angiotensin II** (ATII). Decreased ATII levels result in **decreased aldosterone** levels which decrease Na^+ and H_2O retention. Decreased ATII concentrations also result in ↑ renin release and the formation of angiotensin I. ACE inhibitors increase levels of bradykinin by preventing its degradation. Bradykinin increases the synthesis of prostaglandins which are vasodilators. $t_{1/2}$ = 2 hrs Given PO	**Hypertension** (mild to moderate): in young, white patients with high plasma renin. Often combined with a thiazide diuretic. **Congestive heart failure** **Scleroderma renal crisis** Left ventricular systolic dysfunction following a myocardial infarction Diabetic nephropathy: increases the length of time until end stage renal disease	Dry cough Headache Fatigue Hypotension (often with 1st dose) Skin rash Dysgeusia (altered taste) Hyperkalemia may occur in patients with renal insufficiency or who are also taking K^+ sparing diuretics. Acute renal failure due to reduced glomerular filtration Proteinuria ◆ Contraindication: Pregnancy: fetal exposure may cause hypotension, renal failure, anuria, skull hypoplasia, even death.
Enalapril (Vasotec®) Enalaprilat (Vasotec®)	Same MOA as captopril. **Prodrug** hydrolyzed by esterases in the liver to the active metabolite **enalaprilat**. $t_{1/2}$ = 1-2 hrs (enalapril) 11 hrs (enalaprilat) Given PO (enalapril), IV (enalaprilat)	**Hypertension** (mild to moderate): in young, white patients with high plasma renin. Often combined with a thiazide diuretic. **Congestive heart failure** Asymptomatic left ventricular dysfunction.	
Lisinopril (Prinivil®, Zestril®)	Same MOA as captopril. Lysine analog of enalaprilat which is slightly more potent. $t_{1/2}$ = 12 hrs. Given PO	**Hypertension** (mild to moderate): in young, white patients with high plasma renin. Often combined with a thiazide diuretic. **Congestive heart failure**	

Angiotensin II Receptor Antagonist

Drug	MOA & Pharmacokinetics	Clinical Uses	Side Effects
Losartan (Cozaar®)	Nonpeptide angiotensin II receptor (AT_1 subtype) antagonist which inhibits the vasoconstrictor and aldosterone-secreting effects of angiotensin II (ATII). Converted to a 5-carboxylic acid **metabolite** which is 10-40 times more potent and is responsible for most of the pharmacologic activity. Decreased ATII levels results in **decreased aldosterone** levels which decrease Na^+ and H_2O retention. Decreased ATII concentrations also result in ↑ renin release and the formation of angiotensin I. Possesses a uricosuric effect (increases clearance of uric acid). $t_{1/2}$ = 2 hrs (losartan), 6-9 hrs (metabolite) Given PO	**Hypertension** (mild to severe)	Headache Hypotension in patients with high plasma renin Hyperkalemia may occur in patients with renal insufficiency or those who are also taking K^+ sparing diuretics. ◆ Contraindication: Pregnancy: fetal exposure may cause hypotension, renal failure, anuria, skull hypoplasia, even death.

Calcium Channel Blockers

Calcium channel blockers decrease Ca^{2+} influx in vascular smooth muscle and/or cardiac muscle. Of note is the varying specificity of these agents:

Effect on vascular smooth muscle: nifedipine > diltiazem > verapamil
Effect on cardiac muscle: verapamil > diltiazem > nifedipine

Drug	MOA & Pharmacokinetics	Clinical Uses	Side Effects
Nifedipine (Procardia®) Nicardipine (Cardene®)	Dihydropyridine derivatives which inhibit slow, voltage-gated (L-type) **Ca^{2+} channels** resulting in ↓ Ca^{2+} influx. This causes relaxation of **arterial** smooth muscle and ↓ PVR. This causes a reflex increase in sympathetic tone (↑ HR and cardiac output) which may mask negative inotropic effects. Exhibit less effects on SA node automaticity and AV nodal conduction than diltiazem and verapamil. Given PO	**Hypertension** (mild to moderate) especially useful in black and elderly white patients with low renin levels. Efficacy may be enhanced by concomitant use of ACE inhibitors, methyldopa or β-blockers. **Angina**: may be combined with nitrates to treat stable angina. Raynaud's phenomenon	**Headache** **Dizziness** **Peripheral edema** **Tachycardia** **Flushing** **Nausea** Fatigue Constipation Hypotension
Diltiazem (Cardizem®)	Benzothiazepine derivative which binds cardiac L-type Ca^{2+} channels and decreases **SA node** automaticity and **AV nodal conduction** with some negative inotropic effects on the heart. Exhibits mild vasodilatory effects on blood vessels (less than nifedipine). Given PO, IV	**Hypertension** (mild to moderate) especially useful in black and elderly white patients with low renin levels. Efficacy may be enhanced by concomitant use of ACE inhibitors, methyldopa or β-blockers. **Angina** **Supraventricular arrhythmias**	Incidence is infrequent but may include: Skin rash Congestive heart failure Hypotension Peripheral edema Dizziness Flushing Headache ◆ Contraindication: Patients with pre-existing depressed cardiac function.

Drug	MOA & Pharmacokinetics	Clinical Uses	Side Effects
Verapamil (Calan®, Isoptin®, Verelan®) "V for ventricle"	Diphenylalkylamine which binds cardiac L-type Ca^{2+} channels and decreases **SA node** automaticity and **AV nodal conduction** with negative inotropic effects on the heart. Exhibits mild vasodilatory effects on arterioles. This decreases afterload which partially offsets the negative inotropic effects. Given PO, IV	**Hypertension** (mild to moderate) especially useful in black and elderly white patients with low renin levels. Efficacy may be enhanced by concomitant use of ACE inhibitors, methyldopa or β-blockers. **Angina** **Supraventricular arrhythmias** Hypertrophic cardiomyopathy	Incidence is infrequent but may include: Skin rash Bradycardia Congestive heart failure Hypotension Peripheral edema Constipation Dizziness Fatigue Headache ◆ Contraindication: Patients with pre-existing depressed cardiac function.

Hypertensive Emergencies

Drug	MOA & Pharmacokinetics	Clinical Uses	Side Effects
Diazoxide (Hyperstat®)	Activates ATP-sensitive K^+ channels causing hyperpolarization of arteriolar smooth muscle cells. This results in arteriolar vasodilation. Stimulates reflex sympathetic tone resulting in ↑ cardiac output, HR and contractility. The major compensatory responses are salt and H_2O retention. Onset of action: 1 minute Peak effect: 2-5 minutes Given IV	**Hypertensive emergencies**: used in combination with a diuretic to decrease sodium retention and a β-blocker to prevent reflex tachycardia.	Edema Tachycardia Hyperglycemia due to its ability to inhibit insulin secretion from pancreas. Hypotension
Sodium nitroprusside (Nitropress®)	Metabolized by red blood cells and smooth muscle cells to its active metabolite, **nitric oxide** (NO, EDRF), which leads to the formation of **cGMP**. The ↑ cGMP leads to ↓ Ca^{2+} ions in **arteriolar** and **venous** vessels, causing vasodilation. This results in a ↓ preload and afterload. A toxic metabolite, **cyanide**, is converted in the liver to a less toxic metabolite, **thiocyanate,** which undergoes renal elimination. Onset of action: ~30 seconds Effects disappear: within 3 minutes Given IV	**Hypertensive emergencies** **Congestive heart failure** Controlled hypotension during surgical procedures	Hypotension Arrhythmias Cyanide toxicity may occur in patients with hepatic dysfunction or after prolonged administration. Thiocyanate toxicity may occur in patients with renal dysfunction or after prolonged administration.

Drug	MOA & Pharmacokinetics	Clinical Uses	Side Effects
Trimethaphan (Arfonad®)	A ganglionic blocking agent which competitively antagonizes postsynaptic acetylcholine receptors. This reduces both arterial blood pressure and the upslope of the arterial pressure wave in the aorta. The latter effect is responsible for the drug's efficacy to treat acute dissecting aneurysms. Other effects include direct peripheral vasodilation and release of histamine. Onset of action: immediate Duration of action: 10-15 minutes Given IV	**Hypertensive emergencies**: especially in patients with acute **dissecting aortic aneurysm** and in patients with pulmonary edema secondary to pulmonary hypertension. Controlled hypotension during surgical procedures	Orthostatic hypotension Constipation Urinary retention Blurred vision Dry mouth Impotence
Labetalol (Normodyne®) Labetalol: **l**oss of **a**lpha and **b**eta receptor activity.	A mixed adrenergic antagonist which is composed of 4 stereoisomers, one of which antagonizes α_1-receptors, one of which nonselectively blocks β-receptors and possesses intrinsic sympathomimetic activity and two of which are inactive. The α_1-receptor blockade prevents the reflex vasoconstriction seen with other β-blockers. Blockade of β_1 receptors also contributes to a decrease in blood pressure by blunting reflex sympathetic stimulation of the heart. Given PO, IV	**Hypertensive emergencies**: IV administration **Hypertension** (severe) most useful in elderly and black patients.	Orthostatic hypotension Dizziness Other side effects are related to α- and β-adrenergic receptor blockade.

Notes

Antianginal Drugs

The most common symptom of chronic ischemic heart disease is chest pain (**angina pectoris**). Myocardial ischemia which produces angina results from imbalances in myocardial oxygen supply-demand relationship such as decreased oxygen supply and/or increased oxygen demand. Therapeutics aim at restoring this imbalance by increasing oxygen supply, decreasing oxygen demand or both. The three classes of antianginal agents are nitrates, Ca^{2+}-channel blockers and β-adrenergic blockers.

Agents which ↓ O_2 demand and ↑ O_2 supply		Agents which ↓ O_2 demand
Nitrates	Ca^{2+}-channel blockers	β-blockers
Nitroglycerin Isosorbide dinitrate Amyl nitrate	Nifedipine Nicardipine Diltiazem Verapamil	Propanolol Timolol Metoprolol Atenolol

There are three types of angina pectoris:

Type	Other names	Description	Drug therapy
Stable	Atherosclerotic Classic Exertional Fixed	Usually caused by atherosclerotic obstruction in coronary arteries. These episodes are usually precipitated by exercise, excitement, cold or consumption of a heavy meal.	Nitrates Ca^{2+}-channel blockers β-blockers
Variant	Prinzemetal's Vasospasmic	Usually due to vasospasm of coronary vessels. These episodes may occur at any time, not only during exercise.	Nitrates Ca^{2+}-channel blockers
Unstable	Crescendo	Usually results from a combination of atherosclerotic lesions, platelet aggregation, thrombotic processes and vasospasm. Such an episode is a direct precursor to a myocardial infarction and is considered a medical emergency.	Nitrates Ca^{2+}-channel blockers

Nitrates

Drug	MOA & Pharmacokinetics	Clinical Uses	Side Effects
Nitroglycerin Isosorbide dinitrate (Isordil®, Sorbitrate®) Amyl nitrite (Aspirols®, Vaporole®)	Metabolized by smooth muscle cells to their active metabolite, nitric oxide (**NO**) which activates guanylate cyclase and increases **cGMP**. This increase in cGMP results in the dephosphorylation of myosin light chains and the subsequent relaxation of smooth muscle. Relaxes venous (predominant effect) and arterial smooth muscle leading to peripheral vasodilation resulting in ↓ preload, afterload and cardiac output. Overall this results in ↓ myocardial O_2 demand and consumption. Also causes a redistribution of blood flow to subendocardial regions of the heart which ↑ myocardial O_2 supply. May inhibit platelet aggregation. Tolerance develops after 8 hrs. Therefore, rest periods are necessary with long acting formulations. Nitroglycerin is available in buccal, sublingual, PO, transdermal or topical formulations depending on the desired onset of action, duration of action and potency. Isosorbide dinitrate is available sublingual, PO. Amyl nitrate is available as an inhalant.	**Angina pectoris** **Myocardial infarction** (MI) Congestive heart failure Hypertension Controlled hypotension during surgical procedures. Cyanide poisoning: nitrates convert Fe^{2+} in hemoglobin to Fe^{3+} yielding methemoglobin. Methemoglobin competes CN^- away from its target, cytochrome oxidase. Amyl nitrate is the nitrate of choice in treating cyanide poisoning.	**Headache** **Tachycardia** (reflex) **Postural hypotension** leading to dizziness, weakness Rash **Monday disease**: describes occupational toxicity in which munition workers developed tolerance to nitrates during the work week, lost tolerance during the weekend and experienced headache, tachycardia and dizziness the following Monday.

Calcium Channel Blockers

Calcium channel blockers decrease Ca^{2+} influx in vascular smooth muscle and/or cardiac muscle. Of note is the varying specificity of these agents:

Effect on vascular smooth muscle: nifedipine > diltiazem > verapamil
Effect on cardiac muscle: verapamil > diltiazem > nifedipine

Drug	MOA & Pharmacokinetics	Clinical Uses	Side Effects
Nifedipine (Procardia®) Nicardipine (Cardene®)	Dihydropyridine derivatives which inhibit slow, voltage-gated (L-type) **Ca^{2+} channels** resulting in ↓ Ca^{2+} influx. This causes relaxation of **arterial** smooth muscle and ↓ PVR. This causes a reflex increase in sympathetic tone (↑ HR and cardiac output) which may mask negative inotropic effects. Exhibit less effects on SA node automaticity and AV nodal conduction than diltiazem and verapamil. Given PO	**Hypertension** (mild to moderate) especially useful in black and elderly white patients with low renin levels. Efficacy may be enhanced by concomitant use of ACE inhibitors, methyldopa or β-blockers. **Angina**: may be combined with nitrates to treat stable angina. Raynaud's phenomenon	**Headache** **Dizziness** **Peripheral edema** **Tachycardia** **Flushing** **Nausea** Fatigue Constipation Hypotension
Diltiazem (Cardizem®)	Benzothiazepine derivative which binds cardiac L-type Ca^{2+} channels and decreases **SA node** automaticity and **AV nodal conduction** with some negative inotropic effects on the heart. Exhibits mild vasodilatory effects on blood vessels (less than nifedipine). Given PO, IV	**Hypertension** (mild to moderate) especially useful in black and elderly white patients with low renin levels. Efficacy may be enhanced by concomitant use of ACE inhibitors, methyldopa or β-blockers. **Angina** **Supraventricular arrhythmia**	Incidence is infrequent but may include: Skin rash Congestive heart failure Hypotension Peripheral edema Dizziness Flushing Headache ◆ Contraindication: Patients with pre-existing depressed cardiac function.

Drug	MOA & Pharmacokinetics	Clinical Uses	Side Effects
Verapamil (Calan®, Isoptin®, Verelan®) "V for ventricle"	Diphenylalkylamine which binds cardiac L-type Ca^{2+} channels and decreases **SA node** automaticity and **AV nodal conduction** with negative inotropic effects on the heart. Exhibits mild vasodilatory effects on arterioles. This decreases afterload which partially offsets the negative inotropic effects. Given PO, IV	**Hypertension** (mild to moderate) especially useful in black and elderly white patients with low renin levels. Efficacy may be enhanced by concomitant use of ACE inhibitors, methyldopa or β-blockers. **Angina** **Supraventricular arrhythmias** Hypertrophic cardiomyopathy	Incidence is infrequent but may include: Skin rash Bradycardia Congestive heart failure Hypotension Peripheral edema Constipation Dizziness Fatigue Headache ◆ Contraindication: Patients with pre-existing depressed cardiac function.

β-Adrenergic Blockers

Drug	MOA & Pharmacokinetics	Clinical Uses	Side Effects
Propranolol (Inderal®) Note: timolol, another non-selective β-blocker, is also used to treat angina.	Nonselective β_1 and β_2-adrenergic receptor antagonist. Antianginal effect is due to negative inotropic and chronotropic effects which decrease myocardial oxygen demand. Antiarrhythmic effects (Class II): these agents decrease phase 4 (resting potential) depolarization leading to ↓ rate of firing of sinus and ectopic pacemakers and ↓ AV node conduction. Antihypertensive effects may include reduced cardiac output, ↓ sympathetic outflow to peripheral vasculature (↓PVR) and inhibition of renin release by the kidney. Crosses the blood brain barrier. Given PO	**Hypertension** (mild to moderate) especially in young patients with high plasma renin and rapid pulse. Often given in combination with a thiazide diuretic. **Angina**: stable **Arrhythmias** (supraventricular arrhythmia, ventricular tachycardia, digitalis-induced tachyarrhythmia) Myocardial infarction: reduces myocardial ischemia by decreasing myocardial oxygen demand. Hypertrophic cardiomyopathy Pheochromocytoma (adjuvant) Hyperthyroidism Migraine prophylaxis Panic symptoms such as stage fright	Impotence CNS effects: drowsiness, insomnia, fatigue Bronchoconstriction Abrupt withdrawal may result in arrhythmias, heart failure or angina. Hypoglycemia due to a ↓ glucagon secretion and glycogenolysis (use with caution in patients with labile diabetes) Masks hypoglycemia-induced tachycardia Lipidemia due to ↑ plasma triglycerides and ↓ HDL Claudication of peripheral vessels

Drug	MOA & Pharmacokinetics	Clinical Uses	Side Effects
Metoprolol (Lopressor®) Note: atenolol, another β_1-selective blocker, is also used to treat angina.	Selective β_1-adrenergic receptor antagonist (cardioselective). Antianginal effect is due to negative inotropic and chronotropic effects which decrease myocardial oxygen demand. Antiarrhythmic effects (Class II): these agents decrease phase 4 depolarization leading to ↓ rate of firing of sinus and ectopic pacemakers and ↓ AV node conduction. Antihypertensive effects are due to reduced cardiac output, ↓ sympathetic outflow to peripheral vasculature (↓PVR) and inhibition of renin release by the kidney.	**Hypertension** in patients with asthma or diabetes. **Angina**: stable Arrhythmias Myocardial infarction: used to reduce myocardial ischemia by decreasing myocardial oxygen demand.	Bradycardia CNS effects: sedation, fatigue Bronchospasm, hypoglycemia, peripheral vasoconstriction and hyperlipidemia, but less than non-selective β-blockers. Congestive heart failure may occur due to the reduction of cardiac output.

Congestive Heart Failure Drugs

Congestive heart failure (CHF) occurs when cardiac output is insufficient to meet the body's requirements. Clinically, CHF manifests as vascular congestion in either the pulmonary (left heart failure) or the systemic (right heart failure) circulation. Pharmacologically, there are various approaches to treating CHF which are listed below:

Drug class	Examples	Pharmacologic mechanism
Cardiac glycosides	Digoxin Digitoxin	(+) inotropic effect
Diuretics	Loop diuretics Thiazide diuretics	↓ Na^+ and H_2O retention
Vasodilators	Hydralazine Minoxidil Sodium nitroprusside	↓ preload and afterload
ACE inhibitors	Captopril Enalapril Lisinopril	↓ afterload ↓ Na^+ and H_2O retention
Angiotensin II receptor antagonist	Losartan	↓ afterload ↓ Na^+ and H_2O retention
β-adrenergic agonist	Dobutamine	(+) inotropic effect
Phosphodiesterase inhibitors	Amrinone Milrinone	(+) inotropic effect ↓ preload and afterload

Cardiac Glycosides

Drug	MOA & Pharmacokinetics	Clinical Uses	Side Effects
Digoxin (Lanoxin®) Digitoxin (Crystodigin®) These agents are derived from the foxglove (digitalis) plant.	Binds to and inhibits the **Na^+-K^+ ATPase** in myocardial cell membranes thereby increasing exchange of intracellular Na^+ for extracellular Ca^{2+} by the Na^+-Ca^{2+} exchanger. This increased intracellular Ca^{2+} is stored in the sarcoplasmic reticulum and upon release results in a positive inotropic effect. **Antiarrhythmic effects**: indirectly alters autonomic outflow by ↑ parasympathetic and ↓ sympathetic tone. This results in a ↓ conduction time and ↑ refractory period of the AV node.	**Congestive heart failure** **Supraventricular arrhythmias**: especially atrial fibrillation and flutter.	**Atrial** or **ventricular dysrhythmias**: can be precipitated by **hypokalemic** states. GI effects: **nausea**, **vomiting**, **diarrhea** CNS effects: visual disturbances, drowsiness, confusion, delirium, headache and fainting. Selected Drug Interactions: K^+-depleting (loop and thiazide) diuretics Quinidine: ↓ renal clearance of digoxin Ca^{2+}-channel blockers (particularly verapamil): additive depression of AV node conduction (bradycardia) **Overdose** is observed as cardiac depression leading to cardiac arrest. Treatment of overdose: withdrawal of drug, correction of electrolyte imbalances, administration of antiarrhythmic drugs and **digoxin antibodies** (F'ab fragments).

Summary of differences between digoxin and digitoxin:

	Digoxin	Digitoxin
Routes of administration	PO, IV, IM	PO
Oral bioavailability	70-80 % (tablets) 85-100 % (elixir)	~ 100 %
$t_{1/2}$	36-48 hrs	4-8 days
Route of elimination	renal	hepatic
Duration of action	6 days	14 days
Plasma protein bound	20-30 %	> 90 %
Therapeutic blood level	0.5-2 μg/L	10-25 μg/L
Toxic blood level	2-3 μg/L	>35 μg/L

Figure 4.1: Action of cardiac glycosides

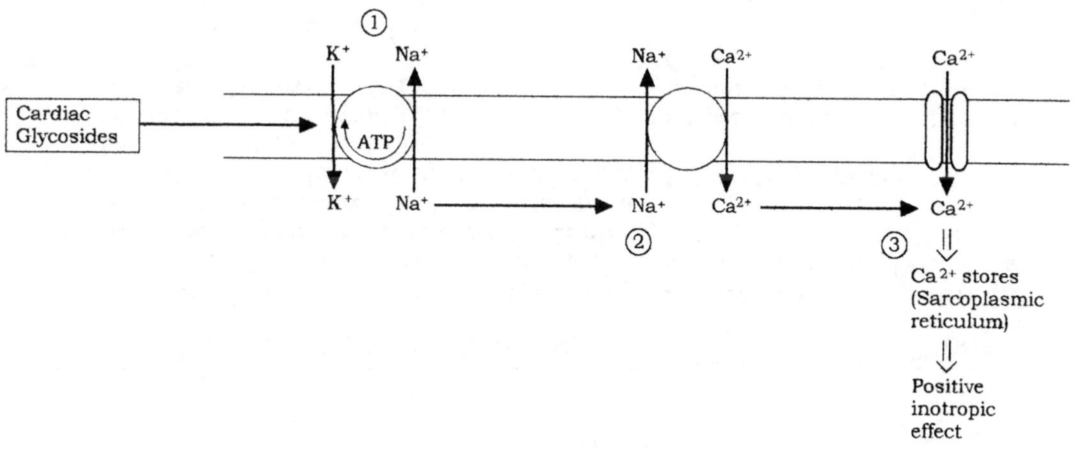

Diuretics

Loop Diuretics

Drug	MOA & Pharmacokinetics	Clinical Uses	Side Effects
Furosemide (Lasix®) Note: loop diuretics are the most efficacious diuretics available and are thus called "high ceiling diuretics." The name lasix comes from "lasts six" hours.	**Sulfonamide** derivative which inhibits the **Na^+- K^+- $2Cl^-$ symporter** in the luminal membrane of the **thick ascending limb of the loop of Henle** (TALH) by interfering with the Cl^- binding site of this symporter. Delivery of these electrolytes to distal regions of the nephron results in secretion of K^+ and H^+ (hypokalemic alkalosis). A decrease in the TALH membrane potential inhibits the reabsorption of Ca^{2+} and Mg^{2+}. Antihypertensive effect results from an initial decrease in blood volume and thus cardiac output. Eventually, cardiac output returns to normal but is accompanied by a decrease in peripheral resistance which maintains the hypotensive effects. Very short $t_{1/2}$ Given PO, IV	**Edema**: associated with CHF, liver and renal disease (including nephrotic syndrome) **Pulmonary edema** **Hypertension**: usually reserved for patients refractory to other diuretics. **Hypercalcemia**: due to the stimulation of tubular Ca^{2+} secretion	Hypokalemic metabolic alkalosis Hyponatremia Hypochloremia Hypomagnesemia Hyperuricemia leading to gouty attacks Hypercalciuria: leading to kidney stone formation Orthostatic hypotension (hypovolemia) Ototoxicity occurs especially with ethacrynic acid and the concurrent use of other ototoxic drugs Allergic reactions occur with the sulfonamide derivatives: furosemide, bumetanide, torsemide
Bumetanide (Bumex®)	Sulfonamide derivative with activity similar to furosemide, but is 10 to 40 times more potent.		
Torsemide (Demadex®)	A newer sulfonamide derivative with activity similar to furosemide, but has a longer $t_{1/2}$ (due to an active metabolite).		
Ethacrynic acid (Edecrin®)	**Non**-sulfonamide derivative which possesses activity and potency similar to furosemide. Useful in patients allergic to sulfa drugs.		

Thiazide Diuretics

Drug	MOA & Pharmacokinetics	Clinical Uses	Side Effects
Hydrochlorothiazide (HydroDIURIL®) Chlorthalidone (Hygroton®) Indapamide (Lozol®) Metolazone (Mykrox®) Note: Thiazide diuretics have a synergistic effect when combined with loop diuretics.	Sulfonamide derivatives which inhibit the **Na^+-Cl^- symporter** on the luminal side of the epithelial cells in the early **distal convoluted tubules** (DCT) resulting in decreased reabsorption of NaCl. This decrease in Na^+ reabsorption promotes Na^+-Ca^{2+} exchange which leads to hypercalcemia and H_2O excretion. Delivery of Na^+ to distal regions of the nephron results in secretion of K^+ and H^+ (hypokalemic alkalosis). These agents are only moderately efficacious since most of the filtered load is reabsorbed before reaching the DCT. Possess a mild antidiuretic effect resulting from Na^+ and H_2O depletion which leads to increased reabsorption of the glomerular filtrate in the PCT. Antihypertensive effect results from an initial decrease in blood volume and thus cardiac output. Eventually, cardiac output returns to normal but is accompanied by a decrease in peripheral resistance which maintains the hypotensive effects. Indapamide possesses the strongest vasodilatory effects of the thiazide diuretics. Given PO	**Hypertension** (mild to severe) in black and elderly patients with low plasma renin and increased plasma volume. **Edema** associated with **CHF**, hepatic disease, renal disease and corticosteroid therapy. Nephrogenic diabetes insipidus: thiazide diuretics decrease urine volume due to volume contraction which leads to increased proximal tubular reabsorption. Calcium nephrolithiasis	Hypokalemic metabolic alkalosis Hyponatremia Hypochloremia Hypomagnesemia Hypercalcemia Hyperuricemia leading to gouty attacks Hyperglycemia: ↓ insulin release Hyperlipidemia: ↑ cholesterol and triglycerides Orthostatic hypotension Allergic reactions Photosensitivity Drug Interactions: May increase the toxicity of lithium by decreasing its renal clearance. May enhance digitalis toxicity associated with hypokalemia.

Vasodilators

Drug	MOA & Pharmacokinetics	Clinical Uses	Side Effects
Hydralazine (Apresoline®)	Direct vasodilator of **arteriolar** smooth muscle resulting in a significant ↓PVR. This action elicits a compensatory sympathetic response including ↑ HR and stroke volume (↑ cardiac output) and fluid retention. Because of the sympathetic responses, hydralazine is often combined with a diuretic and/or a β-blocker. Increases renal blood flow. Given PO, IV, IM	**Hypertension** (moderate to severe): used in combination with a diuretic to decrease sodium retention and a β-blocker to prevent reflex tachycardia. Congestive heart failure	Headache Nausea Diarrhea Cardiovascular effects: hypotension, palpitations, tachycardia and angina pectoris **Lupus-like syndrome**: especially in slow acetylators Edema ◆ Contraindications: Dissecting aortic aneurysm Coronary artery disease
Minoxidil (Loniten®) Note: also available as a topical formulation (Rogaine®) which is used to treat alopecia androgenetica (male pattern baldness).	**Prodrug** metabolized to minoxidil N-O sulfate which is an **arteriolar** smooth muscle vasodilator. Minoxidil sulfate ↑ K^+ efflux by opening K^+ channels causing hyperpolarization and relaxation of smooth muscle. The vasodilatory activity results in a ↓PVR. This action elicits a compensatory sympathetic response including ↑ HR and stroke volume (↑ cardiac output) and fluid retention. Because of these sympathetic responses, minoxidil is often combined with a diuretic and/or a β-blocker. More potent than hydralazine. Given PO	**Hypertension**: used in patients with symptomatic or organ damaging hypertension refractory to other antihypertensive medications. Used in combination with a diuretic to decrease sodium retention and a β-blocker to prevent reflex tachycardia.	Edema Reflex tachycardia Flushing Hypertrichosis (increased hair growth)

Drug	MOA & Pharmacokinetics	Clinical Uses	Side Effects
Sodium nitroprusside (Nitropress®)	Metabolized by red blood cells and smooth muscle cells to its active metabolite, **nitric oxide** (NO, EDRF), which leads to the formation of **cGMP**. The ↑ cGMP leads to a ↓ of Ca^{2+} ions in **arteriolar** and **venous** vessels, causing vasodilation. This results in a ↓ preload and afterload. A toxic metabolite, **cyanide**, is converted in the liver to a less toxic metabolite, **thiocyanate**, which undergoes renal elimination. Onset of action: ~30 seconds Effects disappear: within 3 minutes Given IV	**Hypertensive emergencies** **Congestive heart failure** Controlled hypotension during surgical procedures	Hypotension Arrhythmias Cyanide toxicity may occur in patients with hepatic dysfunction or after prolonged administration. Thiocyanate toxicity may occur in patients with renal dysfunction or after prolonged administration.

ACE (Angiotensin Converting Enzyme) Inhibitors

Drug	MOA & Pharmacokinetics	Clinical Uses	Side Effects
Captopril (Capoten®)	Reversibly inhibits angiotensin converting enzyme (ACE, kininase II) preventing the conversion of angiotensin I into the vasoconstrictor **angiotensin II** (ATII). Decreased ATII levels results in decreased **aldosterone** levels which decrease Na^+ and H_2O retention. Decreased ATII concentrations also result in ↑ renin release and the formation of angiotensin I. ACE inhibitors increase levels of bradykinin by preventing its degradation. Bradykinin increases the synthesis of prostaglandins which are vasodilators. $t_{1/2}$ = 2 hrs Given PO	**Hypertension** (mild to moderate) in young, white patients with high plasma renin. Often combined with a thiazide diuretic. **Congestive heart failure** **Scleroderma renal crisis** Left ventricular systolic dysfunction following a myocardial infarction Diabetic nephropathy: increases the length of time until end stage renal disease	Dry cough Headache Fatigue Hypotension (often with 1st dose) Skin rash Dysgeusia (altered taste) Hyperkalemia may occur in patients with renal insufficiency or who are also taking K^+ sparing diuretics. Acute renal failure due to reduced glomerular filtration Proteinuria ◆ Contraindication: Pregnancy: fetal exposure may cause hypotension, renal failure, anuria, skull hypoplasia, even death.
Enalapril (Vasotec®) Enalaprilat (Vasotec®)	Same MOA as captopril. **Prodrug** hydrolyzed by esterases in the liver to the active metabolite **enalaprilat**. $t_{1/2}$ = 1-2 hrs (enalapril) 11 hrs (enalaprilat) Given PO (enalapril), IV (enalaprilat).	**Hypertension** (mild to moderate) in young, white patients with high plasma renin. Often combined with a thiazide diuretic. **Congestive heart failure** Asymptomatic left ventricular dysfunction.	
Lisinopril (Prinivil®, Zestril®)	Same MOA as captopril. Lysine analog of enalaprilat which is slightly more potent. $t_{1/2}$ = 12 hrs Given PO	**Hypertension** (mild to moderate) in young, white patients with high plasma renin. Often combined with a thiazide diuretic. **Congestive heart failure**	

Angiotensin II Receptor Antagonist

Drug	MOA & Pharmacokinetics	Clinical Uses	Side Effects
Losartan (Cozaar®)	Nonpeptide angiotensin II receptor (AT_1 subtype) antagonist which inhibits the vasoconstrictor and aldosterone-secreting effects of angiotensin II (ATII). Converted to a 5-carboxylic acid **metabolite** which is 10-40 times more potent and is responsible for most of the pharmacologic activity. Decreased ATII levels results in **decreased aldosterone** levels which decrease Na^+ and H_2O retention. Decreased ATII concentrations also result in ↑ renin release and the formation of angiotensin I. Possesses a uricosuric effect (increases clearance of uric acid). $t_{1/2}$ = 2 hrs (losartan), 6-9 hrs (metabolite) Given PO	**Hypertension** (mild to severe)	Headache Hypotension in patients with high plasma renin Hyperkalemia may occur in patients with renal insufficiency or those who are also taking K^+ sparing diuretics. ◆ Contraindication: Pregnancy: fetal exposure may cause hypotension, renal failure, anuria, skull hypoplasia, even death.

β-Adrenergic Agonist

Drug	MOA & Pharmacokinetics	Clinical Uses	Side Effects
Dobutamine (Dobutrex®)	Stimulates **β_1-receptors** on the heart to ↑ contractility (**inotropic**) and stroke volume. Also ↓ ventricular filling pressure and facilitates AV nodal conduction. May have chronotropic effects at high doses. Maintains blood flow to the kidney. $t_{1/2}$ = 2 min Given IV	**Congestive heart failure** Shock	Tachycardia Angina Arrhythmias Hypokalemia

Phosphodiesterase (PDE) Inhibitors

Drug	MOA & Pharmacokinetics	Clinical Uses	Side Effects
Amrinone (Inocor®)	Bypyridine derivative which inhibits cAMP phosphodiesterase (PDE III) in cardiac and smooth muscle. This increase in cAMP results in a (+) **inotropic** effect and **vasodilation** (↓ preload and afterload). $t_{1/2}$ = 2-3 hrs Given IV	**Congestive heart failure**: used for short-term management when there has been an inadequate response to digitalis, diuretics and/or vasodilators.	Arrhythmias Hypotension, dizziness Abdominal pain Fever Nausea and vomiting Thrombocytopenia (rare) Hepatotoxicity ◆ Contraindications: Severe aortic or pulmonic valvular disease.
Milrinone (Primacor®)	Same MOA as amrinone. Greater selectivity for PDE III isoenzymes. More potent, less severe side effects and more commonly used than amrinone. $t_{1/2}$ = 30-60 min Given IV		

Antiarrhythmic Drugs

Antiarrhythmic drugs can be classified according to their predominant effects on the action potential. They work primarily by reducing ectopic pacemaker activity and/or altering conduction in reentrant circuits. The following table summarizes the antiarrhythmic agents described in this section.

Class I (Na^+ channel blockers)	Class II (β-blockers)	Class III (K^+ channel blockers)	Class IV (Ca^{2+} channel blockers)	Miscellaneous
Class IA: Quinidine Procainamide Disopyramide Class IB: Lidocaine Tocainide Mexiletine Phenytoin Class IC: Flecainide Propafenone Moricizine	Propranolol Metoprolol Esmolol Sotalol	Amiodarone Bretylium	Diltiazem Verapamil	Adenosine Digitalis Magnesium sulfate

Arrhythmias are generally classified as supraventricular or ventricular in origin. These two categories can be further subdivided, as summarized below.

Supraventricular Arrhythmias	Ventricular Arrhythmias
Atrial tachycardia Paroxysmal tachycardia Multifocal atrial tachycardia Atrial fibrillation Atrial flutter	Wolff-Parkinson-White (preexcitation syndrome) Ventricular tachycardia Ventricular fibrillation Premature ventricular contraction

The action potential

The following table summarizes the major electrophysiological events during slow and fast cardiac action potentials.

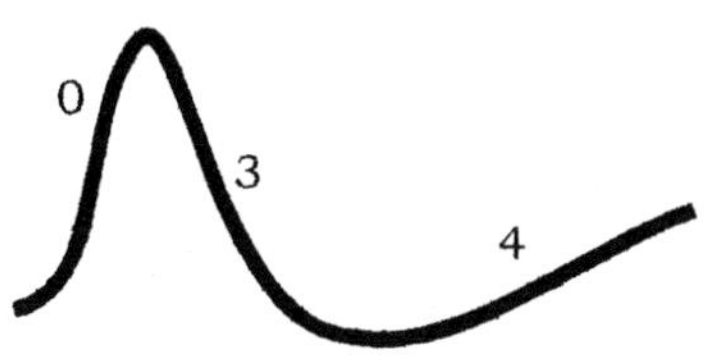

Slow cardiac action potentials are usually observed in the SA and AV nodes and can be broken down into 3 phases: 4, 0 and 3.

Phase 4: Unstable resting potential produces the **pacemaker** automaticity and is due to the influx of Ca^{2+} through **slow Ca^{2+} channels**. An increase in Na^{+} influx and a decrease in K^{+} efflux contribute to this phase.

Phase 0: Depolarization is also due to the influx of Ca^{2+} through **slow Ca^{2+} channels**. A decrease in K^{+} efflux contributes to this phase.

Phase 3: Repolarization results from **K^{+} efflux** as K^{+} conductance increases.

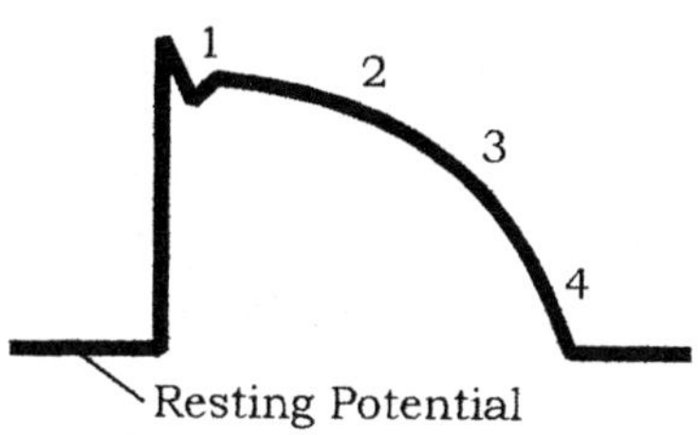

Fast cardiac action potentials are usually observed in the atria, Bundle of His, Purkinje fibers and the ventricles and can be divided into 5 phases: 4, 0, 1, 2 and 3.

Phase 4: The resting membrane potential is maintained by **high K^{+} efflux** and low Na^{+} and Ca^{2+} influx.

Phase 0: Rapid depolarization results from opening of **fast Na^{+} channels**.

Phase 1: Limited repolarization is due to inactivation of fast Na^{+} channels. An increase in K^{+} efflux and Cl^{-} influx also contribute to this phase.

Phase 2: Plateau results from **Ca^{2+} influx** through slow Ca^{2+} channels.

Phase 3: Rapid repolarization results from inactivation of slow Ca^{2+} channels and K^{+} efflux.

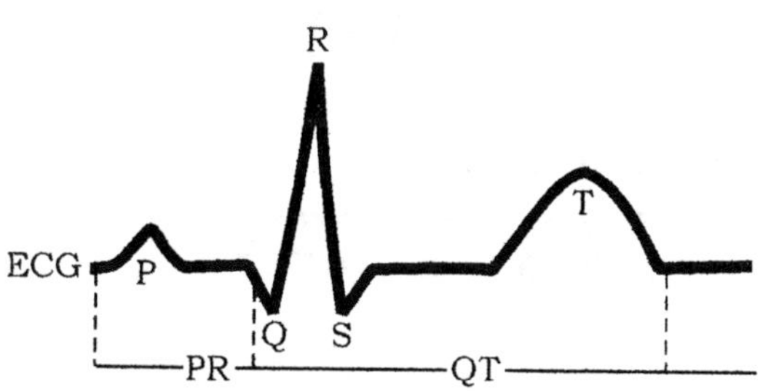

The electrocardiogram (ECG) is divided into various waves, segments and intervals. The major electrophysiological events occurring during these phases include:

P-wave:	atrial depolarization
PR interval:	atrial depolarization and conduction through the AV node.
QRS complex:	ventricular depolarization
QT interval:	ventricular action potential including ventricular depolarization and repolarization.
T-wave:	ventricular repolarization

Class I Drugs (Na^+ Channel Blockers)

Class IA Drugs

Drug	MOA & Pharmacokinetics	Clinical Uses	Side Effects
Quinidine (Quinaglute®, Quinidex®)	Binds to **open Na^+ channels** preventing Na^+ influx thus decreasing the slopes of phase 0 and phase 4 (↑ QRS complex). Inhibits K^+ currents, resulting in an ↑ repolarization time and action potential duration (↑ QT interval). Also blocks muscarinic and α-adrenergic receptors. $t_{1/2}$ = 6 hrs Given PO, IM	Ventricular arrhythmias Supraventricular arrhythmias Malaria	**Diarrhea** Nausea and vomiting Hypersensitivity reactions: fever, skin rash, thrombocytopenia Cinchonism: blurred vision, dizziness, headache, tinnitus Torsades de pointes is exacerbated by hypokalemia or hypomagnesemia. Treatment includes IV administration of $MgSO_4$. Drug Interaction: Decreases clearance of **digoxin**.
Procainamide (Procan-SR®, Pronestyl®)	Similar to quinidine except that it does not block muscarinic or α-adrenergic receptors. Metabolized to N-acetyl procainamide (NAPA) which no longer possesses Na^+ channel blocking activity but still blocks K^+ channels (class III agent). $t_{1/2}$ = 3-4 hrs Given PO, IV	Ventricular arrhythmias Supraventricular arrhythmias	Hypotension Diarrhea **Lupus syndrome**: more common with long term use and in slow acetylators. Initially seen as rash and small-joint arthralgia. Torsades de pointes
Disopyramide (Norpace®)	Similar to quinidine except that it possesses stronger antimuscarinic effects and does not block α-adrenergic receptors. Has a significant negative inotropic effect. $t_{1/2}$ = 7 hrs Given PO, IV	Ventricular arrhythmias Supraventricular arrhythmias	**Anticholinergic effects**: dry mouth, urinary retention, constipation and acute glaucoma CHF Torsades de pointes

Class IB Drugs

Drug	MOA & Pharmacokinetics	Clinical Uses	Side Effects
Lidocaine (Xylocaine®)	Blocks **activated** and **inactivated** Na^+ channels but exerts greater effects on inactivated channels. This blockade decreases the phase 0 slope. Also shortens the action potential duration. Given IV	**Ventricular arrhythmias**: **DOC** for acute management Local anesthetic	CNS effects: drowsiness, numbness, slurred speech, dizziness, confusion, convulsions, seizures, paresthesias Nystagmus is an early sign of toxicity.
Tocainide (Tonocard®)	An orally active analog of lidocaine which possesses similar activity. Given PO Renal excretion	Ventricular arrhythmias: often combined with quinidine to increase efficacy and reduce adverse effects.	Anorexia CNS effects: dizziness, tremor Nausea Blood dyscrasias and **pulmonary fibrosis** (rare)
Mexiletine (Mexitil®)	An orally active analog of lidocaine which possesses similar activity. Given PO Hepatic metabolism	Ventricular arrhythmias: often combined with quinidine to increase efficacy and reduce adverse effects.	CNS effects: dizziness, nervousness, trembling Nausea and vomiting Blood dyscrasias (rare)
Phenytoin (Dilantin®)	Anticonvulsant drug which binds to inactivated Na^+ channels and prolongs the inactivated state. Shortens action potential duration. Given PO, IV	Ventricular arrhythmias: especially drug-induced (**digitalis**, tricyclic antidepressants) Epilepsy: generalized tonic-clonic, partial seizures and status epilepticus.	CNS effects: nystagmus, ataxia, confusion Gingival hyperplasia Enzyme induction: P_{450} system Hypersensitivity reactions: fever, rash, lymphadenopathy Hypotension

Class IC Drugs

Drug	MOA & Pharmacokinetics	Clinical Uses	Side Effects
Flecainide (Tambocor®) In the CAST (Cardiac Arrhythmias Suppression Trial, 1989) study, flecainide was associated with excessive mortality when compared with placebo in patients with non-life threatening arrhythmias who suffered a recent MI.	Blocks Na^+ channels thus decreasing the phase 0 slope. In Purkinje cells, flecainide blocks late-opening Na^+ channels thus shortening the action potential duration. However, flecainide also blocks K^+ channels in ventricular myocytes which prolongs the action potential duration. The net effect is no change in the action potential duration. Exhibits a negative inotropic effect. Given PO	Supraventricular arrhythmias in patients without structural heart disease Ventricular arrhythmias	**Pro-arrhythmogenic** CNS effects: blurred vision, dizziness, headache, nausea, fatigue and tremor.
Propafenone (Rythmol®)	Same MOA as flecainide, but has some β-adrenergic blocking properties. Given PO	Supraventricular arrhythmias Ventricular arrhythmias	**Pro-arrhythmogenic** β-adrenergic blockade: blurred vision, bradycardia, bronchospasm Other cardiovascular effects: AV nodal block, exacerbation of CHF Drug Interactions: Increases serum **digoxin** and **warfarin** levels.
Moricizine (Ethmozine®) In the CAST II study (1991), moricizine was associated with excessive mortality when compared with placebo in patients with non-life threatening arrhythmias who suffered a recent MI.	Same MOA as flecainide. The effect on the action potential duration is unclear; some studies indicate that moricizine increases the action potential duration while others report a decrease. Exhibits some anticholinergic effects. Given PO	Ventricular arrhythmias	**Pro-arrhythmogenic** Anticholinergic effects: blurred vision, constipation Other cardiovascular effects: AV nodal block, exacerbation of CHF

Class II Drugs (β-Adrenergic Blockers)

Drug	MOA & Pharmacokinetics	Clinical Uses	Side Effects
Propranolol (Inderal®) Note: timolol, another non-selective β-blocker, is also used to treat arrhythmias.	Nonselective β_1 and β_2-adrenergic receptor antagonist. Antianginal effect is due to negative inotropic and chronotropic effects which decrease myocardial oxygen demand. Antiarrhythmic effects (Class II): these agents decrease phase 4 (resting potential) depolarization leading to ↓ rate of firing of sinus and ectopic pacemakers and ↓ AV node conduction. Antihypertensive effects may include reduced cardiac output, ↓ sympathetic outflow to peripheral vasculature (↓PVR) and inhibition of renin release by the kidney. Crosses the blood brain barrier. Given PO	**Hypertension** (mild to moderate) especially in young patients with high plasma renin and rapid pulse. Often given in combination with a thiazide diuretic. **Angina**: stable **Arrhythmias** (supraventricular arrhythmia, ventricular tachycardia, digitalis-induced tachyarrhythmia) Myocardial infarction: reduces myocardial ischemia by decreasing myocardial oxygen demand. Hypertrophic cardiomyopathy Pheochromocytoma (adjuvant) Hyperthyroidism Migraine prophylaxis Panic symptoms such as stage fright	Impotence CNS effects: drowsiness, insomnia, fatigue Bronchoconstriction Abrupt withdrawal may result in arrhythmias, heart failure or angina. Hypoglycemia due to a ↓ glucagon secretion and glycogenolysis (use with caution in patients with labile diabetes) Masks hypoglycemia-induced tachycardia Lipidemia due to ↑ plasma triglycerides and ↓ HDL Claudication of peripheral vessels

Drug	MOA & Pharmacokinetics	Clinical Uses	Side Effects
Metoprolol (Lopressor®)	Selective β_1-adrenergic receptor antagonist (cardioselective). Antianginal effect is due to negative inotropic and chronotropic effects which decrease myocardial oxygen demand. Antiarrhythmic effects (Class II): these agents decrease phase 4 depolarization leading to ↓ rate of firing of sinus and ectopic pacemakers and ↓ AV node conduction. Antihypertensive effects are due to reduced cardiac output, ↓ sympathetic outflow to peripheral vasculature (↓PVR) and inhibition of renin release by the kidney.	**Hypertension** in patients with asthma or diabetes. **Angina**: stable Arrhythmias Myocardial infarction: used to reduce myocardial ischemia by decreasing myocardial oxygen demand.	Bradycardia CNS effects: sedation, fatigue Bronchospasm, hypoglycemia, peripheral vasoconstriction and hyperlipidemia, but less than non-selective β-blockers. Congestive heart failure may occur due to the reduction of cardiac output.
Esmolol (Brevibloc®)	Selective β_1-adrenergic receptor antagonist (cardioselective). Decreases phase 4 depolarization leading to a decreased rate of firing of sinus and ectopic pacemakers and ↓ AV node conduction. $t_{1/2}$ = 8 min Given IV	Supraventricular arrhythmias: used to control ventricular rate perioperatively or in emergency situations. Perioperative hypertension: not a first-line agent	**Hypotension** CNS effects: anxiety, confusion, headache, drowsiness
Sotalol (Betapace®) Note: due to its K^+ channel blocking activity, Sotalol is also considered a **Class III** antiarrhythmic agent.	**Non-selective** β-adrenergic receptor antagonist. Decreases phase 4 depolarization leading to a decreased rate of firing of sinus and ectopic pacemakers and ↓ AV node conduction. Inhibits K^+ currents, resulting in an increase in action potential duration. Given PO	Supraventricular arrhythmias Ventricular arrhythmias	Torsades de pointes: exacerbated by hypokalemia Other side effects are related to β-adrenergic receptor blockade: especially bradycardia.

Class III Drugs (K^+ Channel Blockers)

The class III agents include amiodarone, bretylium and sotalol. **Sotalol** also exhibits β-adrenergic activity and therefore was discussed in the class II antiarrhythmic drug section

Drug	MOA & Pharmacokinetics	Clinical Uses	Side Effects
Amiodarone (Cordarone®)	A structural analog of thyroid hormone which exhibits Class I, II, III and IV antiarrhythmic activity. The dominant antiarrhythmic effect is due to K^+ channel blockade resulting in a prolonged refractory period and action potential duration. Also non-competitively blocks α-adrenergic receptors resulting in coronary and peripheral vasodilation. $t_{1/2}$ = 7 wks Given PO	Supraventricular arrhythmias Ventricular arrhythmias Note: due to its side effects, amiodarone is used when other less toxic agents have failed.	Neurotoxicity: proximal muscle weakness, peripheral neuropathy, tremors, ataxia Photosensitivity Pneumonitis: may progress to pulmonary fibrosis Nausea Corneal microdeposits Hypotension Hypo/hyperthyroidism Hepatic dysfunction Drug interactions: Increases serum levels of digoxin, other antiarrhythmics and warfarin
Bretylium (Bretylol®)	Blocks K^+ channels prolonging the action potential duration. Replaces norepinephrine in presynaptic sympathetic nerve terminals to produce a sympathectomy which also contributes to bretylium's antiarrhythmic activity. Given IV, IM	Ventricular arrhythmias	Hypotension May produce a transient hypertension and arrhythmia due to an initial release of norepinephrine.

Class IV Drugs (Calcium Channel Blockers)

Calcium channel blockers decrease Ca^{2+} influx in vascular smooth muscle and/or cardiac muscle. Of note is the varying specificity of these agents:

Effect on vascular smooth muscle: nifedipine > diltiazem > verapamil
Effect on cardiac muscle: verapamil > diltiazem > nifedipine

Drug	MOA & Pharmacokinetics	Clinical Uses	Side Effects
Diltiazem (Cardizem®)	Benzothiazepine derivative which binds cardiac L-type Ca^{2+} channels and decreases **SA node** automaticity and **AV nodal conduction** with some negative inotropic effects on the heart. Exhibits mild vasodilatory effects on blood vessels (less than nifedipine). Given PO, IV	**Hypertension** (mild to moderate) especially useful in black and elderly white patients with low renin levels. Efficacy may be enhanced by concomitant use of ACE inhibitors, methyldopa or β-blockers. **Angina** **Supraventricular arrhythmias**	Incidence is infrequent but may include: Skin rash Congestive heart failure Hypotension Peripheral edema Dizziness Flushing Headache ◆ Contraindication: Patients with pre-existing depressed cardiac function.
Verapamil (Calan®, Isoptin®, Verelan®) "V for ventricle"	Diphenylalkylamine which binds cardiac L-type Ca^{2+} channels and decreases **SA node** automaticity and **AV nodal conduction** with negative inotropic effects on the heart. Exhibits mild vasodilatory effects on arterioles. This decreases afterload which partially offsets the negative inotropic effects. Given PO, IV	**Hypertension** (mild to moderate) especially useful in black and elderly white patients with low renin levels. Efficacy may be enhanced by concomitant use of ACE inhibitors, methyldopa or β-blockers. **Angina** **Supraventricular arrhythmias** Hypertrophic cardiomyopathy	Incidence is infrequent but may include: Skin rash Bradycardia Congestive heart failure Hypotension Peripheral edema Constipation Dizziness Fatigue Headache ◆ Contraindication: Patients with pre-existing depressed cardiac function.

Miscellaneous Drugs

Drug	MOA & Pharmacokinetics	Clinical Uses	Side Effects
Adenosine (Adenocard®) Adenosine causes temporary asystole (chemical defibrillation).	Binds to G-protein coupled adenosine receptors resulting in activation of acetylcholine sensitive K^+ channels in the SA and AV nodes. This increase in conductance results in shortened action potential duration, hyperpolarization and decreased automaticity. Also inhibits Ca^{2+} channels resulting in ↑ AV nodal refractoriness. Extremely short $t_{1/2}$ (seconds). Given IV	**Supraventricular arrhythmias**: **DOC** for acute termination	Flushing Headache Dyspnea Chest pain
Digoxin (Lanoxin®) Digitoxin (Crystodigin®) These agents are derived from the foxglove (digitalis) plant.	Binds to and inhibits the **Na^+-K^+ ATPase** in myocardial cell membranes thereby increasing exchange of intracellular Na^+ for extracellular Ca^{2+} by the Na^+-Ca^{2+} exchanger. This increased intracellular Ca^{2+} is stored in the sarcoplasmic reticulum and upon release results in a positive inotropic effect. **Antiarrhythmic effects:** indirectly alters autonomic outflow by ↑ parasympathetic and ↓ sympathetic tone. This results in a ↓ conduction time and ↑ refractory period of the AV node.	**Congestive heart failure** **Supraventricular arrhythmias**: especially atrial fibrillation and flutter	**Atrial** or **ventricular dysrhythmias**: can be precipitated by **hypokalemic** states. GI effects: **nausea**, **vomiting**, **diarrhea** CNS effects: visual disturbances, drowsiness, confusion, delirium, headache and fainting. Selected Drug Interactions K^+-depleting (loop and thiazide) diuretics Quinidine: ↓ renal clearance of digoxin Ca^{2+}-channel blockers (particularly verapamil): additive depression of AV node conduction (bradycardia) **Overdose** is observed as cardiac depression leading to cardiac arrest. Treatment of overdose: withdrawal of drug, correction of electrolyte imbalances, administration of antiarrhythmic drugs and **digoxin antibodies** (F'ab fragments).

Drug	MOA & Pharmacokinetics	Clinical Uses	Side Effects
Magnesium sulfate	Antiarrhythmic mechanism is unclear but may be related to stabilizing cardiac cell membranes. Given IV	**Torsades de pointes** Digitalis-induced arrhythmias	Bradycardia Flushing Headache Respiratory paralysis

Notes

Diuretic Drugs

Diuretics cause an **increase in the volume of urine** produced and affect the pH, ionic composition and concentration of urine and blood. Clinically, they are used to manage edema, hypertension and electrolyte imbalances (e.g. hypercalcemia, hyperkalemia and hyponatremia). The efficacy of these drugs as well as the region of the nephron at which they act varies considerably among the different classes of diuretic drugs. They are listed below in the order in which they act on the nephron.

Drug	Site of action	Mechanism	Excretory Effects					
			H_2O	Na^+	K^+	Cl^-	HCO_3^-	Ca^{2+}
Carbonic Anhydrase Inhibitor: Acetazolamide	Proximal convoluted tubule	Inhibits carbonic anhydrase	↑↑	↑	↑↑	↑	↑↑	-
Osmotic Diuretic: Mannitol	Proximal convoluted tubule and the loop of Henle	Osmotic agent	↑↑	↑↑	↑	↑	↑	↑
Loop Diuretics: Furosemide, Bumetanide, Torsemide, Ethacrynic acid	Thick ascending limb of the loop of Henle	Inhibit the Na^+- K^+- $2Cl^-$ symporter	↑↑↑	↑↑	↑↑	↑↑	↑	↑↑
Thiazides: Hydrochlorothiazide, Chlorthalidone, Indapamide, Metolazone	Distal convoluted tubule	Inhibit the Na^+-Cl^- symporter	↑↑	↑	↑↑	↑	↑	V
Potassium Sparing Diuretics: Spironolactone, Amiloride, Triamterene	Distal convoluted tubule	Aldosterone receptor antagonist (spironolactone) or inhibit Na+ channels (amiloride, triamterene)	↑	↑	↓	↑	-	I

↑ = increase urinary excretion; ↓ = decrease urinary excretion (reabsorption); V = variable; I = insufficient data; - = no effect

Figure 4.2 Sites of action of diuretic agents

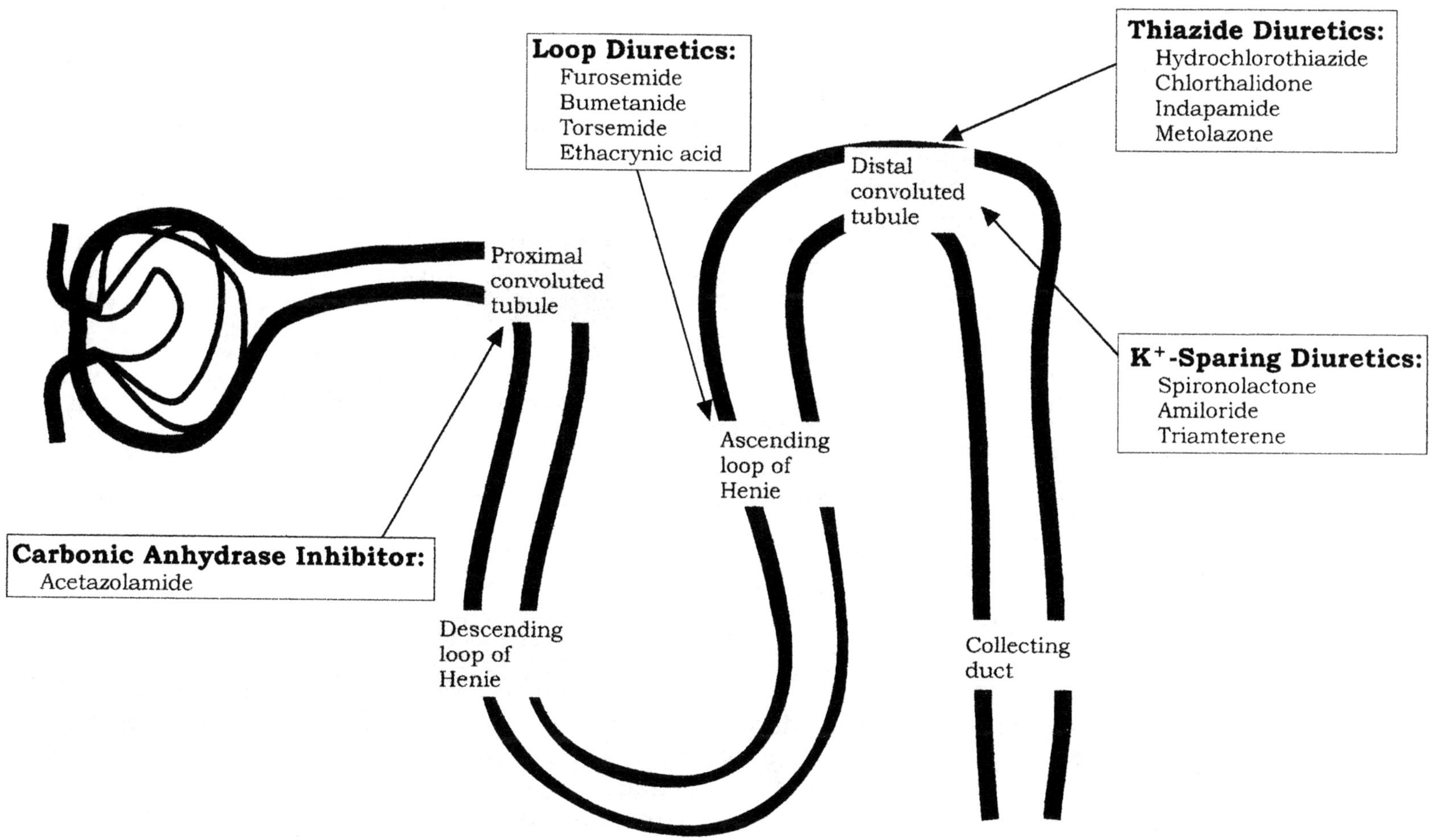

Carbonic Anhydrase Inhibitor

Drug	MOA & Pharmacokinetics	Clinical Uses	Side Effects
Acetazolamide (Diamox®)	Sulfonamide derivative which acts primarily on the **proximal convoluted tubule** to inhibit carbonic anhydrase. This results in decreased reabsorption of Na^+ and HCO_3^- in the proximal convoluted tubule; however, some of the Na^+ is reabsorbed in the loop of Henle. Furthermore, the increased delivery of Na^+ to more distal regions of the nephron results in exchange of K^+ for Na^+ leading to hypokalemia. The major effects of **HCO_3^- loss** are urinary alkalinization and hyperchloremic metabolic acidosis. The diuretic effects are self-limited (2-3 days) due to metabolic acidosis. Decreases renal blood flow and glomerular filtration rate by ↑ afferent arterial resistance. Given PO	**Glaucoma**: lowers intraocular pressure by decreasing production of aqueous humor. **Altitude sickness**: increases respiratory rate as a compensatory response to metabolic acidosis. Epilepsy Familial periodic paralysis	Drowsiness Paresthesias Metabolic acidosis Renal calculus Sulfonamide-like toxicities: bone marrow depression, skin rash, renal lesions, allergic reactions.

Osmotic Diuretics

Drug	MOA & Pharmacokinetics	Clinical Uses	Side Effects
Mannitol (Osmitrol®) * Remember, mannitol does it all (excretes everything)! Others: Glycerin Isosorbide Urea	Acts as an osmotic agent by increasing plasma osmolality thus drawing fluid from tissue to plasma. As a result cerebral edema, elevated intracranial and intraocular pressure are reduced. Acts at the **proximal tubule** and **loop of Henle** to promote diuresis. Because mannitol is not reabsorbed, the osmolality of the glomerular filtrate is increased. This results in the excretion of H_2O and inhibits the reabsorption of Na^+, Cl^- and other solutes. Given IV	**Edema**: adjuvant to fluid replacement for prevention of acute tubular necrosis or in the treatment of oliguria in acute renal failure Cerebral edema, elevated intracranial pressure Glaucoma (acute attacks) Preoperative reduction of intraocular pressure Used to promote urinary excretion of and prevent renal damage due to toxic substances	Headache Nausea and vomiting Dehydration Electrolyte imbalance Pulmonary edema in patients with heart failure

Loop Diuretics

Drug	MOA & Pharmacokinetics	Clinical Uses	Side Effects
Furosemide (Lasix®) Note: loop diuretics are the most efficacious diuretics available and are thus called "high ceiling diuretics." The name lasix comes from "lasts six" hours.	**Sulfonamide** derivative which inhibits the **Na^+- K^+- $2Cl^-$ symporter** in the luminal membrane of the **thick ascending limb of the loop of Henle** (TALH) by interfering with the Cl^- binding site of this symporter. Delivery of these electrolytes to distal regions of the nephron results in secretion of K^+ and H^+ (hypokalemic alkalosis). A decrease in the TALH membrane potential inhibits the reabsorption of Ca^{2+} and Mg^{2+}. Antihypertensive effect results from an initial decrease in blood volume and thus cardiac output. Eventually, cardiac output returns to normal but is accompanied by a decrease in peripheral resistance which maintains the hypotensive effects. Very short $t_{1/2}$ Given PO, IV	**Edema**: associated with CHF, liver and renal disease (including nephrotic syndrome) **Pulmonary edema** **Hypertension**: usually reserved for patients refractory to other diuretics. **Hypercalcemia**: due to the stimulation of tubular Ca^{2+} secretion	Hypokalemic metabolic alkalosis Hyponatremia Hypochloremia Hypomagnesemia Hyperuricemia leading to gouty attacks Hypercalciuria: leading to kidney stone formation Orthostatic hypotension (hypovolemia) Ototoxicity occurs especially with ethacrynic acid and the concurrent use of other ototoxic drugs Allergic reactions occur with the sulfonamide derivatives: furosemide, bumetanide, torsemide
Bumetanide (Bumex®)	Sulfonamide derivative with activity similar to furosemide, but is 10 to 40 times more potent.		
Torsemide (Demadcx®)	A newer sulfonamide derivative with activity similar to furosemide, but has a longer $t_{1/2}$ (due to an active metabolite).		
Ethacrynic acid (Edecrin®)	**Non**-sulfonamide derivative which possesses activity and potency similar to furosemide. Useful in patients allergic to sulfa drugs.		

Thiazide Diuretics

Drug	MOA & Pharmacokinetics	Clinical Uses	Side Effects
Hydrochlorothiazide (HydroDIURIL®) Chlorthalidone (Hygroton®) Indapamide (Lozol®) Metolazone (Mykrox®) Note: Thiazide diuretics have a synergistic effect when combined with loop diuretics.	Sulfonamide derivatives which inhibit the **Na^+-Cl^- symporter** on the luminal side of the epithelial cells in the early **distal convoluted tubules** (DCT) resulting in decreased reabsorption of NaCl. This decrease in Na^+ reabsorption promotes Na^+-Ca^{2+} exchange which leads to hypercalcemia and H_2O excretion. Delivery of Na^+ to distal regions of the nephron results in secretion of K^+ and H^+ (hypokalemic alkalosis). These agents are only moderately efficacious since most of the filtered load is reabsorbed before reaching the DCT. Possess a mild antidiuretic effect resulting from Na^+ and H_2O depletion which leads to increased reabsorption of the glomerular filtrate in the PCT. Antihypertensive effect results from an initial decrease in blood volume and thus cardiac output. Eventually, cardiac output returns to normal but is accompanied by a decrease in peripheral resistance which maintains the hypotensive effects. Indapamide possesses the strongest vasodilatory effects of the thiazide diuretics. Given PO	**Hypertension** (mild to severe) in black and elderly patients with low plasma renin and increased plasma volume. **Edema** associated with **CHF**, hepatic disease, renal disease and corticosteroid therapy. Nephrogenic diabetes insipidus: thiazide diuretics decrease urine volume due to volume contraction which leads to increased proximal tubular reabsorption. Calcium nephrolithiasis	Hypokalemic metabolic alkalosis Hyponatremia Hypochloremia Hypomagnesemia Hypercalcemia Hyperuricemia leading to gouty attacks Hyperglycemia: ↓ insulin release Hyperlipidemia: ↑ cholesterol and triglycerides Orthostatic hypotension Allergic reactions Photosensitivity Drug Interactions: May increase the toxicity of lithium by decreasing its renal clearance. May enhance digitalis toxicity associated with hypokalemia.

Potassium Sparing Diuretics

These drugs are rarely used alone and are often combined with thiazide or loop diuretics to offset urinary K^+ loss.

Drug	MOA & Pharmacokinetics	Clinical Uses	Side Effects
Spironolactone (Aldactone®)	**Aldosterone antagonist** at mineralocorticoid receptors in the late distal tubule and collecting ducts leading to decreased synthesis of Na^+ channels and Na^+/K^+-ATPase. This activity causes an increase in Na^+ clearance and a decrease in K^+ and H^+ excretion in the distal nephron. Antihypertensive effect results from an initial decrease in blood volume and thus cardiac output. Eventually, cardiac output returns to normal but is accompanied by a decrease in peripheral resistance which maintains the hypotensive effects. Antiandrogenic effect is due to both antagonism at androgen receptors and inhibition of steroid biosynthesis. Given PO	**Edematous states** including those associated with secondary hyperaldosteronism such as cardiac failure, hepatic cirrhosis, ascites and nephrotic syndrome. **Hypertension** (mild to severe) especially useful when combined with thiazide and loop diuretics. **Primary hyperaldosteronism** (Conn's syndrome) Hirsutism	**Hyperkalemia** Metabolic acidosis Endocrine effects: impotence, gynecomastia and menstrual irregularities CNS effects: drowsiness, lethargy, ataxia, confusion and headache GI effects: diarrhea, gastritis, gastric bleeding and peptic ulcers ◆Contraindication: Conditions predisposing to hyperkalemia especially renal insufficiency
Amiloride (Midamor®) Triamterene (Dyrenium®)	Block Na^+ channels in the late distal convoluted tubule and collecting ducts. This activity causes an increase in Na^+ clearance and a decrease in K^+ and H^+ excretion in the distal nephron. Given PO	**Edematous states** including those associated with secondary hyperaldosteronism such as cardiac failure, hepatic cirrhosis, ascites and nephrotic syndrome. **Hypertension** (mild to severe) especially useful when combined with thiazide and loop diuretics.	**Hyperkalemia** Metabolic acidosis Headache GI effects: nausea, vomiting, diarrhea Megaloblastic anemia: triamterene ◆Contraindication: Conditions predisposing to hyperkalemia especially renal insufficiency

Antidiuretic Drugs

Drug	MOA & Pharmacokinetics	Clinical Uses	Side Effects
Vasopressin (ADH) (Pitressin®, Pressyn®) ADH: Adds hydration to the body	Activates $\mathbf{V_2}$ receptors on the renal tubule cells to increase the number of water channels in the kidney collecting tubules. This results in the increased reabsorption of water and the formation of a concentrated urine. It interacts with $\mathbf{V_1}$ receptors on vascular smooth muscle cells to cause smooth muscle contraction. Increases the release of Factor VIII and von Willebrand factor. Given IV or intranasally	**Central diabetes insipidus** Variceal bleeding or colonic diverticular bleeding: causes the cessation of bleeding because of its vasoconstrictive properties.	Headache, nausea, abdominal cramps Hyponatremia due to antidiuretic effect Hypertension Bradycardia
Desmopressin acetate (DDAVP®)	Long acting **synthetic analog** of **vasopressin** which activates V_2 receptors on the renal tubule cells to increase the number of water channels in the kidney collecting tubules. This increases the reabsorption of water and the formation of a concentrated urine. Minimal activity at V_1 receptors. Increases the release of Factor VIII and von Willebrand factor. Given IV, SC or intranasally	**Central diabetes insipidus**: **DOC** Nocturnal enuresis Hemophilia A von Willebrand's disease	Headache, nausea, abdominal cramps Hyponatremia at high doses

Notes

Antithrombotics

There are three classes of drugs designed to treat thrombosis: **antiplatelet**, **anticoagulant** and **thrombolytics** drugs. They work by various mechanisms to inhibit thrombus formation or to enhance thrombus dissolution. Antiplatelet drugs prevent clot formation by inhibiting platelets. Anticoagulants inhibit the coagulation cascade to prevent fibrin deposition. Thrombolytic agents enhance the activity of plasmin to break down thrombi.

Antiplatelet Drugs	Anticoagulants	Thrombolytics
Aspirin Ticlopidine Dipyramidole Sulfinpyrazone	Heparin Warfarin	Streptokinase Eminase Tissue plasminogen activator Urokinase

Antiplatelet Drugs

These drugs increase bleeding time by inhibiting platelet aggregation.

Drug	MOA & Pharmacokinetics	Clinical Uses	Side Effects
Aspirin (Acetylsalicylic acid, ASA) (Bayer®, Bufferin®)	**Irreversibly** inhibits cyclooxygenase decreasing the production of prostaglandins and thromboxane. Due to its irreversibility, the antiplatelet activity of aspirin lasts for the life-span of the platelet (7-10 days). Patients undergoing elective surgery should stop administration 1 week prior to their procedure. **Salicylic acid**, a metabolite of aspirin, also contributes to the drug's activity by **reversibly** inhibiting cyclooxygenase. Exhibits a uricosuric effect at high doses (5000 mg/day). Given PO; $t_{1/2}$ = 2-3 hrs Hepatic metabolism Renal excretion; alkalinization of the urine significantly increases the rate of excretion.	Myocardial infarction: DOC Antiplatelet (<300 mg/day) Analgesia: low to moderate pain (300-2400 mg/day) Antipyretic: only in febrile patients (300-2400 mg/day) Anti-inflammatory (2400-4000 mg/day)	Bleeding complications Gastric intolerance Hypersensitivity reactions Renal toxicity Hepatotoxicity **Reye's Syndrome**: a fatal, fulminating hepatitis and cerebral edema seen in children with fever caused by viral illness who are given aspirin. Children with fever should be given acetaminophen. **Salicylate poisoning**: characterized by hyperventilation (respiratory alkalosis), metabolic acidosis, hyperpyrexia, coma, renal, vasomotor and respiratory failure, tinnitus and vertigo. Treatment of overdose includes induction of emesis, correction of electrolyte imbalance, alkalinization of the urine and dialysis. ◆ Contraindications: Pregnancy Peptic ulcer disease Hemophilia Children with fever caused by viral illnesses (associated with **Reye's Syndrome**)

Drug	MOA & Pharmacokinetics	Clinical Uses	Side Effects
Ticlopidine (Ticlid®)	Inhibits ADP-induced binding of fibrinogen to the platelet membrane at the glycoprotein IIb/IIIa complex.	**Stroke**: initial or recurrent Especially useful in patients who cannot tolerate aspirin.	**GI effects**: diarrhea, nausea Skin rash Leukopenia, agranulocytosis Bleeding due to thrombocytopenia
Dipyramidole (Dipridacot®, Persantine®)	Not fully elucidated but may increase adenosine levels resulting in coronary vasodilation and inhibition of platelet aggregation and activation.	**Thromboemboli**: prophylaxis in patients with **prosthetic heart valves**.	**Angina pectoris** **CV effects**: hypotension, tachycardia **GI effects**: nausea, diarrhea **Dizziness**, **headache**
Sulfinpyrazone (Anturan®, Anturane®)	Weak antiplatelet effects mediated through a sulfide metabolite which inhibits platelet adherence to the subendothelium and the release of platelet factors. Inhibits uric acid absorption in the proximal tubule.	Chronic gout Hyperuricemia Recurrent MI: may reduce the risk of a reinfarction (rarely indicated except in patients who cannot tolerate aspirin)	**Renal calculi** **Acute gouty arthritis** GI disturbances: nausea, vomiting Hypersensitivity

Anticoagulants

Anticoagulants fall into two categories. One type, heparin, increases the rate of destruction of clotting factors, acts within minutes and is injectable. The second type, oral anticoagulants (warfarin, dicumarol) inhibits the synthesis of new clotting factors and may take days to confer anticoagulant activity.

Drug	MOA & Pharmacokinetics	Clinical Uses	Side Effects
Heparin (MW= 5-20kDa) Low molecular weight fractions of heparin are also currently in use.	Enhances the proteolytic actions of **antithrombin III** which inactivates factors **IIa** (thrombin), **IXa**, **Xa**, **XIa** and **XIIa**. Does not cross the placenta. Highly protein bound. Given SC, IV	**Anticoagulant**: DOC during pregnancy **Deep vein thrombosis** **Pulmonary thromboembolism** Prevention of blood clotting during dialysis and cardiac surgery. Thromboembolism Stroke	**Bleeding**: Thrombocytopenia Osteoporosis: with long term use Alopecia: with long term use Treatment of overdose: **Protamine** ◆ Contraindications: Hypersensitivity to heparin Bleeding dyscrasias
Warfarin (Coumadin®) Dicumarol is another coumarin derivative used for anticoagulation.	A coumarin derivative which inhibits the synthesis of **vitamin K** and thus prevents vitamin K-mediated **γ-carboxylation** of the procoagulant factors **II** (prothrombin), **VII**, **IX** and **X**, as well as the anticoagulant factors **C** and **S**. Exhibits a delayed effect related to the $t_{1/2}$ of pre-existing clotting factors. Crosses the placenta. $t_{1/2}$ = 2 days Given PO	**Deep vein thrombosis** **Pulmonary thromboembolism** Thromboembolism associated with chronic atrial fibrillation (due to prosthetic heart valves, rheumatic mitral stenosis) or myocardial infarction.	**Hemorrhage** Skin rash GI effects: nausea, diarrhea Skin necrosis: in patients with protein C deficiency Treatment of overdose: **Vitamin K, fresh frozen plasma** ◆ Contraindication: Pregnancy: warfarin can interfere with fetal bone development when administered early in the pregnancy.

Thrombolytics

Thrombolytic drugs convert plasminogen to plasmin either indirectly (streptokinase and eminase) or directly (t-PA and urokinase). Plasmin, the protease responsible for dissolution of thrombi, degrades fibrin, fibrinogen and factors V and VIII. These drugs should be given IV within several hours of thrombosis.

Drug	MOA & Pharmacokinetics	Clinical Uses	Side Effects
Streptokinase (Streptase®, Kabikinase®)	An **indirect** thrombolytic which combines with plasminogen to form an **activator complex** which converts free and fibrin-bound plasminogen to plasmin. Derived from *Streptococcus* (antigenic). $t_{1/2}$ of the activator complex = 23 min.	Acute myocardial infarction Pulmonary thromboemboli Acute arterial thromboembolism	**Systemic bleeding**: treated with aminocaproic acid, an inhibitor of plasminogen activation. **Antigenicity**: fever, hypersensitivity with repeated doses.
Eminase (Anistreplase®)	An anisoylated streptokinase (prodrug) which combines with plasminogen to form an **activator complex** which converts free and fibrin-bound plasminogen to plasmin. $t_{1/2}$ of the activator complex = 90 min. The longer half-life (compared to streptokinase) is due to the slow metabolism of the anisoyl group.	Acute myocardial infarction	**Systemic bleeding**: treated with aminocaproic acid, an inhibitor of plasminogen activation. **Antigenicity**: fever, hypersensitivity with repeated doses.
Tissue Plasminogen Activator (t-PA) (Alteplase®)	**Directly** converts only fibrin-bound plasminogen to plasmin. More selective than urokinase. Produced by human endothelial cells.	Acute myocardial infarction Acute pulmonary thromboembolism: generally administered with heparin	Incidence of stroke and cerebral hemorrhages greater than with other thrombolytic agents.
Urokinase (Abbokinase®)	**Directly** converts plasminogen, both free and fibrin-bound, to plasmin. Produced by human kidney cells. $t_{1/2}$ = 20 min.	Acute pulmonary thromboembolism	**Systemic bleeding**: treated with aminocaproic acid, an inhibitor of plasminogen activation.

Notes

Antihyperlipidemics

Antihyperlipidemics are used for the treatment of elevated serum lipids (hyperlipidemias). Hyperlipidemia is associated with a higher risk of coronary heart disease (CHD) and cerebrovascular disease, two major causes of death in the United States. Lipids are transported around the body by particles called lipoproteins. These lipoproteins are further classified as high, intermediate and low-density lipoproteins (HDL, IDL and LDL respectively). Clinically, the absolute and relative amounts of these lipoprotein classes are used to assess the risk of an individual for CHD. Guidelines for serum cholesterol level classification are summarized on the following table:

Classification	Total Cholesterol (mg/dl)	LDL cholesterol (mg/dl)	Triglycerides
Desirable	<200	<130	<200
Borderline high	200-239	130-159	200-400
High	>240	>160	400-1000

Antihyperlipidemic drugs act on various aspects of lipid absorption and metabolism and can be classified as the following:

HMG-CoA Reductase Inhibitors	Bile Acid Sequestrants (Resins)	Vitamin	Miscellaneous
Lovastatin Simvastatin Pravastatin Fluvastatin	Cholestyramine Colestipol	Niacin (Vitamin B3)	Gemfibrozil Clofibrate Probucol

Figure 4.3: Lipid metabolism

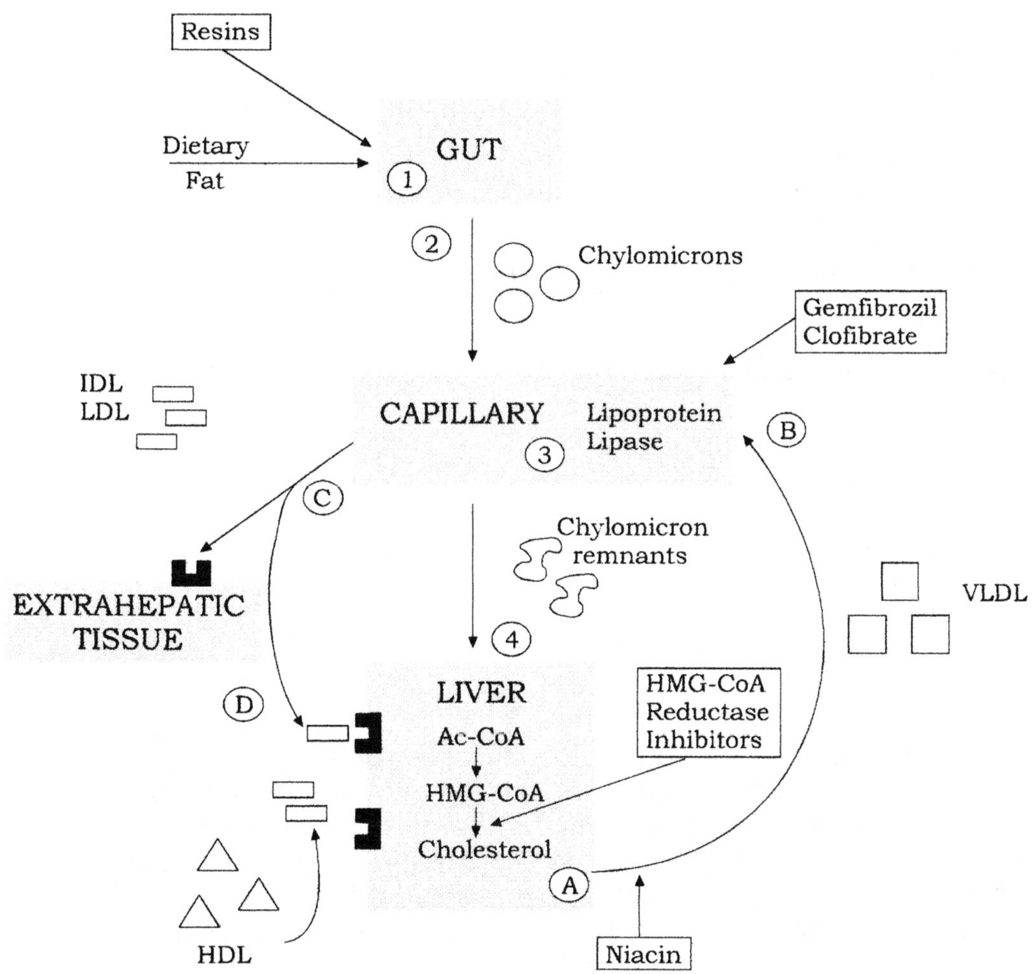

Exogenous Pathway:

1. Dietary triglycerides and cholesterol are taken up by intestinal cells and formed into chylomicrons.

2. Chylomicrons are released into the vascular system and are hydrolyzed by lipoprotein lipase in adipose tissue and muscle.

3. The action of lipoprotein lipase liberates triglycerides and releases chylomicron remnants.

4. Chylomicron remnants are taken up by the liver and cleaved, resulting in free cholesterol.

Endogenous Pathway:

A. The liver synthesizes very low density lipoproteins (VLDLs).

B. VLDLs are released into the bloodstream and cleaved by lipoprotein lipase. This results in the liberation of triglycerides and intermediate density lipoproteins.

C. IDLs can either be taken up by LDL-receptors on the liver or further hydrolyzed to release triglycerides and form LDLs.

D. LDLs bind their receptors on extrahepatic or hepatic tissues.

E. HDLs are formed by peripheral cells and serve to transport cholesterol to the liver.

Types of Hyperlipidemia

In general, **primary hyperlipidemia** results from a single gene defect or from both genetic and environmental factors. In contrast, secondary hyperlipidemia may be secondary to general metabolic disorders such as diabetes mellitus, hypothyroidism, obstructive liver disease, alcoholism, cirrhosis, renal disease and oral contraceptives.

Primary hyperlipidemia can be further subcategorized as follows:

Type	Lab Findings	Cause	Drug
I Familial Hyperchylomicronemia	↑ chylomicrons	Deficiency of lipoprotein lipase or deficiency of apoprotein CII	
IIa Familial Hypercholesterolemia	↑ LDL	Absence of or defective LDL receptors	HMG CoA reductase inhibitor, resin, niacin, probucol
IIb Familial Combined Hyperlipidemia	↑ LDL ↑ VLDL	↑ secretion of VLDL (biochemical cause unknown)	Niacin, gemfibrozil, resin, HMG CoA reductase inhibitor
III Familial Dysbetalipoproteinemia	↑ IDL ↑ chylomicrons ↓ LDL ↓ HDL	↑ production or ↓ utilization of IDL (defect in ApoEII)	Niacin, gemfibrozil
IV Familial Hypertriglyceridemia	↑ VLDL	↑ secretion of VLDL (biochemical cause unknown)	Niacin, gemfibrozil
V Familial Mixed Hypertriglyceridemia	↑ VLDL ↑ chylomicrons	↑ production or ↓ removal of VLDL and chylomicrons (biochemical cause unknown)	Drug therapy if necessary

HMG-CoA Reductase Inhibitors

Drug	MOA & Pharmacokinetics	Clinical Uses	Side Effects
Lovastatin (Mevacor®) Simvastatin (Zocor®) Pravastatin (Pravachol®) Fluvastatin (Lescol®)	**Reversibly** and **competitively inhibit HMG-CoA reductase**, the enzyme which catalyzes the rate limiting step in cholesterol biosynthesis (HMG CoA → mevalonate). This results in an increase of LDL receptors in the liver and a subsequent increase in the catabolism of LDL. Lovastatin and simvastatin are **prodrugs**. Pravastatin and fluvastatin are **not prodrugs**. Given PO. Extensive first-pass effect.	**Type IIa** and **Type IIb** hyperlipidemias	GI effects: constipation, diarrhea, stomach pain, nausea Myalgia, myositis and/or rhabdomyolysis may occur in patients with renal insufficiency or with concomitant use of gemfibrozil, niacin, cyclosporin or erythromycin. Increase in liver enzymes such as serum transaminases. ◆ Contraindications: Hepatic disease Pregnant and nursing women Children

Resins

Drug	MOA & Pharmacokinetics	Clinical Uses	Side Effects
Cholestyramine (Questran®, Cholybar®) Colestipol (Colestid®)	Promote the excretion of bile salts by forming an insoluble complex in the small intestine. This increases the conversion of cholesterol to bile acids and increases the number of LDL receptors in the liver which results in increased removal of LDL from the plasma.	**Type IIa** and **IIb** hyperlipidemias Pruritus associated with biliary obstruction	**GI effects**: **constipation**, steatorrhea, stomach pain **Decreased absorption** of fat soluble vitamins and certain drugs

Vitamin

Drug	MOA & Pharmacokinetics	Clinical Uses	Side Effects
Niacin (Nicotinic acid, Vitamin B3)	Decreases production of VLDL resulting in ↓LDL. Increases HDL via an unknown mechanism. Given PO with a meal	**Type IIa**, **IIb**, **III**, **IV** and **V** hyperlipidemias Niacin deficiency Pellagra	**Intense cutaneous flush**: prevented by prior administration of aspirin. Pruritus GI effects: nausea, vomiting ◆ Contraindications: Hepatic disease Diabetes Peptic ulcer disease Gout

Miscellaneous

Drug	MOA & Pharmacokinetics	Clinical Uses	Side Effects
Gemfibrozil (Lopid®) Clofibrate (Atromid-S®)	Decreases serum triglycerides by decreasing hepatic secretion of VLDL and increasing lipoprotein lipase activity in capillary endothelial cells. 95% bound to plasma albumin. Given PO with a meal	**Type IIb**, III, **IV** and **V** hyperlipidemias Note: clofibrate is used less due to increased toxicity	GI distress: stomach pain, gas Rash, gallstones, myositis (rare) GI and hepatobiliary neoplasms (clofibrate) Drug Interaction: Potentiates antiplatelet effects of **anticoagulants**
Probucol (Lorelco®, Bifenabid®)	Lowers serum cholesterol by increasing LDL catabolism. Given PO with a meal	**Type IIa** hyperlipidemia	GI distress: nausea, diarrhea Arrhythmias: prolonged QT Eosinophilia

Notes

Antimicrobial Drugs

Page	Topic

Antimicrobial Drugs

Antibiotics are chemical substances produced by certain microorganisms (bacteria, fungi, actinomycetes) that may either inhibit the growth of other microorganisms (static) or kill them (cidal). Synthetic antibacterial agents, those not produced by microbes, also exist and includes the sulfonamides and quinolones. Listed below are the antimicrobial classes and agents which will be discussed in this section.

Cell Wall Synthesis Inhibitors and β-Lactamase Inhibitors	Protein Synthesis Inhibitors	Nucleic Acid Synthesis and Replication Inhibitors	Metabolic Inhibitors	Antimycobacterial Agents
Penicillins Cephalosporins Carbapenams Monobactams Vancomycin Cycloserine β-Lactamase Inhibitors	Aminoglycosides Tetracyclines Chloramphenicol Macrolides Lincosamides	Fluoroquinolones Rifampin	Sulfonamides Trimethoprim	Rifampin Isoniazid (INH) Pyrazinamide Ethambutol Streptomycin

Resistance: refers to bacterial growth which is not reduced by an antimicrobial agent. General mechanisms of resistance include:

1) Failure of the antibiotic to permeate the microorganism.
2) Decreased affinity of the drug for its target binding site (e.g. a ribosomal subunit, a cell membrane).
3) Inactivation of the drug by microbial enzymes.

Cross-resistance: refers to resistance of organisms to drugs of similar structure and mechanisms of action.

Spectrum: refers to the range of antimicrobial activity which a certain agent covers. The spectrum of an agent may be narrow, extended or broad.

Bacteriostatic vs. bactericidal: bacteriostatic drugs arrest the growth and replication of bacteria while drugs which are bactericidal kill bacteria and decrease the total number of viable organisms.

Selection of antimicrobial agents:

1. Identification of the organism and sensitivity of it to a particular agent.
2. The safety of the agent and toxic effects it may have on a particular patient.
3. The site of infection may limit the use or determine how an agent should be administered.

Figure 5.1: Site of action of various antimicrobials.

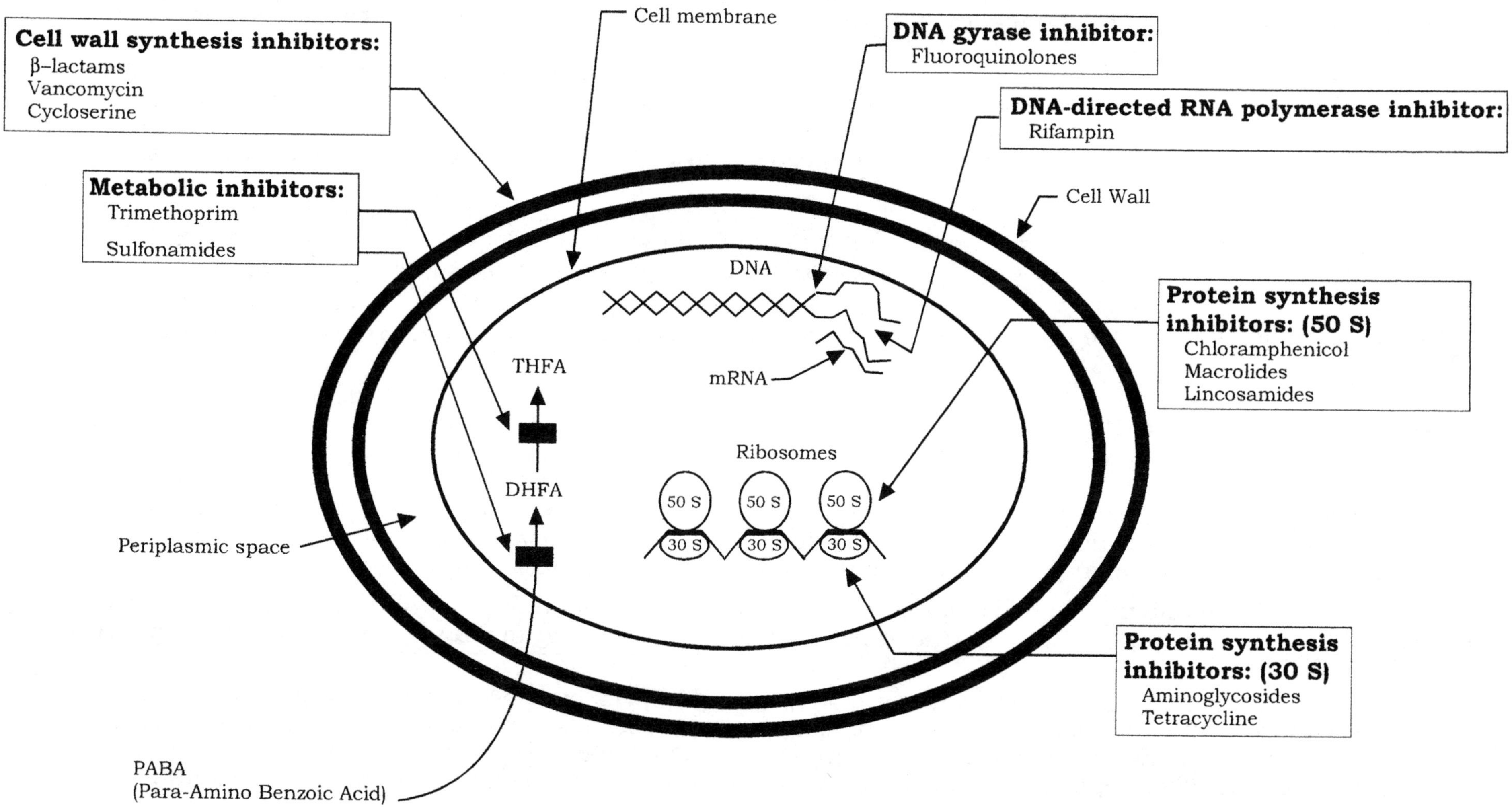

Antibiotic Classification

Class	Agent(s)	Mechanism of Action	Effect
Cell Wall Synthesis Inhibitors	β-lactams Penicillins Cephalosporins Carbapenams Monobactams	• Bind to specific receptors (penicillin-binding proteins), within the bacterial cytoplasmic membrane. • Inhibit the last **transpeptidation** reaction (third step of murein synthesis) in peptidoglycan cross-linking. • Activate autolytic enzymes within the bacteria.	Cidal
	Vancomycin	Inhibits the second step of **murein** synthesis.	Cidal
	Cycloserine	Inhibits the enzyme **alanine racemase** (first stage of murein synthesis), since it is structurally similar to D-alanine. This blocks the production of the pentapeptide.	Cidal
β-Lactamase Inhibitors	Clavulanic acid Sulbactam Tazobactam	Inhibit **β-lactamases** and prevent them from destroying the antibiotics which are their normal substrates. They have little antibacterial activity when given alone.	—
Protein Synthesis Inhibitors	Aminoglycosides	Inhibit protein synthesis by binding irreversibly to the **30S** ribosomal subunit, however, some aminoglycosides may also bind to the 50S subunit.	Cidal
	Tetracyclines	Inhibit the binding of **aminoacyl tRNA** by binding to the **30S** ribosomal subunit.	Static
	Chloramphenicol	Inhibits the enzyme **peptidyl transferase** and the formation of peptide bonds by binding to the **50S** prokaryotic ribosomal subunit.	Static
	Macrolides Lincosamides	Inhibit the enzyme **peptidyl transferase** and the translocation reactions by binding to the **50S** prokaryotic ribosomal subunit.	Static in most cases
Nucleic Acid Synthesis and Replication Inhibitors	Fluoroquinolones	Inhibit replication by binding **DNA gyrase**.	Cidal
	Rifampin	Inhibits transcription by binding **DNA-dependent RNA polymerase**.	Cidal
Metabolic Inhibitors	Sulfonamides	Competitively inhibit **PABA** (Para-Amino Benzoic Acid). This disrupts the prokaryotic **folate** synthesis pathway.	Static
	Trimethoprim	Competitively inhibits **dihydrofolate reductase**.	Static

Figure 5.2: Bacterial wall synthesis

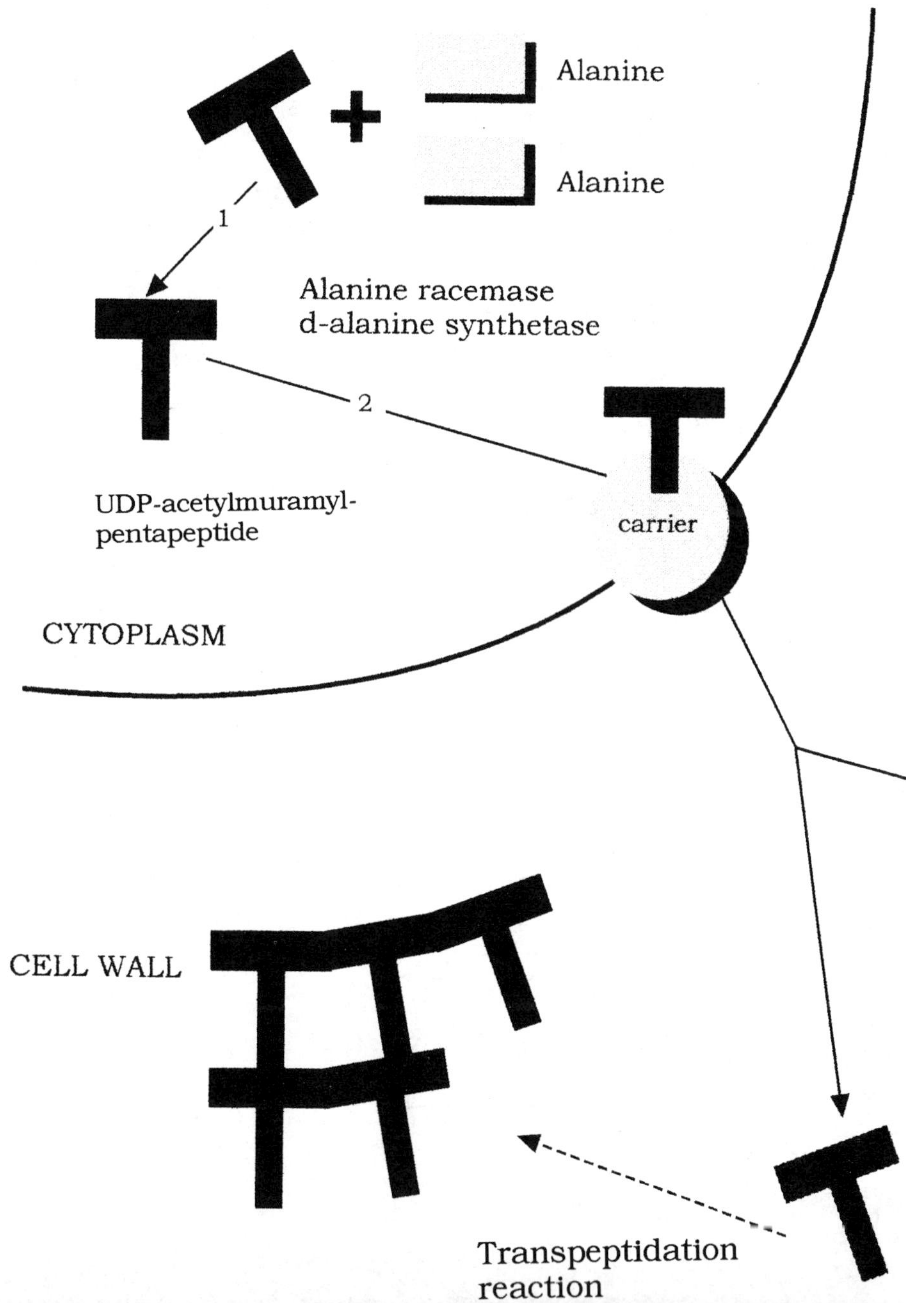

Bacterial cell walls are vital for the normal growth and development of bacteria. Peptidoglycan (murein) is the essential component of the cell wall providing rigid support and maintaining cell shape. It is composed of glycan chains which are linear strands of two alternating amino sugars (NAG and NAM) that are cross-linked by peptide chains.

Bacterial cell wall/peptidoglycan synthesis involves approximately thirty bacterial enzymes, but for simplicity it may be considered in the following three stages:

1) The cytoplasmic precursor molecule is joined by a dipeptide, D-alanyl-D-alanine, resulting in UDP-acetylmuramyl-pentapeptide. The reaction is catalyzed by alanine racemase which is inhibited by cycloserine.

2) UDP-acetylmuramyl-pentapeptide is transported across the plasma membrane by a carrier protein and linked to UDP-acetylglucosamine forming a long polymer.

3) The carrier protein is recycled and completion of the cross-linking is accomplished by a transpeptidation reaction occurring outside the cell membrane. The final step is inhibited by the β-lactams.

Cell Wall Synthesis Inhibitors and β-Lactamase Inhibitors

Cell wall synthesis inhibitors are **bactericidal**; they kill bacteria by selectively interfering with either the synthesis or repair of the cell wall. The cell wall is a rigid outer layer that is unique to bacteria. It surrounds the cytoplasmic cell membrane, maintains the shape of the cell and protects bacteria, which possess a high internal osmotic pressure (hyperosmolar), from absorbing water and exploding.

The cell wall contains a cross-linked polymer of glycan known as **peptidoglycan** (murein, mucopeptide). Peptidoglycan chains are synthesized in the cytoplasm, cross the plasma membrane and join other peptidoglycan chains resulting in a rigid cross-linked barrier surrounding the bacteria (see *Figure 5.2*). The peptidoglycan layer found in gram-positive cell walls in thicker than the cell wall seen in gram-negative bacteria. This important difference allows the gram stain to separate most bacteria into two groups: the gram-positive bacteria which stain blue, and the gram-negative bacteria which stain red.

Eukaryotic cells lack cell walls and are therefore unaffected by inhibitors of cell wall synthesis. This is why penicillins and cephalosporins have relatively few side effects. Vancomycin and cycloserine, however, are quite toxic suggesting that they work by a different mechanism. In order for these agents to be most effective, they require bacteria to be actively proliferating. They have relatively little or no effect on microorganisms which are not growing.

β-lactamase Inhibitors such as clavulanic acid are used in combination with a variety of penicillins to extend their spectrum and protect them from β-lactamases. Alone, they are ineffective antibacterial agents.

Penicillins	Cephalosporins	Carbapenams and Monobactams	Others	β-Lactamase Inhibitors
Natural Antistaphylococcal Aminopenicillins Antipseudomonal	First Generation Second Generation Third Generation	Imipenem Aztreonam	Vancomycin Cycloserine	Clavulanic acid Sulbactam Tazobactam

Penicillins

The **penicillins** are among the most important β-lactam antibiotics. They originated from a mold of the genus *Penicillium* whose antibiotic properties were first witnessed by Alexander Fleming in 1928. However, an effective quantity of penicillin was not produced until 1940 by Florey, Chain and Abraham. Since their discovery, numerous other effective antimicrobial agents have been produced, however, penicillin and newer derivatives of the basic penicillin nucleus (6-Aminopenicillanic acid) continue to be the drug of choice for many infectious diseases.

Natural Penicillins	Antistaphylococcal Penicillins	Aminopenicillins	Antipseudomonal Penicillins
Penicillin G Penicillin V Penicillin G procaine Penicillin G benzathine	Methicillin Nafcillin Oxacillin Dicloxacillin Cloxacillin	Ampicillin Amoxicillin	Mezlocillin Piperacillin Azlocillin Carbenicillin Ticarcillin

Mechanism of Resistance (resistance continues to increase at a rapid rate):

- Production of enzymes (e.g. β-lactamases) by certain organisms that break the beta-lactam ring of penicillin. This is common with *S. aureus, H. influenzae, N. gonorrhoeae* and many gram-negative bacilli.
- Removal or alteration of specific receptors (penicillin binding proteins) to which the antimicrobials bind.
- Decreased permeability to the drug preventing it from reaching its target binding receptors.
- Inhibition of cell wall autolytic enzymes.
- Organisms that lack a cell wall (e.g. mycoplasma) or that are metabolically inactive (e.g. L-forms) are not susceptible to penicillins or other cell wall inhibitors because they do not synthesize peptidoglycan.

Penicillin Binding Proteins (PBP's): refer to bacterial enzymes located on the bacterial cytoplasmic membrane which are involved in synthesis of the cell wall and in the maintenance of the bacterial morphology. They are the initial receptors for penicillins and other cell wall synthesis inhibitors.

Transpeptidases: refer to bacterial enzymes responsible for the final step in cell wall synthesis by cross-linking linear peptidoglycan chains.

β-Lactamases: refer to a family of bacterial enzymes which hydrolyze the cyclic amide bond of the β-lactam ring common to penicillins, cephalosporins and other β-lactam antibiotics.

Natural Penicillins

Drug	MOA & Pharmacokinetics	Clinical Uses	Side Effects
Penicillin G (Pfizerpen®) Penicillin V (V-Cillin K®) Penicillin G procaine (Duracillin A.S.®) Penicillin G benzathine (Bicillin L-A®)	Attach to specific penicillin binding proteins and inhibit cell wall synthesis by **blocking transpeptidation** of **peptidoglycan**. Activate or disinhibit intracellular cytotoxic "autolysins." Bactericidal if active peptidoglycan synthesis takes place. Lower drug levels are found in the eye, prostate and the CNS. However, with inflammation of the meninges, as in bacterial meningitis, penicillins reach effective levels in the CSF. **Penicillin V** is more acid-stable than penicillin G and is therefore more easily absorbed from the GI tract and has a higher bioavailability. Given PO, IV, IM, IT	Spectrum: gram(+), gram(-), spirochetes, many anaerobes. **Pneumonia** due to *Strep. pneumoniae* (pneumococcal) ***Strep. pyogenes*** (group-A β-hemolytic) infections including : pharyngitis, scarlet fever, pneumonia, arthritis, meningitis and endocarditis. ***Neisseria meningitidis*** (meningococcal) infections **Gingivostomatitis** due to *Leptotrichia buccalis* and spirochetes present in the mouth. **Syphilis** due to *Treponema pallidum* **Actinomycosis** due to *Actinomyces israelii* **Diphtheria** due to *Corynebacterium diphtheria* **Anthrax** due to *Bacillus anthracis* **Gas Gangrene** due to *Clostridium perfringens*	**Hypersensitivity reactions** are the most common adverse side effect and may occur at any dose. This allergic reaction presents with: fever, maculopapular rash, urticarial rash, bronchospasm, vasculitis, serum sickness, exfoliative dermatitis, Steven-Johnson Syndrome, anaphylaxis. **Positive Coombs' reaction** often occurs during prolonged therapy, but hemolytic anemia is rare. Eosinophilia occasionally occurs during other allergic reactions to penicillin. May potentiate the effects of anticoagulants. Sodium salts of some penicillins are a problem with CHF patients, since sodium promotes fluid retention. **Seizures** may occur with intrathecal administration or high doses of penicillin G because penicillins are irritating to the CNS and increase the excitability of neurons by inhibiting GABA (inhibitory neurotransmitter). Drug Interactions: **Probenecid** increases serum concentrations by decreasing tubular secretion into the proximal convoluted tubule.

Antistaphylococcal Penicillins (Penicillinase resistant)

Drug	MOA & Pharmacokinetics	Clinical Uses	Side Effects
Methicillin (Staphcillin®) Nafcillin (Unipen®) Oxacillin (Bactocill®) Dicloxacillin (Dynapen®) Cloxacillin (Tegopen®)	Cell wall synthesis inhibitors All are **highly protein bound** (95-98%) but unlike sulfonamides they don't displace bilirubin from plasma proteins and are safe for neonates. Generally the high protein binding translates into decreased potency. **Methicillin** and **dicloxacillin** are the most resistant to β–lactamases. All are relatively acid-stable and well absorbed from the gut. Methicillin, oxacillin, dicloxacillin and cloxacillin are excreted by the kidneys. **Nafcillin** is excreted 80% by the **liver** and is the best antistaphylococcal PCN for patients in renal failure.	Spectrum: narrow; *Staphylococcus* **Penicillinase producing *Staphylococci***: DOC Some activity against *Streptococcus* Note: these agents are ineffective against gram(-) organisms.	**Methicillin** has the most nephrotoxicity, so much so that **acute interstitial nephritis** has limited its utility. Methicillin, nafcillin and other penicillins occasionally cause **granulocytopenia**, especially in children.

Aminopenicillins (Extended spectrum)

Drug	MOA & Pharmacokinetics	Clinical Uses	Side Effects
Ampicillin (Omnipen®) Amoxicillin (Amoxil®) Note: Aminopenicillins are often combined with β-lactamase inhibitors in the following combinations: Ampicillin plus sulbactam (Unasyn®) Amoxicillin plus clavulanic acid (Augmentin®)	Cell wall synthesis inhibitors Ampicillin and amoxicillin only differ in absorption, not in their spectrum of activity. **Ampicillin** and **amoxicillin** are acid stable, but amoxicillin is better absorbed. As a result amoxicillin has a decreased incidence of pseudomembranous colitis and diarrhea compared to ampicillin. Inactivated by β-lactamases unless combined with a **β-lactamase inhibitor**.	Spectrum: gram(-) bacteria **Upper respiratory infections** due to *Strep. pyogenes*, *Strep. pneumoniae* and *H. influenzae* **Urinary tract infection** due to Group-D *Enterococci* **Bacterial meningitis** due to *Listeria monocytogenes* **Invasive *Salmonella*** (blood culture positive) infections Acute gastroenteritis (shigellosis) due to *Shigella* can be treated more successfully with ampicillin than amoxicillin	**Hypersensitivity reactions** **Nausea**, **vomiting** and **diarrhea** **Skin rashes**, urticaria, some of which are not allergic in nature (e.g., a maculopapular rash occurs > 95% of the time in patients with mononucleosis who take aminopenicillins).

Antipseudomonal penicillins

Drug	MOA & Pharmacokinetics	Clinical Uses	Side Effects
Mezlocillin (Mezlin®) Piperacillin (Pipracil®) Azlocillin (Azlin®) Carbenicillin (Geopen®) Ticarcillin (Ticar®)	Cell wall synthesis inhibitors **Destroyed** by **β-lactamases**. **Ticarcillin** is more potent than carbenicillin and is the prototype for this class.	Spectrum: gram(-) bacilli Serious *Pseudomonas* infections: in combination with aminoglycosides Other gram(-) bacilli	Decreased platelet agglutination **Eosinophilia** and leukopenia with mezlocillin and piperacillin Carbenicillin causes **hypokalemic alkalosis** and **serum transaminase elevation**. It can also induces abnormal platelet aggregation leading to a bleeding tendency

Cephalosporins

Cephalosporins are β-lactam antibiotics which are related structurally and chemically to the penicillins, however the cephalosporins show greater resistance to β-lactamases than penicillins. The majority of cephalosporins are produced synthetically and there has been an explosive growth in use of these agents in the last decade. The cephalosporins are classified largely by their antimicrobial activity and by their resistance to β-lactamases and are designated as first, second and third generation drugs. There is now a fourth generation cephalosporin (cefepime), however, it is not yet available in the United States.

First Generation	Second Generation	Third Generation
Cephalothin	Cefamandole	Ceftriaxone
Cephapirin	Cefaclor	Ceftazidime
Cephradine	Cefoxitin	Cefotaxime
Cephalexin	Cefotetan	Ceftizoxime
Cefazolin	Cefonicid	Moxalactam
Cefadroxil	Cefprozil	Cefixime
	Cefuroxime	Cefoperazone
	Cefpodoxime proxetil	

Mechanism of Resistance: similar to penicillins.

The cephalosporins are ineffective against methicillin-resistant *Staphylococcus aureus* (MRSA), *Listeria monocytogenes* and *Clostridium difficile.*

Generational Differences: as you go from 1st to 3rd generation cephalosporin, the drugs show:

1) decreased gram-positive activity
2) increased gram-negative activity
3) increased resistance to β-lactamases
4) increased CNS penetration
5) increased potency and broader spectrum of activity
6) increased cost

Probenecid (uricosuric agent) delays the tubular secretion of most cephalosporins, except moxalactam, and results in elevated plasma drug concentrations. This interaction is also observed with many penicillins.

1st Generation Cephalosporins

Drug	MOA & Pharmacokinetics	Clinical Uses	Side Effects
Cephalothin (Keflin®) Cephapirin (Cefadyl®) Cephradine (Velosef®) Cephalexin (Keflex®) Cefazolin (Ancef®) Cefadroxil (Duricef®)	Cell wall synthesis inhibitors which work in a manner similar to the penicillins. Penetrate most tissues well (except the CNS) and are therefore an excellent choice for surgical prophylaxis. Do **not** penetrate the CNS and should not be used to treat meningitis. Less expensive than 2nd or 3rd generation cephalosporins. Given PO (cefadroxil, cephalexin and cephradine) Given IV (cephalothin, cephapirin and cefazolin)	Spectrum: excellent gram(+), poor gram(-), poor anaerobic coverage **Surgical prophylaxis** (DOC) *Streptococci* infections except for some penicillin-resistant strains. **Endocarditis** due to severe *Staphylococcus aureus* infections may be treated with *cephalothin* because it is less likely to be penetrated by *staph.* β-lactamase. Note: Methicillin-resistant (MRSA) strains are **not** sensitive to the cephalosporins. Urinary tract infections due to: *E. coli, Proteus and Klebsiella.* Pneumonia due to *Klebsiella pneumoniae.* *Proteus mirabilis* (Indole-negative) Anaerobic cocci infections due to: *Peptococcus* and *Peptostreptococcus*, however, *B. fragilis* is **not** sensitive to the 1st generation cephalosporins.	**Hypersensitivity reactions** are the most common adverse side effects and may be caused all cephalosporins. It is identical to the hypersensitivity reaction caused by the penicillins. Patients who are allergic to penicillin may also be allergic to a cephalosporin (cross-reactivity). **Nephrotoxicity** with *cephalothin.* Cephalosporins are not as toxic to the kidney as the aminoglycosides, however, high doses of *cephalothin* may cause acute tubular necrosis. Positive Coombs' reaction is common at high doses of cephalosporins, however, hemolysis is rare.

2nd Generation Cephalosporins

Drug	MOA & Pharmacokinetics	Clinical Uses	Side Effects
Cefamandole (Mandol®) Cefaclor (Ceclor®) Cefoxitin (Mefoxin®) Cefotetan (Cefotan®) Cefonicid (Monocid®) Cefprozil (Cefzil®) Cefuroxime (Ceftin®) Cefpodoxime proxetil (Vantin®)	Cell wall synthesis inhibitors. Most second generation cephalosporins have limited CNS penetration, however, some may cross the blood brain barrier, when the meninges are inflamed. **Cefuroxime**, however, does not appear to require inflamed meninges to enter the CNS. **Cefpodoxime proxetil** shows decreased absorption when given with H_2 blockers or antiacids. Given PO (cefaclor, cefpodoxime, cefprozil and cefuroxime) Given IV (all others including cefuroxime)	Spectrum: increased gram(-), decreased gram(+) coverage, some anaerobes. **Sepsis** or **peritonitis** due to *B. fragilis* (anaerobic) can be treated with ***cefotetan*** and ***cefoxitin***. **Meningitis** due to *H. influenzae, Neisseria meningitidis* and *Strep. pneumoniae* is successfully treated with ***cefuroxime*** because it penetrates the CNS well. Urinary tract infections Sinusitis and otitis media Bone and soft tissue infections *Enterobacter aerogenes* *Proteus mirabilis* (Indole-positive) *E. coli* *Klebsiella pneumonia* *Serratia* nosocomial infections may be treated with *cefoxitin* or *cefotetan*.	**Hypersensitivity reactions** are the most common adverse side effects and may be caused by all cephalosporins. It is identical to the hypersensitivity reaction caused by the penicillins. Patients who are allergic to penicillin may also be allergic to a cephalosporin (cross-reactivity). **Alcohol intolerance** (disulfiram-like reaction) has been noted with *cefamandole* and *cefotetan* because they block the second step in alcohol oxidation resulting in elevated levels of acetaldehyde. **Serious bleeding** due to hypoprothrombinemia or platelet dysfunction is associated with *cefamandole* and *cefotetan*. This problem is usually seen in the elderly, poorly nourished and those with renal insufficiency. Treated with Vitamin K. Superinfection caused by gram(+) bacteria and fungi due to limited coverage of these organisms. This is more commonly seen with third generation cephalosporins.

3rd Generation Cephalosporins

Drug	MOA & Pharmacokinetics	Clinical Uses	Side Effects
Ceftriaxone (Rocephin®) Ceftazidime (Fortaz®) Cefotaxime (Claforan®) Ceftizoxime (Cefizox®) Moxalactam (Moxam®) Cefixime (Suprax®) Cefoperazone (Cefobid®)	Cell wall synthesis inhibitors All have good CNS penetration, except **cefoperazone**. Ceftriaxone and cefotaxime possess exhibit the greatest CNS penetration. Most expensive group of cephalosporins. **Ceftriaxone** has the longest $t_{1/2}$ (6-8 hrs). Given PO (cefixime), IV (all others) **Cefoperazone** and **ceftriaxone** are excreted through bile into feces.	Spectrum: broad gram(-), but decreased gram(+) coverage, moderate anaerobic and some aerobic activity. Particularly effective against: H. *influenzae*, *Neisseria gonorrhoeae* and *Enterobacter*. **Meningitis** due to: H. *influenzae*, *Neisseria meningitidis*, *Strep. pneumoniae*. *Ceftriaxone* is DOC. **Pneumonia** and **sinusitis** due to *Strep. pneumoniae.* **Gonorrhea** due to *N. gonorrhoeae.* The DOC is *ceftriaxone* with penicillinase-producing Neisseria. **Lyme disease (stage 2)** due to *Borrelia burgdorferi* is treated with *ceftriaxone.* **Chancroid** due to *H. ducreyi* **Urinary tract infections** due to *Pseudomonas aeruginosa, Proteus,* and *Klebsiella.* *Bacteroides fragilis* *Salmonella* infections *Serratia* nosocomial infections.	**Hypersensitivity reactions** are the most common adverse side effects and may be caused by all cephalosporins. It is identical to the hypersensitivity reaction caused by the penicillins. Patients who are allergic to penicillin may also be allergic to a cephalosporin (cross-reactivity). **Diarrhea**: may be more frequent with ***cefoperazone*** because of its greater biliary excretion. **Alcohol intolerance** (disulfiram-like reaction) has been noted with *moxalactam and cefoperazone.* **Serious bleeding** due to hypoprothrombinemia or platelet dysfunction is associated with ***moxalactam***, but also with *cefoperazone*. It is usually seen in the elderly, poorly nourished and those with renal insufficiency. Treated with Vitamin K. Superinfection caused by gram(+) bacteria and fungi due to limited coverage of these organisms.

Carbapenems and Monobactams

Imipenem is a carbapenem derived from *Streptococcus cattleya.* Imipenem, a β-lactam, acts identically to penicillins and cephalosporins. However, imipenem is resistant to β-lactamases, active against an extremely **broad spectrum** of bacteria and is combined with **cilastatin** to increase its plasma half-life and to prevent the formation of imipenem's nephrotoxic metabolite.

Aztreonam is a monobactam produced by *Chromobacterium violaceum.* It is extremely resistant to β-lactamases, but has a limited and **narrow spectrum** of antibacterial activity and is primarily use against aerobic gram-negative rods. *Enterobacter* and *Pseudomonas aeruginosa* are particularly susceptible, while gram-positive bacteria and anaerobes are resistant to aztreonam.

Carbapenems

Drug	MOA & Pharmacokinetics	Clinical Uses	Side Effects
Imipenem/Cilastatin (Primaxin®) Note: Imipenem is smaller than most β-lactams and can penetrate through membrane pores.	Imipenem is a cell wall synthesis inhibitor Cilastatin inhibits the enzyme dehydropeptidase in the proximal convoluted tubules. This inhibits the cleavage of imipenem which has a nephrotoxic metabolite. Good CNS and tissue penetration. Resistant to β-lactamases. Given IV, IM Excreted unmetabolized in the urine.	Spectrum: **broadest spectrum β-lactam antibiotic currently available**. Active against aerobic and anaerobic gram(+) and gram(-) organisms. Covers *P. Aeruginosa* and *B. fragilis*, but **not** methicillin-resistant *S. aureus* (MRSA).	High doses may cause **seizures** and caution is advised in those with renal insufficiency. Individuals allergic to penicillins are at high risk of also being allergic to imipenem due to cross-sensitivity. ◆ Contraindication: Epilepsy due to a decreased seizure threshold.

Monobactams

Drug	MOA & Pharmacokinetics	Clinical Uses	Side Effects
Aztreonam (Azactam®)	Cell wall synthesis inhibitor Resistant to β-lactamases. Given IV, IM	Spectrum: gram(-) aerobic rods including *P. aeruginosa* and *Serratia.* **Not** active against gram(+) bacteria or anaerobes. Resembles aminoglycosides in spectrum of activity.	Superinfections with *Streptococci* and *Enterococci* Occasional skin rashes and elevations in serum transaminases occur. Penicillin-allergic patients can tolerate aztreonam without allergic reactions.

Vancomycin

Vancomycin is a large and complex tricyclic glycopeptide antibiotic produced by *Streptomyces orientalis.* It is active against **gram-positive** bacteria, particularly *staphylococci.* Due to its large size it cannot penetrate the outer membrane of gram-negative bacteria. It is **bactericidal** and can act synergistically with aminoglycosides against certain enterococci and other gram-positive bacteria. Resistance is now relatively rare, but is a growing concern, because it is the last line of defense against some infections.

Mechanisms of Resistance:
- Plasmid mediated (Van A) especially with *enterococci* (group D streptococcus).
- Decreased binding to receptor molecules.

Drug	MOA & Pharmacokinetics	Clinical Uses	Side Effects
Vancomycin (Vancocin®)	Bactericidal cell wall inhibitor that binds to the **D-alanyl D-alanine** terminus of gram(+) cell wall precursors preventing **transpeptidation**; a step earlier than penicillin. Penetrates CNS only if the meninges are inflamed. Poorly absorbed from the GI tract and is given orally only for the treatment of antibiotic-associated enterocolitis due to *C. difficile.* Given PO for colitis, IV (slow push) Renally excreted	Spectrum: gram(+) organisms: methicillin-resistant *S. aureus* (MRSA), multidrug resistant *Staph. epidermidis* (MRSE), *Enterococcus faecalis* (group D streptococcus). **Pseudomembranous colitis** caused by *C. difficile.* The only oral indication for vancomycin. Serious gram(+) infections resistant to β-lactam antibiotics. Prophylaxis in patients with prosthetic heart valves undergoing dental procedures. Not active against gram(-) organisms.	**Hearing loss**: dose related ototoxicity and cochlear damage. **Nephrotoxicity**: potentiated by other nephrotoxic drugs such as aminoglycosides, amphotericin B and cisplatin. **Red man syndrome**: rapid IV infusion of vancomycin causes histamine release which leads to hypotension and a red pruritic rash on the patient's torso. Patients may be pre-treated with H_1-receptor antagonists and aspirin to avoid this uncomfortable but not life-threatening side effect.

Cycloserine

Cycloserine is a broad-spectrum bactericidal antibiotic produced by *Streptococcus orchidaceus*. It is an analogue of D-alanine and inhibits alanine racemase. It is an effective inhibitor of many strains of tubercle bacilli, however, due to its severe toxicity it is only used when first-line agents have failed.

Drug	MOA & Pharmacokinetics	Clinical Uses	Side Effects
Cycloserine (Seromycin®)	Structural analog of D-alanine which **antagonizes D-alanine** by inhibiting alanine racemase and preventing bacterial cell-wall synthesis. Rapidly absorbed and distributed in all tissues and fluids. It penetrates the CNS well; CSF concentrations are approximately the same as those in plasma. Toxic concentrations may accumulate in patients with renal insufficiency. Poorly metabolized and much of it is excreted unchanged in the urine. Given PO	Spectrum: gram(+), gram(-), but primarily mycobacteria **Tuberculosis**: most commonly used in combination with other tuberculostatic drugs for pulmonary and extrapulmonary Tb in patients who have failed first line medications. Note: the clinical use of cycloserine is limited because of its serious **toxicity**.	**CNS effects**: drowsiness, headache, confusion, loss of memory, hyperirritability, aggression, convulsions, tremor. Seizures induced by large doses of cycloserine or concurrent ingestion of alcohol. Drug Interactions: Isoniazid may potentiate CNS side effects. Ethanol may increase the risk of seizures. ◆ Contraindication: Epilepsy

β-Lactamase Inhibitors

Drug	MOA & Pharmacokinetics	Clinical Uses	Side Effects
Clavulanic acid Sulbactam Tazobactam Note: these agents are known as "suicide " inhibitors.	Irreversibly bind to and **inactivate β-lactamases** preventing them from destroying β-lactam antibiotics. Contain a β-lactam ring, but have little antibacterial affect when given alone. Therefore, these agents are always administered in combination with other β-lactam antibiotics. Given PO, IV	**Protect** hydrolyzable penicillins such as ampicillin, amoxicillin, ticarcillin and piperacillin from inactivation. **Extend the spectrum** of certain β-lactam agents.	Toxicity is similar to other β-lactam agents.

Protein Synthesis Inhibitors

Protein synthesis inhibitors work by targeting bacterial ribosomes. Mammalian (eukaryotic) cells have 80S ribosomes composed of 60S and 40S subunits, whereas bacteria (prokaryotic cells) have 70S ribosomes composed of 50S and 30S subunits. These differences explain how this group of drugs inhibit bacterial protein synthesis without any major effects on mammalian cells. However, the mitochondria found in mammalian cells are susceptible to some of these agents such as chloramphenicol and tetracycline because they contain ribosomes which resemble those found in bacterial.

Aminoglycosides	Tetracyclines	Chloramphenicol	Macrolides	Lincosamides
Streptomycin Gentamicin Tobramycin Amikacin Netilmicin Neomycin Kanamycin	Tetracycline Doxycycline Minocycline Demeclocycline Oxytetracycline	Chloramphenicol	Erythromycin Clarithromycin Azithromycin	Clindamycin Lincomycin

The protein synthesis inhibitors listed above work on different ribosomal subunits within bacteria and vary in their bactericidal and bacteriostatic nature.

30S Inhibitors:
Aminoglycosides are bactericidal.
Tetracyclines are bacteriostatic.

50S Inhibitors:
Chloramphenicol is bacteriostatic.
Macrolides are bacteriostatic, however, at high doses erythromycin can be bactericidal.
Lincosamides are bacteriostatic.

Aminoglycosides

Aminoglycosides are a group of **bactericidal** drugs which **inhibit protein synthesis**. The search for antibacterial substances was prompted by the discovery of penicillin, and in 1943 the aminoglycosides were obtained from various *Streptomyces* species. They contain amino sugars linked to an aminocyclitol ring by glycosidic bonds and are more active at alkaline than at acid pH. All aminoglycosides bind irreversibly to the **30S** ribosomal subunit and interfere with protein synthesis in susceptible bacteria. They are highly **polar** compounds and their uptake is often facilitated by concurrent use with cell wall inhibitors such as β-lactams and vancomycin. A disadvantage of aminoglycosides is the development of multiple types of resistance.

The aminoglycosides remain important agents, and are used to treat infections caused by severe **aerobic gram-negative** bacteria, however, due to their highly **toxic** effects, their use is now more restricted. Some of their former indications have been replaced by safer agents such as cephalosporins, fluoroquinolones and imipenem/cilastatin. Most all aminoglycosides are given parenterally because they are poorly absorbed when administered orally. They do **not** cover anaerobes because **oxidative metabolism** is required for their uptake.

Mechanisms of Resistance:

- Plasmid-mediated synthesis of aminoglycoside-inactivating enzymes such as acetyltransferase, nucleotidyltransferase and phosphotransferase which modify and inactivate these drugs. Amikacin and netilmicin are less vulnerable to these enzymes.
- Changes in the 30S ribosomal subunit resulting in decreased affinity between the drug and 30S subunit.
- Decreased membrane permeability: transport of aminoglycosides across the cytoplasmic membrane is an oxygen-dependent, active process. Anaerobic, hyperosmolar and/or a low pH environment would effectively block the active transport process required for aminoglycosides to enter the cytoplasm.

Drug	MOA & Pharmacokinetics	Clinical Uses	Side Effects
Streptomycin Note: streptomycin, as well as the other aminoglycosides are frequently used in combination with other antibiotics, particularly the penicillins and cephalosporins.	**Bactericidal** agent which inhibits protein synthesis by binding irreversibly to the **30S** ribosomal subunit. Crosses the outer membrane and enters the periplasmic space of gram(-) bacteria by diffusing through aqueous channels formed by porin proteins. Crosses the inner cytoplasmic membrane by an **oxygen-dependent active transport** system which is inactivated by cations (Ca^{2+}, Mg^{2+}), low pH and anaerobic conditions. Poor CNS penetration. Highly polar compound which is poorly absorbed in the GI tract. Given IV, IM, IT	Spectrum: aerobic gram(-) bacilli, some gram(+) and mycobacteria. **Tuberculosis**: due to *M. tuberculosis* in combination with other first-line agents **Bubonic plague** due to *Yersinia pestis* Bacterial endocarditis caused by *enterococci* (group D streptococci) and oral *Strep. viridans*: in combination with penicillin G. Tularemia due to *Francisella tularensis* Brucellosis due to *Brucella* species	**Ototoxicity**: may be irreversible. Patients taking loop diuretics are at higher risk. **Nephrotoxicity**: usually reversible. Neuromuscular blockade: patients with myasthenia gravis are particularly at risk. Allergic skin reactions: most common with neomycin
Gentamicin (Garamycin®) Tobramycin (Nebcin®) Amikacin (Amikin®) Netilmicin (Netromycin®)	Similar MOA to streptomycin. **Amikacin** has a broad spectrum of activity and has a unique resistance to the inactivating enzymes. Given IV, IM, topically (gentamicin)	**Pneumonia** caused by *Pseudomonas aeruginosa* **Urinary tract infections** due to *E. coli, Enterobacter, Proteus, Klebsiella* and *Pseudomonas* Bacterial endocarditis caused by *enterococci* (group D streptococci) and oral *Strep. viridans*: in combination with penicillin G.	
Neomycin (Mycifradin®) Kanamycin (Kantrex®)	Similar MOA to streptomycin. **Neomycin** has a broad spectrum of activity. Given PO, topically	**Bowel sterilization** in preparation for surgery: neomycin in combination with erythromycin. Skin infections with *Staph. aureus* Hepatic coma adjunctive therapy	

Tetracyclines

The **tetracyclines** are a large group of related agents which consist of four fused rings possessing one to two conjugated double bonds. They are the prototypical broad-spectrum antimicrobial drugs which are effective against both **aerobic** and **anaerobic** gram-positive and gram-negative bacteria, as well as, **rickettsiae**, **mycoplasmas** and **chlamydiae**. They can cross the placenta, however, they have poor CNS penetration. Due to the emergence of resistance in the last decade their effectiveness against some organisms has declined.

Mechanisms of Resistance:

Microorganisms often exhibit cross-resistance to the tetracyclines. Resistance usually results from acquisition of an **R-factor** which may code for the following:

- Active efflux mechanism that pumps drug out of the microorganism.
- Loss of cytoplasmic transport proteins which are required for entry into susceptible organisms.
- Changes in membrane permeability to the drug.

Drug	MOA & Pharmacokinetics	Clinical Uses	Side Effects
Tetracycline (Achromycin®) Doxycycline (Vibramycin®) Minocycline (Minocin®) Demeclocycline (Declomycin®) Oxytetracycline (Terramycin®)	Bacteriostatic agents which bind to the **30S** ribosomal subunit and block binding of **aminoacyl-tRNA** to the acceptor (A) site on the mRNA-ribosomal complex. Absorption is severely impaired by food, milk, Ca^{2+}, Mg^{2+}, Al^{3+} and Fe^{2+} salts. This absorption interaction is less common with **doxycycline**. **Minocycline** can penetrate the CNS. Given PO (demeclocycline and oxytetracycline), all others are given PO, IV. Tetracycline undergoes renal excretion. **Doxycycline** is excreted in the stool.	Spectrum: broad; aerobic and anaerobic gram(+) and gram(-) bacteria. **Rickettsial diseases** including: Rocky Mountain Spotted Fever, Q-Fever and typhus infections. **Chlamydial diseases** including: lymphogranuloma venereum, trachoma, pneumonia and psittacosis. **Pneumonia** due to *Mycoplasma pneumoniae* and *Ureaplasma* **Lyme disease** due to *Borrelia* Amebiasis due to *Entamoeba histolytica* Acne and rosacea Cholera due to *Vibrio cholera* Brucellosis due to *Brucella* Tularemia due to *Francisella* Meningococcal meningitis prophylaxis with **minocycline**.	**GI irritation**: epigastic burning, nausea, vomiting and diarrhea. **Tooth** and **bone discoloration** **Pseudo tumor cerebri** (benign intra-cranial hypertension). Photosensitivity and onycholysis with doxycycline, demeclocycline. **Hepatic toxicity** resulting in jaundice, azotemia, acidosis, shock. **Renal toxicity**: azotemia and possibly **Fanconi syndrome** with ingestion of outdated drug **Vestibular problems**: vertigo and dizziness with minocycline. ◆ Contraindications: **Children ≤ 8 yrs old** due to tooth and bone discoloration. **Pregnant** or lactating women due to **teratogenic** effects.

Chloramphenicol

Chloramphenicol is a broad spectrum antibiotic which was first isolated from cultures of *Streptomyces venezuelae* in 1947. It is a unique natural compound which contains a nitrobenzene nucleus. Chloramphenicol **inhibits protein synthesis** in bacteria by binding to the **50S** ribosomal subunit, but may also interfere with mitochondrial protein synthesis in mammalian bone marrow cells. It remains an important drug for life-threatening infections such as meningitis, typhoid fever and some rickettsial diseases, however, because of its potential to cause **anemia** it is **not** a first-line agent.

Mechanisms of Resistance: resistance of gram-negative bacteria to this drug is usually caused by a plasmid acquired by conjugation which may code for the following:

- R-factors coding for Acetyl-CoA transferase, which inactivates chloramphenicol.
- Decreased ability to penetrate the organism.

Drug	MOA & Pharmacokinetics	Clinical Uses	Side Effects
Chloramphenicol (Chloromycetin®) Note: Chloramphenicol is often used in conjunction with other antibiotics such as the penicillins, however, it competitively inhibits macrolides and clindamycin because they bind the 50S ribosomal subunit in a similar location.	Bacteriostatic agent which binds **reversibly** to the **50S** ribosomal subunit preventing the action of **peptidyl transferase** which is necessary to synthesis new peptide bonds and chain elongation. Irreversibly inhibits $\mathbf{P_{450}}$ enzymes which may prolong the life of other drugs. **Hepatic failure** may lead to chloramphenicol toxicity but renal failure is not as significant because the glucuronide metabolite is non-toxic. Penetrates the CNS well Given PO, IV	Spectrum: broad; anaerobic and aerobic gram(+) and gram(-) bacteria. **Typhoid fever** due to *Salmonella typhi* **Bacterial meningitis** due to *H. influenzae*, as well as, *Neisseria meningitidis* and *Strep. pneumoniae* in those allergic to β-lactams. **Rickettsial** diseases in children and pregnant women since tetracycline is contraindicated in these patients. **Psittacosis** due to *Chlamydia psittaci* Anaerobic infections due to: *Bacteroides*, as well as, brain abscesses, abdomen, pelvic and bowel infections. Brucellosis due to *Brucella* when tetracycline is contraindicated.	**Anemia** due to toxic effect on bone marrow resulting in aplastic anemia (not dose-related), and hemolytic anemia in patients with Glucose-6-phosphate dehydrogenase (G6PD) deficiency. **Gray Baby Syndrome**: observed as cyanosis, vomiting, green stools and vasomotor collapse (40% fatal). It is caused by the accumulation of unmetabolized drug, since the neonatal liver has yet to synthesize sufficient **glucuronidase** enzymes to detoxify many drugs. Nausea, vomiting, diarrhea and perineal irritation. Drug Interactions: Increases levels of drugs metabolized by the P_{450} system.

Macrolides

The **macrolides** are a group of closely related compounds characterized by a macrocyclic lactone ring to which sugars are attached. The prototype drug, erythromycin, was obtained in 1952 from *Streptomyces erythreus*. Clarithromycin and azithromycin are newer derivatives of erythromycin.

Mechanisms of Resistance:

- Plasmids coding for specific enzymes (erythromycin esterases) which inactive these drugs.
- Methylation of an adenine residue on the 23S rRNA binding site leads to decreased affinity for the 50S ribosomal subunit (the target binding site for the macrolides).
- Defective uptake of the drug by the microbe.

Macrolides

Drug	MOA & Pharmacokinetics	Clinical Uses	Side Effects
Erythromycin Base (E-Mycin®), Estolate (Ilosone®), Ethyl succinate (EES®) Lactobionate **Clarithromycin** (Biaxin®) **Azithromycin** (Zithromax®)	Bacteriostatic inhibitor of protein synthesis which binds reversibly to the 23S rRNA of the **50S** ribosomal subunit and interferes with translocation. Poor CNS penetration. Active against **intracellular organisms**: can enter macrophages, neutrophils and fibroblasts. **Inhibit P_{450}** enzymes. **Clarithromycin** is metabolized to a 14-OH metabolite that has greater activity against *H. influenzae* than the parent compound. **Azithromycin** is eliminated slowly with a $t_{1/2}$ of 2-4 days. The others are eliminated rapidly ($t_{1/2}$ = 2-4 hrs). Given PO, IV	Spectrum: aerobic gram(+) cocci and bacilli. **Pneumonia** due to *Mycoplasma pneumoniae* **Legionnaires' disease** due to *Legionella pneumophila* **Pertussis** (whooping cough) due to *Bordetella pertussis* **Diphtheria** due to *Corynebacterium diphtheriae* Pneumonia and urogenital infections caused by *Chlamydia* Atypical mycobacterial infections especially in AIDS patients; treat with clarithromycin. Chancroid due to *H. ducreyi* Urethritis due to *Ureaplasma urealyticum.* Tetanus due to *Clostridium tetani* in penicillin-allergic patients Gastroenteritis due to *Campylobacter jejuni*	**GI effects**: nausea, vomiting, diarrhea **Cholestatic hepatitis** Drug Interactions: Chloramphenicol binds to the same site as erythromycin and may decrease activity when given together. Digoxin: macrolides kill the gut bacteria needed for the metabolism of digoxin. Increases levels of drugs metabolized by the P_{450} system. ◆ Contraindication: Erythromycin is contraindicated in patients with hepatic dysfunction.

Lincosamides

Lincomycin is the original compound elaborated by *Streptomyces lincolnensis*, but it is rarely used today. **Clindamycin** is a chlorine-substituted congener of lincomycin, but is more potent and shares a similar activity with erythromycin. It is used effectively against **anaerobic** bacteria such as ***B. fragilis***, but is also indicated for many aerobic gram-positive cocci, as well as, *Chlamydia, Pneumocystis,* and *Toxoplasma.* It has little or no effect against aerobic gram-negative bacilli; *Enterococci, Haemophilus* and *Mycoplasma* are often resistant (in contrast to erythromycin). The lincosamides **inhibit protein synthesis** by binding to the **50S** ribosomal subunit which is significant because chloramphenicol and erythromycin also bind to this site, despite their unrelated structures, resulting in competitive inhibition when used concurrently.

Mechanisms of Resistance:

- Methylation of an adenine residue on the 23S rRNA ribosomal binding site leading to decreased affinity for the 50S ribosomal subunit (the target site for clindamycin).
- Defective uptake of the drug by the microbe.

Drug	MOA & Pharmacokinetics	Clinical Uses	Side Effects
Lincomycin (Lincocin®) Clindamycin (Cleocin®)	Bacteriostatic agents which bind to the **50S** ribosomal subunit and inhibit protein synthesis by interfering with translocation (similar to erythromycin). **Lincomycin** penetrates bone. Poor CNS penetration Given PO, IV, IM, topically	<u>Spectrum</u>: few clinical uses; aerobic gram(+) cocci, anaerobes **Anaerobic infections** including *B. fragilis, Clostridium* species (**not** *C. perfringens*) Acne due to *Acne vulgaris* Encephalitis due to *Toxoplasma gondii*: clindamycin in conjunction with pyrimethamine Pneumonia due to *Pneumocystis carinii* (PCP) in AIDS patients. Gram(+) organisms (e.g., *Staph, Strep.*) in patients with severe allergies to penicillins. **No** activity against most gram(-) organisms.	**Pseudomembranous colitis**: lincosamides destroy the normal intestinal flora which allows *C. difficile* to grow and secrete its toxin, causing a bloody diarrhea. Treatment includes oral vancomycin or metronidazole. *C. difficile* is usually resistant to clindamycin. Diarrhea, nausea Skin rashes Erythema multiforme Granulocytopenia and thrombocytopenia Inhibition of neuromuscular transmission

Nucleic Acid Synthesis and Replication Inhibitors

The nucleic acid synthesis and replication inhibitors are a bactericidal broad spectrum group of antibiotics which have many therapeutic uses without many side effects. The **quinolones** such as nalidixic acid were used for many years in the treatment of urinary tract infections, however, due to the rapid development of resistance, these agents have limited use today. The newer members of this class of synthetic agents, the **fluoroquinolones**, are of great therapeutic value and are slow to develop resistance.

Rifampin is a bactericidal drug that inhibits RNA synthesis in prokaryotic microorganisms. It is primarily used against intracellular and extracellular mycobacteria including *M. tuberculosis* and *M. leprae*, as well as prophylactically against meningitis from *N. meningitidis* and *H. influenzae*. When used alone resistance develops quickly; therefore rifampin is usually administered in combination with other antibiotics.

Fluoroquinolones	Rifampin
Ciprofloxacin Ofloxacin Norfloxacin	Rifampin

Fluoroquinolones

The **fluoroquinolones** are a group of bactericidal, synthetic, fluorinated analogues of nalidixic acid. They inhibit **DNA gyrase** which is important for DNA replication and transcription. A similar enzyme, DNA topoisomerase II is present in eukaryotic cells. The quinolones and fluoroquinolones may inhibit eukaryotic DNA topoisomerase II at high concentrations.

Mechanisms of Resistance: resistance to the fluoroquinolones is slow to develop, but can occur by:
- Modifications of DNA gyrase decreasing the affinity for the fluoroquinolones.
- Decreased accumulation in the bacterial cell due to reduction of the porin proteins in the outer membrane or by the energy-dependent efflux system of the inner membrane.

Drug	MOA & Pharmacokinetics	Clinical Uses	Side Effects
Ciprofloxacin (Cipro®) Ofloxacin (Floxin®) Norfloxacin (Noroxin®)	Bactericidal agents which prevent the replication of bacterial DNA by inhibiting **DNA gyrase**. **Ciprofloxacin** and **ofloxacin** have excellent tissue penetration and are used for systemic infections. **Norfloxacin** is found in high levels in the urine, however, serum levels are low. Thus norfloxacin is not used for systemic infections. Poor CNS penetration, however, ofloxacin may enter the CNS well enough to treat infections. Given PO, IV; norfloxacin only PO.	Spectrum: broad; aerobic gram(+), gram(-) bacteria, but **not** anaerobes. **Urinary tract infections** due to *Pseudomonas, Klebsiella, Proteus* **Sexually transmitted diseases**: gonorrhea, chlamydia and chancroid **Prostatitis** **Respiratory infections** caused by *H. influenzae, M. catarrhalis, Strep. pneumoniae* and *M. pneumoniae* **Nosocomial infections** due to *Pseudomonas aeruginosa* **GI. infections** due to *E. coli, vibrio, Shigella, salmonella* and *C. jejuni* **Chronic bone infections** due to *Pseudomonas* and *Staph. aureus* Diabetic foot infections	Generally well tolerated Nausea, dizziness and headaches **Arthralgias** and joint swelling when given to children. May cause cartilage damage and arrest of growth plates. Rashes including photosensitivity Drug Interactions: Fluoroquinolone absorption is reduced when ingested with Mg^{2+}, Al^{3+}, and Fe^{3+} salts in antiacids or supplements. ◆ Contraindications: Pregnant women Neonates

Rifampin

Rifampin is a synthetic derivative of the soil mold *Streptomyces rifampin* or *mediterranei*. It is a **bactericidal** agent which blocks prokaryotic transcription by **inhibiting RNA synthesis**. It binds to the β-subunit of **DNA-dependent RNA polymerase** resulting in suppression of the initiation step of RNA synthesis. When used alone resistance develops quickly; therefore rifampin is usually administered in combination with other antibiotics.

Mechanisms of Resistance:

- Modifications of **DNA dependent RNA polymerase** decreasing the affinity for rifampin.
- Decreased permeability to the drug.

Drug	MOA & Pharmacokinetics	Clinical Uses	Side Effects
Rifampin (Rifadin®, Rimactane®) Note: due to the rapid development of resistance, rifampin is always used in combination with other antibiotics.	**Inhibits DNA-dependent RNA polymerase** by blocking the β-subunit and suppressing chain initiation in RNA synthesis. Penetrates into all fluids and tissues including the CNS. Metabolized by and induces the P_{450} system. Taken up by the liver and undergoes enterohepatic circulation. Given PO	Spectrum: gram(+) and gram(-) bacteria. **Tuberculosis**: **DOC** in combination with isoniazid **Meningitis, prophylaxis** DOC, caused by *N. meningitidis* and *H. influenzae* Endocarditis and osteomyelitis caused by staphylococcus. Treat with rifampin plus a β-lactam antibiotic or vancomycin. **Leprosy** due to *M. leprae*. Treat with dapsone plus rifampin. Methicillin-resistant *S. aureus* (MRSA) infections when combined with other antibiotics Legionnaires' disease due to *Legionella pneumophila*. Treat with erythromycin plus rifampin.	Generally well tolerated **Red-orange** colored secretions: sweat, tears, saliva, urine and feces Rash, fever, nausea and vomiting Hepatitis may occur in patients with chronic liver disease, old age or those suffering from alcoholism. **Flu-like syndrome** with fever, chills and myalgias in patients who use rifampin intermittently. May lead to eosinophilia, interstitial nephritis, tubular necrosis and anemia. Drug Interactions: Decreases the level of drugs metabolized by the P_{450} system

Figure 5.3: Action of metabolic inhibitors.

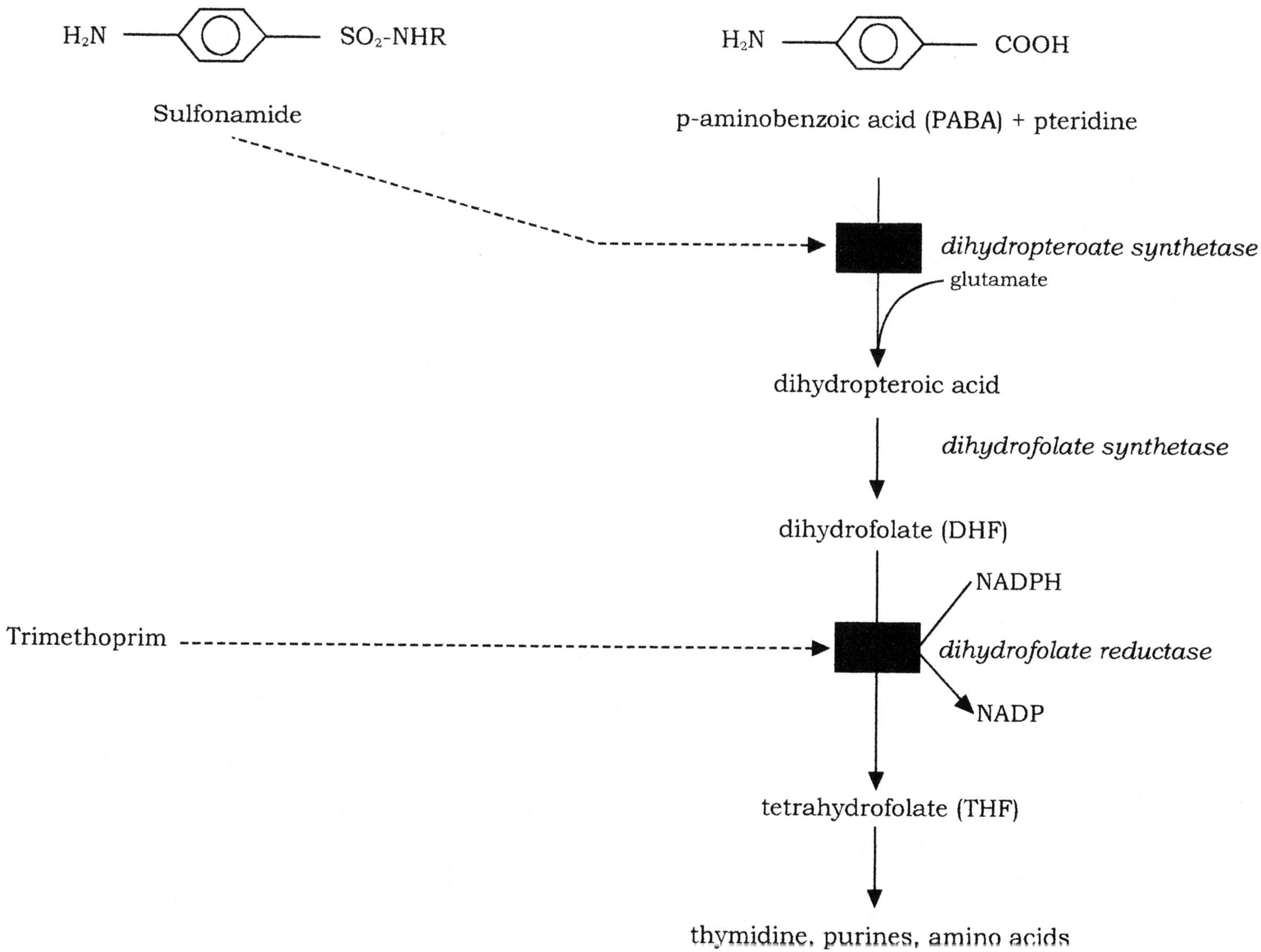

Metabolic Inhibitors

The **metabolic inhibitors** are bacteriostatic agents that **inhibit folic acid coenzymes**. These enzymes, dihydropteroate synthase and dihydrofolate reductase are required for the formation of purines and pyrimidines which are the precursors of RNA, DNA and other compounds necessary for bacterial growth and replication. Bacterial cells make folic acid endogenously to form nucleotides, whereas mammalian cells must rely on external supplies of folic acid and are therefore unaffected by these agents.

The **sulfonamides** were first discovered in 1932 from the azo dye, *prontosil*. They inhibit **dihydropteroate synthetase** and were the first antibacterial drugs to be used systemically. However, due to the emergence of resistant strains and the advent of penicillins in the 1940s, the use of sulfonamides declined. It was not until the 1970s that their use, in combination with trimethoprim, was revitalized.

Trimethoprim is a potent inhibitor of **dihydrofolate reductase** and has an antibacterial spectrum similar to that of the sulfonamides, however, trimethoprim is approximately 20 to 100 times more potent than the sulfonamides. Trimethoprim is most commonly combined with sulfamethoxazole (co-trimoxazole) providing greater antimicrobial activity and decreased resistance than either agent used alone. Co-trimoxazole is bactericidal to some organisms.

Mechanisms of resistance:

Cross resistance may occur and resistance factors are often encoded on plasmids.

- Increased concentration of PABA thereby overwhelming the drug's competitive inhibition.
- Modification of the folic acid coenzyme leading to decreased affinity of the drug for the enzyme.
- Decreased uptake of the drug into the microbial cells.

Sulfonamides	Trimethoprim
Sulfisoxazole Sulfamethoxazole Sulfadiazine Sulfamethizole Sulfasalazine Sulfadoxine Sulfacetamide Silver sulfadiazine Mafenide	Trimethoprim Trimethoprim/Sulfamethoxazole

Sulfonamides

The sulfonamides are listed below with the shortest acting drugs first.
In addition there is a separate group of sulfonamides which have important clinical indications when given topically.

Drug	MOA & Pharmacokinetics	Clinical Uses	Side Effects
Sulfisoxazole (Gantrisin®) Sulfamethoxazole (Gantanol®) Sulfadiazine Sulfamethizole (Proklar®, Thiosulfil®) Sulfasalazine (Azaline®) Sulfadoxine Note: sulfonamides are commonly used in conjunction with other antibiotics, especially **trimethoprim** and **pyrimethamine**.	Bacteriostatic agents which are competitive antagonists of **dihydropteroate synthase**, the enzyme responsible for incorporating para-aminobenzoic acid (PABA) into dihydropteroic acid, the precursor to **folic acid**. Mammalian cells do **not** make folic acid and are not affected. **Cross the placenta** and secreted in breast milk and should not be given to pregnant women. Highly bound to plasma proteins, especially **albumin**. Penetrate the CNS well Because the sulfonamides have solubility limitations, three of them may be combined to reduce precipitation. This combination is known as a **triple sulfa**. Given PO, IV (occasionally)	Spectrum: gram(+), gram(-) **Toxoplasmosis** due to *Toxoplasma gondii* in combination with pyrimethamine. **Ulcerative colitis**, enteritis and granulomatous colitis is best treated with sulfasalazine (most poorly absorbed sulfonamide). **Urinary tract infections** due to *E. coli* and *Klebsiella*, but not *Pseudomonas* Nocardiosis due to *Nocardia*. Chlamydial infections Chancroid due to *H. ducreyi* Malaria due to *Plasmodium falciparum*; treated with the longest acting sulfonamide, sulfadoxine-pyrimethamine.	**Hypersensitivity reactions**: rashes, Steven-Johnson syndrome, skin eruptions and ulcers **Photosensitivity** **GI effects**: nausea, vomiting Hematopoietic disorders: hemolytic anemia may occur in individuals with glucose-6-phosphate dehydrogenase (G6PD) deficiency. Crystalluria and nephrotoxicity with less soluble sulfonamides. Treatment includes adequate hydration and urine alkalization. **Kernicterus** in newborns due to displaced bilirubin from binding sites on albumin. The free bilirubin can then enter the CNS. ◆ Contraindications: Pregnancy Newborns ≤ 2 months old
Sulfacetamide (Isoptocetamide®) Silver sulfadiazine (Silvadene®) Mafenide (Sulfamylon®)	Sulfacetamide penetrates ocular tissues and fluids at high concentrations. Given **topically**	**Ocular infections** due to *Chlamydia trachomatis*: sulfacetamide **Burn infections** due to bacteria and fungi: silver sulfadiazine or mafenide.	Pain upon application, urine alkalization and metabolic acidosis has restricted the use of **mafenide**.

Trimethoprim

Drug	MOA & Pharmacokinetics	Clinical Uses	Side Effects
Trimethoprim (Trimpex®, Proloprim®) Note: trimethoprim is most commonly combined with sulfamethoxazole (below).	Bacteriostatic agent which inhibits **dihydrofolate reductase**. More lipid soluble and greater distribution than sulfonamides. Found in high concentrations in prostatic and vaginal fluids. Given PO	Spectrum: similar to sulfa drugs, gram(+), gram(-). Acute urinary tract infections Bacterial prostatitis	Folate deficiency problems including: anemia, leukopenia and granulocytopenia
Trimethoprim/ Sulfamethoxazole (Bactrim®, Septra®) Also known as co-trimoxazole and TMP-SMX. Advantages of this combination: • Increased potency • Increased spectrum • Decreased incidence of resistance	Synergistically active antimicrobial agent which blocks two sequential steps in the obligate enzymatic reaction in bacteria preventing the formation of nucleotides. **Sulfamethoxazole** competitively inhibits the incorporation of PABA into folic acid and **trimethoprim** inhibits dihydrofolate reductase preventing the reduction of dihydrofolate to tetrahydrofolate. Exhibits selective toxicity because mammalian cells utilize dietary folate while bacteria must synthesize their own folic acid. Trimethoprim is more potent, more lipid soluble and has a greater volume of distribution than the sulfa drugs. Penetrates the CNS well. Given PO, IV in a 1:5 ratio (1 part trimethoprim to 5 parts sulfa drug).	Spectrum: broad; gram(+) and gram(-) bacteria. **Urinary tract infections** both chronic and recurrent due to *E. coli, Proteus* and *Klebsiella.* **Pneumonia** due to *Pneumocystis carinii*: DOC in patients with AIDS **Gonorrhea** and **bacterial prostatitis** **Acute chronic bronchitis** due to *H. influenza* and *Strep. pneumoniae* **Acute otitis media** in children and acute maxillary sinusitis in adults due to *H. influenza* and *Strep. pneumoniae* Chancroid due to *H. ducreyi* Shigellosis due to *Shigella* Typhoid fever due to *Salmonella* Nocardiosis due to *Nocardia*	**Dermatologic effects** **GI effects**: glossitis, stomatitis, nausea, vomiting Headache, depression and hallucinations Hematologic reactions including aplastic, hemolytic and macrocytic anemia, coagulation disorders. Renal impairment in patients with renal disease. AIDS patients are more sensitive to developing rashes and/or hematological effects.

Notes

Antimycobacterial Drugs

Tuberculosis is caused by *Mycobacterium tuberculosis*. It is a devastating and often fatal disease affecting almost every tissue or organ of the body, however, the lungs are the most commonly affected. In the 1960s it was thought that the disease would be completely eradicated in the United States by the year 2000. However, the past decade has shown a significant increase in the number of cases. This resurgence in tuberculosis has been witnessed primarily in AIDS patients and in the homeless. Tuberculosis is a difficult disease to treat because the infections are often chronic and the organism is frequently **intracellular** and has the ability to develop resistance to most single agent therapies. Today, tuberculosis is treated with multiple drug regimes to delay resistance, however, it remains the leading cause of death from infectious disease worldwide.

First-line agents: rifampin, isoniazid, pyrazinamide, ethambutol and streptomycin.

Drug	MOA & Pharmacokinetics	Clinical Uses	Side Effects
Rifampin (Rifadin®, Rimactane®) Note: due to the rapid development of resistance, rifampin is always used in combination with other antibiotics.	**Inhibits DNA-dependent RNA polymerase** by blocking the β-subunit and suppressing chain initiation in RNA synthesis. Penetrates into all fluids and tissues including the CNS. Metabolized by and induces the P_{450} system. Taken up by the liver and undergoes enterohepatic circulation. Given PO	Spectrum: gram(+) and gram(-) bacteria. **Tuberculosis**: **DOC** in combination with isoniazid **Meningitis**, **prophylaxis** DOC, caused by *N. meningitidis* and *H. influenzae* Endocarditis and osteomyelitis caused by staphylococcus. Treat with rifampin plus a β-lactam antibiotic or vancomycin. **Leprosy** due to *M. leprae*. Treat with dapsone plus rifampin. Methicillin-resistant *S. aureus* (MRSA) infections when combined with other antibiotics Legionnaires' disease due to *Legionella pneumophila*. Treat with erythromycin plus rifampin.	Generally well tolerated **Red-orange** colored secretions: sweat, tears, saliva, urine and feces Rash, fever, nausea and vomiting Hepatitis may occur in patients with chronic liver disease, old age or those suffering from alcoholism. **Flu-like syndrome** with fever, chills and myalgias in patients who use rifampin intermittently. May lead to eosinophilia, interstitial nephritis, tubular necrosis and anemia. Drug Interactions: Decreases the level of drugs metabolized by the P_{450} system

Drug	MOA & Pharmacokinetics	Clinical Uses	Side Effects
Isoniazid (INH) (Laniazid®) Note: INH is the only agent used as a solo prophylactic agent against Tb and remains the most important antimycobacterial agent against Tb worldwide.	The mechanism is unknown, but thought to involve the **inhibition of mycolic acids synthesis**. Mycolic acids are necessary for the cell wall. Diffuses easily into all fluids and tissues including the CNS. It penetrates caseous material. Crosses the placenta and may cause peripheral neuritis in newborns. Although it can by used alone for prophylaxis, it is primarily used in conjunction with at least one other first-line agent. Metabolized in the liver by acetylation; the rate of which shows genetic heterogenicity among humans. Given PO, IV	**Tuberculosis** due to *M. tuberculosis*. Administered with at least one other first-line agent to which the bacteria is sensitive. Prophylaxis for tuberculosis when used alone. *M. kansasii* in combination with other first-line agents Note: the standard treatment includes isoniazid, rifampin and pyrazinamide for 2 months followed by isoniazid and rifampin for 4 more months. Patients with HIV typically receive more intense treatment consisting of a four-drug regimen involving isoniazid, rifampin, pyrazinamide and ethambutol or streptomycin.	**Peripheral neuritis** thought to be caused by pyridoxine (Vit B6) deficiency. **Hepatotoxicity**: jaundice and hepatitis; thought to be caused by isoniazid's monoacetylhydrazine metabolite. Hypersensitivity reactions: rashes, skin eruptions, and fevers. May precipitate convulsions in patients with seizures disorders. Hematologic reactions: anemia, eosinophilia, thrombocytopenia. Hemolytic anemia in patients with glucose-6-phosphate dehydrogenase deficiency.

Drug	MOA & Pharmacokinetics	Clinical Uses	Side Effects
Pyrazinamide (Pyrazinamide®)	Unknown MOA Penetrates the CNS Given PO Hepatic metabolism	**Tuberculosis** due to *M. Tuberculosis* in combination with other first-line agents.	**Hepatotoxicity** **Gout** due to inhibition of uric acid secretion leading to hyperuricemia. Arthralgia
Ethambutol (Myambutol®)	Unknown MOA Only first-line drug that is **bacteriostatic**. Penetrates the CNS. Given PO	**Tuberculosis** due to *M. tuberculosis* combined with other first-line agents. Other mycobacterial species including *M. avium* and *M. kansasii.*	**Optic neuritis**: blurred vision, eye pain, color vision loss or any loss of vision. **Gout** due to inhibition of uric acid secretion leading to hyperuricemia. Arthralgia
Streptomycin Note: streptomycin, as well as the other aminoglycosides are frequently used in combination with other antibiotics, particularly the penicillins and cephalosporins.	**Bactericidal** agent which inhibits protein synthesis by binding irreversibly to the **30S** ribosomal subunit. Crosses the outer membrane and enters the periplasmic space of gram(-) bacteria by diffusing through aqueous channels formed by porin proteins. Crosses the inner cytoplasmic membrane by an **oxygen-dependent active transport** system which is inactivated by cations (Ca^{2+}, Mg^{2+}), low pH and anaerobic conditions. Poor CNS penetration. Highly polar compound which is poorly absorbed in the GI tract. Given IV, IM, IT	Spectrum: aerobic gram(-) bacilli, some gram(+) and mycobacteria. **Tuberculosis**: due to *M. tuberculosis* in combination with other first-line agents **Bubonic plague** due to *Yersinia pestis* Bacterial endocarditis caused by *enterococci* (group D streptococci) and oral *Strep. viridans*: in combination with penicillin G. Tularemia due to *Francisella tularensis* Brucellosis due to *Brucella* species	**Ototoxicity**: may be irreversible. Patients taking loop diuretics are at higher risk. **Nephrotoxicity**: usually reversible. Neuromuscular blockade: patients with myasthenia gravis are particularly at risk. Allergic skin reactions: most common with neomycin

Notes

Antifungal Drugs

Fungi are single-celled **eukaryotes** that can cause infections known as **mycoses**. They have cell walls comprised of polysaccharides and **chitin** and cell membranes containing **ergosterol** rather than cholesterol found in mammalian plasma membranes. Most antifungal agents, therefore, target ergosterol to destroy the mycotic cell membrane or to inhibit its synthesis.

The polyenes, amphotericin-B and nystatin, are fungicidal because they bind ergosterol and punch holes in the cell membrane. Amphotericin-B is currently the most effective agent against severe systemic mycoses, however, it is difficult to administer and often causes terrible side effects. The antifungal azoles are fungistatic and inhibit the P_{450} enzymes needed for the synthesis of ergosterol. Flucytosine can be used orally for some systemic infections and is often administered concurrently with amphotericin-B. Griseofulvin inhibits mitosis by binding tubulin and is commonly used against dermatophytic infections.

Many mycotic infections involve superficial or subcutaneous layers of the skin, but other more serious fungal infections are systemic mycoses which often become life-threatening. Mycotic infections, in general, are difficult to treat successfully and often run a chronic course. One of the problems in treating fungal infections is that they are eukaryotic and are resistant to the action of standard antibacterial agents. As a result, many of the drugs available to treat mycotic infections, especially system mycoses, have toxic effects which are the primary disadvantages in their use.

Polyenes	Azoles	Miscellaneous
Amphotericin B Nystatin	Ketoconazole Fluconazole Itraconazole Miconazole Clotrimazole	Flucytosine Griseofulvin

Polyene Antifungal Drugs

Drug	MOA & Pharmacokinetics	Clinical Uses	Side Effects
Amphotericin-B (Fungizone®)	Binds ergosterol and punches holes in cell membranes. This increases fungal cell membrane permeability which results in cell death via osmotic disruption. **Basis for selectivity**: affinity for ergosterol, a component of fungal plasma membranes, is greater than that for cholesterol (a component of mammalian plasma membranes). **Fungicidal** Does not cross blood brain barrier, therefore must be given intrathecally to reach the CSF. Given IV, IT	Severe systemic fungal infections: **Aspergillosis** **Blastomycosis** **Systemic candidiasis** **Coccidioidomycosis** **Cryptococcosis** **Histoplasmosis** Cryptococcal meningitis: in combination with flucytosine Sporotrichosis Leishmaniasis Sporotrichosis Mucormycosis	**Acute febrile reactions**: 25% of patients experience fever, chills and vomiting with infusion. **Nephrotoxicity** Hypokalemia which may lead to muscle weakness, muscle aches and cardiac arrhythmias. Anemia
Nystatin (Mycostatin®)	Binds ergosterol and punches holes in cell membranes. This increases fungal cell membrane permeability which results in cell death via osmotic disruption. Not absorbed from GI tract. Oral administration results in "topical" treatment along the GI tract.	Oral and esophageal candidiasis (given orally) Vaginal candidiasis (applied topically)	Few adverse affects reported when administered orally.

Azoles

Drug	MOA & Pharmacokinetics	Clinical Uses	Side Effects
Ketoconazole (Nizoral®)	Blocks ergosterol synthesis by inhibiting the cytochrome P_{450} enzymes. This causes depletion of ergosterol, resulting in disruption of the permeability of the cell membrane. Does not penetrate CNS well. Highly bound to plasma proteins. Given PO. Absorbed better at low pH. A stomach pH of 1 - 1.5 is required for oral absorption. Absorption is decreased by food, antacids or H_2 blockers. Hepatic metabolism	**Blastomycosis** **Oropharyngeal candidiasis** **Coccidioidomycosis** **Histoplasmosis** Paracoccidioidomycosis May be used to treat adrenal tumors due to cortisol lowering effects. Dermatophytes: including griseofulvin-resistant.	GI effects: vomiting, diarrhea May affect host hepatic P_{450} system in mitochondria. This may lead to a decrease in the conversion of lanosterol to cholesterol resulting in lower levels of various hormones including cortisol and testosterone.
Fluconazole (Diflucan®)	Same MOA as ketoconazole. Does not require an acid pH. **Penetrates the CNS** Given PO, IV Renal elimination	**Oropharyngeal candidiasis**: **DOC** **Cryptococcal meningitis**: in immunosuppressed patients. **Coccidioidomycosis** Blastomycosis Histoplasmosis	GI effects: nausea, vomiting Rash

Drug	MOA & Pharmacokinetics	Clinical Uses	Side Effects
Itraconazole (Sporanox®)	Same MOA as ketoconazole. **Requires acid pH for absorption**, therefore can not be given IV. Long half-life. Poor CNS penetration Given PO Hepatic metabolism and excretion	**Blastomycosis: DOC** **Histoplasmosis** Aspergillosis Mucocutaneous candidiasis Coccidioidomycosis Cryptococcosis *Tinea* infections	GI effects: nausea, vomiting, diarrhea Rash
Miconazole (Monostat®) Clotrimazole (Canesten cream®)	Same MOA as ketoconazole. Given IV, topically.	Commonly used for topical mycotic infections	Anemia Flushing Redness

Miscellaneous Antifungal Drugs

Drug	MOA & Pharmacokinetics	Clinical Uses	Side Effects
Flucytosine (Ancobon®)	A narrow spectrum pyrimidine **antimetabolite** which is converted to 5-fluorouracil, an inhibitor of DNA and RNA synthesis. Inside the cell the drug is deaminated to form the active compound **5F-UMP**, an inhibitor of thymidylate synthetase. It inhibits the formation of deoxythymidine monophosphate (dTMP) from deoxyuridine monophosphate (dUMP). **Membrane permease** allows drug to enter fungal cells. Since host cells lack permease there is little effect on host cells. Penetrates CNS well. Given PO Renal elimination	**Cryptococcal infections**: in combination with amphotericin-B. **Candidiasis**: in combination with amphotericin-B. Chromoblastomycosis	**Bone marrow suppression** occurs in 15% of patients. Includes: leukopenia. thrombocytopenia and anemia. Hepatitis GI effects: nausea, vomiting, diarrhea
Griseofulvin (Fulvicin®)	Inhibits mitosis of cells, by disrupting spindle formation. Binds to tubulin involved in mitotic division and arrests cells in metaphase. May also bind to other proteins such as keratin. Primarily **fungistatic** **Deposits in keratin** which results in the clearing of infections from the inner to outer layers of dermis. Works very slowly. Up to 6 months treatment may be required. Given PO. Absorbed better with fatty foods. Excreted unchanged in feces.	**Dermatophytic infections only** of the skin, hair and nails: due to *Epidermophyton*, *Microsporum* and *Trichophyton* species. *Tinea* infections of the hands and beard	**CNS effects**: headache, photosensitivity and mental confusion. GI effects: nausea, vomiting Bone marrow suppression Hepatitis

Notes

Antivirals

Viruses are obligate intracellular parasites consisting of either double-stranded or single stranded DNA or RNA enclosed in a protein coat (capsid). They do not have a cell wall nor a cell membrane and do not carry out metabolic processes alone, so after attaching to and penetrating into a host cell, viruses depend heavily on the DNA, RNA and protein synthetic machinery of the host cell in order to reproduce.

Antiviral agents are designed to disrupt one of the many steps in viral infection and replication. They are often specific for a particular protein or enzyme and if one of these is used by the host cell, then some of the host cell function(s) may be impaired, which could result in significant toxic side effects.

Antiherpetic Drugs	Antiretroviral Drugs	Other Antiviral Drugs
Acyclovir Foscarnet Ganciclovir Idoxuridine Vidarabine	Didanosine Zalcitabine Zidovudine	Amantadine Rimantadine Ribavirin

Antiviral agents usually target one of the following steps in viral infection and replication:

- Adsorption to and penetration of susceptible host cells.
- Uncoating and release of viral genome into host cell nucleus.
- Transcription of early viral mRNA.
- Translation of early, nonstructural proteins, e.g., nucleic acid polymerases.
- Replication of viral genome.
- Translation of late, structural proteins.
- Posttranslational modification(s).
- Assembly (maturation) of virion components.
- Release from the host cell by budding or lysis.

Antiherpetic Drugs

Drug	MOA & Pharmacokinetics	Clinical Uses	Side Effects
Acyclovir (Avirax®, Zovirax®)	A **guanine** analog which is converted to acyclovir monophosphate by the herpes simplex virus encoded enzyme **thymidine kinase**. Acyclovir monophosphate is then converted to the diphosphate and triphosphate forms by cellular enzymes. Acyclovir triphosphate interferes with viral DNA polymerase and inhibits viral DNA replication. Acyclovir triphosphate can also be incorporated into growing chains of DNA by viral DNA polymerase, resulting in termination of DNA synthesis. Given PO, IV, topically Renal excretion	Herpes virus types I and II: • Mucocutaneous herpes • Genital herpes • Herpes encephalitis Varicella-zoster virus: • Varicella (chickenpox) • Zoster (shingles) • Herpes zoster ophthalmicus Not effective against CMV or EBV.	**Nephrotoxicity** at high doses, because acyclovir tends to precipitates in renal tubules. **Neurotoxicity** at high doses. Observed as delirium, tremor and seizures.
Foscarnet (Foscavir®)	A phosphonoformate derivative which does not require phosphorylation or activation by any kinases. Inhibits viral replication by blocking the pyrophosphate binding site of viral DNA polymerase. This prevents the cleavage of pyrophosphate from deoxynucleotide triphosphates and viral DNA chain elongation. Given IV Renal excretion	**CMV retinitis** in AIDS patients. Treatment of HIV patients with acyclovir-resistant strains of herpes virus, including herpes simplex, varicella-zoster and cytomegalovirus	**Nephrotoxicity** (reversible) GI effects: abdominal pain, anorexia, nausea and vomiting Electrolyte imbalances, especially hypocalcemia and hypomagnesemia

Drug	MOA & Pharmacokinetics	Clinical Uses	Side Effects
Ganciclovir (Cytovene®)	A **guanine** analog that is structurally similar to acyclovir. This prodrug is activated when it is converted to its nucleotide triphosphate form. This nucleotide analog inhibits viral DNA polymerase and can also be incorporated into DNA decreasing chain elongation. Given PO, IV Renal excretion	**Cytomegalovirus (CMV)** infections including: **retinitis**, pneumonia, esophagitis. CMV prophylaxis in organ transplant patients.	**Bone marrow suppression**: neutropenia, thrombocytopenia, granulocytopenia Drug Interactions: Concurrent use of AZT may potentate bone marrow depression.
Idoxuridine (IDU) (Stoxil®)	Nucleoside analog of thymidine which is converted by cellular enzymes into its active triphosphate form in cells. Incorporated into both viral and mammalian DNA. Given topically (ophthalmic)	Herpes simplex virus keratitis Vaccinia virus keratitis	Conjunctival irritation Photophobia
Vidarabine (Ara-A) (Vira-A®)	An **adenosine analog** which is converted in the cell to its triphosphate form. This triphosphate nucleotide analog inhibits viral DNA synthesis Also incorporated into viral DNA where is may act as a chain terminator. Given IV, topically (ophthalmic) Renal excretion	Herpes simplex virus keratoconjunctivitis Herpes simplex virus encephalitis Zoster in immunocompromised patients	GI effects: anorexia, nausea, vomiting, diarrhea Paresthesias Tremor

Antiretroviral Drugs

Drug	MOA & Pharmacokinetics	Clinical Uses	Side Effects
Didanosine (Dideoxyinosine, ddI) (Videx®)	An **adenosine** analog which is phosphorylated by cellular enzymes into its triphosphate which inhibits viral reverse transcriptase. Activated ddI is preferentially incorporated into the growing DNA strand, instead of ATP, which terminates strand growth. Given PO Renal excretion	HIV: indicated in patients intolerant to zidovudine or who have disease progression while receiving zidovudine.	**Peripheral neuropathy**: tingling, burning, numbness or pain in the hands or feet **Pancreatitis** CNS toxicity: anxiety, headache, insomnia GI effects: abdominal pain, nausea diarrhea
Zalcitabine (Dideoxycytidine, ddC) (HIVID®)	A **cytosine** analog which is phosphorylated by cellular enzymes into the triphosphate form which inhibits viral reverse transcriptase. The triphosphate form also inhibits viral DNA replication by terminating chain elongation once incorporated into viral DNA. Given PO Renal excretion	Advanced HIV infection. Usually given in combination with zidovudine in patients with CD4 counts < 300 cells per mm^3. Also indicated as monotherapy in patients intolerant to zidovudine or who have disease progression while receiving zidovudine.	**Peripheral neuropathy**: tingling, burning, numbness or pain in the hands or feet GI effects: abdominal pain, diarrhea, nausea Arthralgia/myalgia Ulceration of mouth and throat Skin rash

Drug	MOA & Pharmacokinetics	Clinical Uses	Side Effects
Zidovudine (AZT) (Retrovir®)	A structural analog of **thymidine** which is phosphorylated by cellular enzymes into its triphosphate. Zidovudine triphosphate is then incorporated into viral DNA by reverse transcriptase. Since zidovudine triphosphate lacks a 3' hydroxyl group, viral DNA synthesis is inhibited. Penetrates CNS. Crosses the placenta. Given PO Renal and hepatic excretion	HIV. Initial drug of choice for treatment of HIV is patients with CD4 counts < 500 cells/mm^3. Maternal-fetal HIV transmission: now recommended for HIV+ pregnant females to take from 14 weeks to until delivery and for infants until 6 weeks post partum. This leads to a decrease in the HIV vertical transmission rate from 25% down to about 8%. Although AZT increases short term survival and decreases the number of opportunistic infections, it does not increase long term survival.	**Anemia** **Neutropenia** Neurotoxicity: may lead to seizures Headaches, insomnia or confusion Drugs Interactions: Drugs which compete with AZT for glucuronidation (e.g., probenecid, acetaminophen, aspirin, cimetidine, morphine) will decrease zidovudine's clearance and potentiate toxicity.

Other Antiviral Drugs

Drug	MOA & Pharmacokinetics	Clinical Uses	Side Effects
Amantadine (Symmetrel®) Rimantadine (Flumadine®)	Inhibits uncoating of the **Influenza A** virus after it enters the cell by blocking bidirectionally the viral M2 membrane protein. The M2 protein forms a pump, which moves protons into the endosome and lowers its pH. The low pH facilitates viral uncoating. Rimantadine does not penetrate the CNS as well as amantadine. Amantadine undergoes renal excretion primarily as unmetabolized drug. Given PO	**Influenza type A** virus: used as prophylaxis in the elderly, very young and immunosuppressed. If given within the first 12-24 hours after influenza symptoms appear, the drug will decrease the duration and severity of the illness. Parkinson's disease	**CNS effects**: anxiety, confusion, insomnia. More common in the elderly. **GI effects**: loss of appetite, nausea Anticholinergic effects: dry mouth, blurred vision and urinary retention **Teratogenic**: avoid use in pregnant women
Ribavirin (Virazole®)	A **guanosine** analog whose mechanism of action is not fully defined but is related to a reduction of intracellular guanosine triphosphate pools and inhibition of viral RNA and protein synthesis Requires phosphorylation by human kinases to be activated. Given IV or by aerosol	**Respiratory syncytial virus** Lassa fever Influenza A and B virus	**Anemia** Worsening of respiratory status. Carefully monitor respiratory function during treatment, especially with infants and adults with COPD or asthma.

Antiprotozoals

Pathogenic protozoa cause parasitic infections worldwide and are an especially heavy burden in underdeveloped countries. Therapy for malaria, amebiasis, leishmaniasis and trypanosomiasis will be discussed in this section.

Malaria	Amebiasis	Leishmaniasis	Trypanosomiasis
Chloroquine Quinine Mefloquine Pyrimethamine/sulfadoxine Primaquine	Metronidazole Diloxanide furoate Paromomycin Iodoquinol	Stibogluconate	Suramin Melarsoprol Nifurtimox Pentamidine

Drugs for Malaria

Malaria continues to be one of the worlds most devastating infections claiming the lives of almost three million humans annually. Of the four *Plasmodium* species causing malaria (*P. falciparum, P. malariae, P. vivax* and *P. ovale) **P. falciparum*** is responsible for most of the fatalities; it is the only form able to invade erythrocytes of any age. Humans are the intermediate hosts who acquire the disease primarily by the bite of an infected female ***Anopheles* mosquito**. The parasites enter the circulation from the saliva of the mosquito and quickly localize within hepatocytes where they multiply and develop into tissue schizonts which later rupture and initiate the erythrocytic cycle of the disease.

Antimalarial agents were produced, primarily, on the basis of their effectiveness against the asexual erythrocytic forms of the parasites. They can be differentiated by the stage and species of *Plasmodium* they effect, however, the mechanism of action for most of these agents remains a subject needing clarification. The development of resistance is a common problem and multi-drug regimens are frequently used.

Drug	MOA & Pharmacokinetics	Clinical Uses	Side Effects
Chloroquine (Aralen®)	The mechanism in unknown, however, proposed mechanisms include: 1) DNA intercalation 2) Inhibition of plasmodium hemoglobin (Hb) polymerase, an enzyme that detoxifies heme produced during Hb breakdown. Inhibition of hemoglobin polymerase results in accumulation of these toxic species within plasmodia. 3) Increase in the pH of plasmodia vacuoles. Enters the CNS. Crosses the placenta. $t_{1/2}$ = 7 days High volume of distribution	Spectrum: effective against erythrocytic forms of: *P. vivax, P. ovale, P. malariae* and *P. falciparum*. Malaria due to non-resistant strains of ***P. falciparum* and *P. malariae***: **DOC** for prophylaxis and treatment. Malaria due to P. *vivax* and *P. ovale*: **DOC** for prophylaxis and treatment when used in combination with primaquine. Extra-intestinal amebiasis: due to *E. histolytica* used in combination with diloxanide furoate. Rheumatoid arthritis Systemic lupus erythematosus	There are few toxic side effects when administered properly. Gastrointestinal irritation Headaches and visual disturbances are more common with high doses. Pruritus, especially in dark skinned persons Cardiovascular effects: hypotension, vasodilation, ECG abnormalities are more common with high doses. ◆ Contraindications: G6PD-deficiency: chloroquine may cause acute **hemolytic anemia**. Porphyria Pregnancy Psoriasis

Drug	MOA & Pharmacokinetics	Clinical Uses	Side Effects
Quinine (Quinain®) Quinine is derived from the cinchona tree.	The MOA is unknown but may involve: 1) Inhibition of plasmodium hemoglobin (Hb) polymerase, an enzyme that detoxifies heme produced during Hb breakdown. Inhibition of hemoglobin polymerase results in accumulation of these toxic species within plasmodia. 2) Increase in the pH of plasmodia vacuoles. Long $t_{1/2}$, therefore, it is given weekly. Given PO	Activity: kills erythrocytic forms of *Plasmodia* species. Gametocidal for *P. vivax* and *P. ovale.* Malaria due to chloroquine- or multidrug resistant *P. falciparum*: **DOC** for treatment. Used in combination with pyrimethamine/ sulfadoxine (Fansidar®) Nocturnal leg cramps Babesiosis: used in combination with clindamycin	**Cinchonism**: observed as dose-related symptoms of tinnitus, nausea, headache and visual disturbances initially. With continued administration or higher doses, cardiac disturbances may be observed. **Blackwater fever** (rare): massive RBC lysis leads to hemoglobinuria which causes dark urine. Associated with renal failure, intravascular coagulation and possibly death. ◆ Contraindications: G-6PD deficiency: quinine may cause acute hemolytic anemia.
Mefloquine (Lariam®)	A structural analog of quinine. The MOA is unknown but may involve an increase in the pH of plasmodia vacuoles Given PO	Active against erythrocytic forms of *Plasmodia* species. Malaria due to chloroquine- and multidrug resistant forms of ***P. falciparum***: **DOC** for prophylaxis and treatment. Malaria due to *P. vivax* and *P. ovale*: **DOC** for prophylaxis	GI effects: abdominal pain, nausea, diarrhea CNS Effects: headaches, dizziness ◆ Contraindications: Pregnancy Epilepsy

Drug	MOA & Pharmacokinetics	Clinical Uses	Side Effects
Pyrimethamine/ sulfadoxine (Fansidar®) Note: Sulfa drugs and dihydrofolate reductase inhibitors exhibit synergistic effects because sulfa drugs are bacteriostatic and their effect is delayed until microbial folate stores are depleted. Dihydrofolate reductase inhibitors act immediately in inhibiting the enzyme.	**Pyrimethamine** inhibits **dihydrofolate reductase** which inhibits the synthesis of tetrahydrofolate, a vital cofactor for purine synthesis. Decreased tetrahydrofolate leads to inhibition of DNA synthesis. **Sulfadoxine**, a PABA analog, competitively inhibits dihydropteroate synthase. Dihydropteroate synthase is responsible for incorporating PABA into dihydropteroic acid, the immediate precursor of folic acid. Sulfadoxine is a sulfa drug. Given PO	Active against erythrocytic forms of *P. falciparum*. Gametocidal. **Toxoplasmosis** due to *Toxoplasma gondii* Malaria due to P. *falciparum*: used in combination with quinine.	GI effects Bone marrow suppression **Hypersensitivity reactions**: photosensitization, toxic epidermal necrolysis, Stevens-Johnson syndrome ◆ Contraindications: Lactating mothers Infants ≤ 2 months of age
Primaquine (Primachine®)	The mechanism is unknown but possibly interferes with electron transport within plasmodia. Given PO. Does not distribute well into tissues.	Active against hepatic and tissue forms of *P. vivax*, *P. ovale* and *P. falciparum*. Gametocidal against all four *Plasmodia* species. Malaria due to *P. vivax* and *P. ovale*: prophylaxis and radical cure due to its activity against tissue forms. Used in combination with agents active against erythrocytic forms of the parasite.	GI effects: abdominal discomfort Methemoglobinemia ◆ Contraindications: G-6PD deficiency: primaquine may cause acute hemolytic anemia. Patients with a predisposition to granulocytopenia such as in SLE and rheumatoid arthritis.

Drugs for Amebiasis

Drug	MOA & Pharmacokinetics	Clinical Uses	Side Effects
Metronidazole (Flagyl®)	Acts as an electron acceptor to deprive cells of required reducing equivalents. Antimicrobial activity results from the formation of chemically reactive species which interact with DNA and proteins. Toxic for amebae and anaerobic bacteria. Enters the CNS	**Luminal amebiasis** due to *E. histolytica*: **DOC** when used in combination with diloxanide furoate. **Extraluminal amebiasis** due *E. histolytica*: **DOC** when used in combination with diloxanide furoate. **Giardiasis** due to *Giardia lamblia*: **DOC** ***Trichomonas vaginalis*** Anaerobic bacteria: including *Bacteroides*, *Clostridium* and *Peptostreptococcus*. Bacterial vaginitis due to *Gardnerella*	GI effects: nausea, vomiting, abdominal discomfort CNS effects: dizziness, headache Metallic taste and dry mouth Neuropathy and paresthesias: with long term treatment or high doses. Discoloration of urine Drug Interaction: Alcohol: may cause a disulfiram-like reaction by causing an accumulation of acetaldehyde. ◆ Contraindication: Pregnancy: may be teratogenic
Diloxanide furoate (Furamide®)	The MOA is unknown. Given PO	Asymptomatic amebiasis ("cyst passers"): **DOC** **Luminal amebiasis** due to *E. histolytica*: **DOC** when used in combination with metronidazole. Second line agent in combination with paromomycin. **Extraluminal amebiasis** due *E. histolytica*: **DOC** when used in combination with metronidazole. Second line agent in combination with chloroquine.	Flatulence Vomiting Dry mouth ◆ Contraindications: Lactating mothers Infants ≤ 2 months of age

Drug	MOA & Pharmacokinetics	Clinical Uses	Side Effects
Paromomycin (Humatin®)	An aminoglycoside antibiotic with direct activity against amebae.	Luminal amebiasis due to *E. histolytica*: second line agent in combination with diloxanide furoate.	**GI effects**: diarrhea CNS effects: dizziness, headache
Iodoquinol (Diodiquin®)	The MOA is unknown but acts on trophozoites of *E. histolytica.* Poorly absorbed therefore reaches high concentrations within the intestinal lumen.	Asymptomatic amebiasis ("cyst passers"): second line agent.	GI effects: diarrhea, nausea, vomiting Headache Fever Hypersensitivity reactions

Drugs for Leishmaniasis

Drug	MOA & Pharmacokinetics	Clinical Uses	Side Effects
Stibogluconate (Pentostam®)	Pentavalent antimony compound whose MOA is unclear but is thought to inhibit glycolysis.	**Cutaneous, mucocutaneous, and visceral leishmaniasis: DOC**	GI effects Cardiac arrhythmias

Drugs for Trypanosomiasis

Drug	MOA & Pharmacokinetics	Clinical Uses	Side Effects
Suramin (Antrypol®)	The mechanism is unclear but may involve inhibition of enzymes required for energy metabolism. Does not penetrate into CNS. Given IV	African sleeping sickness **without CNS** involvement due to *T. rhodesiense* or *T. gambiense*: DOC Onchocerciasis due to *Onchocerca volvulus*: used in combination with diethylcarbamazine.	GI effects: nausea, vomiting CNS effects: paresthesias, photophobia
Melarsoprol (Mel B®)	Arsenical compound which inhibits enzymes in parasites more effectively than those of the host. Penetrates the CNS	African sleeping sickness **with CNS** involvement due to *T. rhodesiense* or *T. gambiense*: DOC	CNS effects: encephalopathy Hypersensitivity reactions GI effects
Nifurtimox (Lampit®)	Forms reactive radical species which are toxic to the parasites. Given PO	**American trypanosomiasis** (Chagas' disease) due to *T. cruzi*: DOC	Hypersensitivity reactions GI effects
Pentamidine (Pentam®)	Not well understood. Appears to interfere with nuclear metabolism and inhibit the synthesis of DNA, RNA, proteins and phospholipids. Does not enter the CNS Given IV or aerosol	Pneumonia due to ***Pneumocystis carinii***: as an alternative to trimethoprim-sulfamethoxazole. African sleeping sickness due to *T. rhodesiense* or *T. gambiense*: an alternative to suramin.	Hypotension due to stimulation histamine release and intrinsic sympathoplegic activity. Pancreatic β-cell dysfunction

Notes

Anthelmintics

Helminths (worms) are responsible for parasitic infections (helminthiasis) in over two million people throughout the world and are more frequently acquired in underdeveloped tropical nations. The role of anthelmintics is to reduce or eradicate these parasites from the intestinal tract or other body tissues.

Phylum	Class and Examples	Drugs
Nematode (Roundworms)	**Intestinal Nematodes** *Ascaris lumbricoides* (giant roundworm) *Necator americanus* (hookworm) *Strongyloides stercoralis* (threadworm) *Trichinella spiralis* *Trichuris trichiura* (whipworm) *Enterobius vermicularis* (pinworm) *Ancylostoma* species **Blood and Tissue Nematodes** *Onchocerca volvulus* *Wuchereria bancrofti* *Brugia malayi* *Loa loa* *Dracunculus medinensis* (guinea worm) *Toxocara* species	Pyrantel pamoate Diethylcarbamazine Ivermectin Mebendazole Thiabendazole
Platyhelminths (Flatworms)	**Trematodes** (flukes) *Schistosoma* (blood flukes) *Clonorchis sinensis* (liver fluke) *Paragonimus westermani* (lung fluke)	Praziquantel
	Cestodes (tapeworms) *Taenia solium* (pork tapeworm) *Taenia saginata* (beef tapeworm) *Diphyllobothrium latum* (fish tapeworm) *Hymenolepis nana* (dwarf tapeworm) *Echinococcus granulosus*	Niclosamide

Treatment of Nematodes

Drug	MOA & Pharmacokinetics	Clinical Uses	Side Effects
Pyrantel pamoate (Antiminth®)	Depolarizing neuromuscular blocking agent which results in paralysis of the worm. Also inhibits cholinesterases and stimulates nicotinic receptors.	**Ascariasis** due to *Ascaris lumbricoides* *Necator americanus* *Enterobius vermicularis*	Transient and mild but may include nausea, vomiting and/or headache.
Diethylcarbamazine (Hetrazan®) This drug is a piperazine derivative	MOA is not well understood but diethylcarbamazine is thought to work by decreasing the muscular activity of the organisms and/or by increasing the susceptibility of microfilaria to phagocytosis.	**Filariasis** due to *W. bancrofti* and *B. malayi*: **DOC** Ascariasis due to *Ascaris lumbricoides*. Loiasis due to *Loa loa* . Onchocerciasis due to *Onchocerca volvulus*: second-line agent. Tropical pulmonary eosinophilia	**Mazzotti reaction**: typically occurs in patients with onchocerciasis within a few hours after taking the first dose. This reaction results from the **death of the parasites**. Observed as intense itching, skin rashes, enlarged and tender lymph nodes, sometimes fever, tachycardia, hypotension, arthralgias and headaches.
Ivermectin	Increases GABA mediated neurotransmission in nematodes resulting in paralysis of the parasites.	**River blindness** caused by *Onchocerca volvulus*: **DOC** Lymphatic filariasis caused by *W bancrofti* and *B malayi*: second-line agent.	

Drug	MOA & Pharmacokinetics	Clinical Uses	Side Effects
Mebendazole (Mebendacin®)	Binds to tubulin and inhibits **microtubule** polymerization.	**Pinworm** infections caused by *E. vermicularis*: DOC **Whipworm** infections caused by *T. trichiura*: DOC ***Necator americanus*** Ascariasis due to *A. lumbricoides*: second-line agent	Abdominal pain Diarrhea
Thiabendazole (Triasox®)	Binds to tubulin and inhibits **microtubule** polymerization.	***S. stercoralis***: DOC **Cutaneous larva migrans** caused by *Ancylostoma* species: DOC **Visceral larva migrans** cause by *Toxocara* species: DOC Trichinosis caused by *T. spiralis*	CNS effects: numbness or tingling in the hands and feet GI effects: anorexia, diarrhea, nausea and vomiting Neuropsychiatric toxicity: delirium, disorientation, hallucination, irritability Stevens-Johnson syndrome

Treatment of Trematodes and Cestodes

Drug	MOA & Pharmacokinetics	Clinical Uses	Side Effects
Praziquantel (Biltricide®, Cysticide®)	**Increases calcium permeability** leading to calcium efflux. This causes initial contraction, spasm and eventual paralysis of the worms. CSF penetration	**Schistosomiasis**: DOC for all schistosome species. Other trematodes such as *Clonorchis sinensis* and *Paragonimus westermani.* Cestodes such as *T. saginata, T. solium, D. latum* and *H. nana.* **Cysticercosis** from the ingestion of *T. solium* eggs. Not indicated for ocular cysticercosis due to the risk of causing ocular damage.	CNS effects: dizziness, drowsiness, headache Fever GI effects: abdominal, nausea, vomiting, diarrhea Skin rash
Niclosamide (Niclocide®)	Inhibits oxidative phosphorylation in the mitochondria of cestodes.	**Cestodes**: Niclosamide is the DOC for most cestode infections, including *T. saginata, T. solium, D. latum and H. nana.* It is only effective against these intestinal tapeworms; it is ineffective against cysticercosis (praziquantel is used) and in treating *E. granulosus* (mebendazole is used).	GI effects: abdominal pain, diarrhea, loss of appetite, nausea or vomiting

Cancer Chemotherapy

Page	Topic

Cancer Chemotherapy

Cancer is defined as abnormal and unrestricted cell proliferation resulting in tumor formation. Tumors can arise in virtually any tissue and can be either benign or malignant depending on their ability to invade locally and spread (metastasize) to distant sites. **Benign tumors** grow locally and do not invade or metastasize. The majority of benign tumors are not fatal, however, any tumor located in a critical site (e.g., the brain) may compress local structures and exert lethal effects. **Malignant tumors** invade and destroy neighboring tissues and possess the ability to metastasize to all areas of the body via the blood or lymphatic channels. In contrast to benign tumors, most malignant tumors are fatal.

There are various therapies used in the treatment of cancer such as surgery, radiation therapy and chemotherapy. The choice of treatment depends on the type, grade, stage and location of the tumor, as well as the age and condition of the patient. Below is a list of various chemotherapeutic agents used in the treatment of cancer. They are divided into antimetabolites, alkylating agents, antibiotics, plant alkaloids and endocrine agents.

Antimetabolites	Alkylating Agents	Antibiotics	Plant Alkaloids	Endocrine Agents
6-Mercaptopurine Methotrexate Cytarabine 5-Fluorouracil Hydroxyurea	Nitrogen mustards Mechlorethamine Cyclophosphamide Melphalan Nitrosoureas Lomustine Carmustine Streptozocin Miscellaneous Cisplatin Carboplatin Busulfan Dacarbazine	Dactinomycin Doxorubicin Daunorubicin Bleomycin Mitomycin	Vinblastine Vincristine Paclitaxel Etoposide	Glucocorticoids Flutamide Tamoxifen Leuprolide

The Cell Cycle

The cell cycle is comprised of 5 phases (G_1, S, G_2, M and G_0). The **growth fraction** is the total number of cells in the growth cycle (G_1, S, G_2, M) divided by the total number of cells. It represents the proportion of cells actively proliferating and is important in therapeutic regimens which target a specific phase of the cell cycle.

Chemotherapeutic agents which kill cells during certain phases in the cell cycle are termed **cell cycle specific** (CCS). In contrast, **cell cycle non-specific** (CCNS) agents act at various points of the cell cycle.

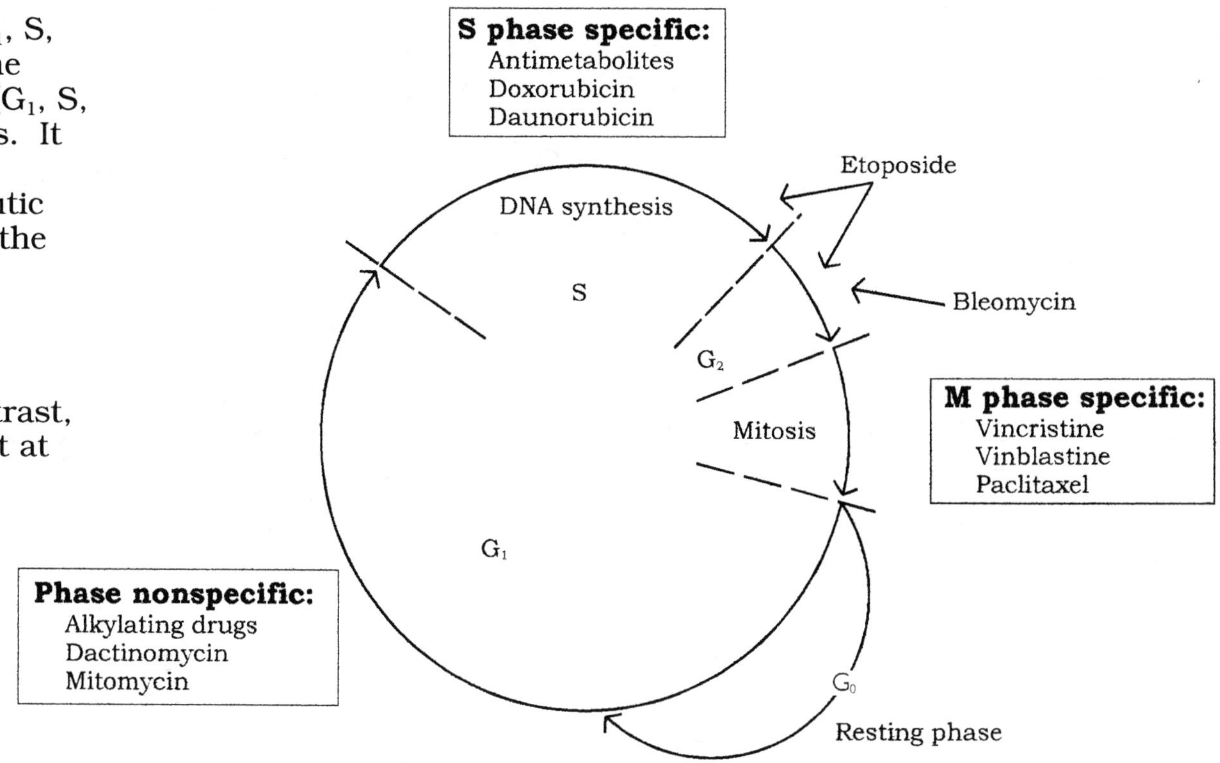

	Definition and Clinical Indication	Examples
Cell cycle specific (CCS)	Agents which selectively kill proliferating cells (i.e., cells which are not in G_0). As such, these agents are used for **high growth fraction** malignancies.	Antimetabolites Plant alkaloids Some antibiotics
Cell cycle non-specific (CCNS)	Agents which kill both proliferating and resting cells. As such, these agents are used to treat both **low** and **high growth fraction** malignancies.	Alkylating agents Some antibiotics

Log Kill Hypothesis & Modes of Resistance

Log kill hypothesis	Cytotoxic drugs exhibit **first-order kinetics**, killing a **constant fraction** of cells rather than a constant number of cells. For example, a 3-log kill dose of a drug will decrease a tumor by 99.9% of the cells. Therefore, if a tumor contains 10^9 cells, 10^6 cells would still remain.
Modes of resistance	A major problem in chemotherapy is the development of drug resistance. The most common mechanisms by which cancer cells gain resistance include: • Decreased drug activation or increased drug inactivation • Increased efflux or decreased uptake • Changes in target enzymes: altered binding or increased amount of substrate • Increased DNA repair • Alternative metabolic pathways

Combination Therapy

Many cancers are treated with multiple chemotherapeutic agents to increase the log kill and reduce the impact of drug resistance to a single agent. Listed below are some of the major combination regimens.

	Agents	Clinical Uses
A **B** **V** **D**	Adriamycin® (doxorubicin) Bleomycin Vinblastine Dacarbazine	Hodgkin's lymphoma
M **O** **P** **P**	Mechlorethamine Oncovin® (vincristine) Procarbazine Prednisone	Hodgkin's lymphoma
C **H** **O** **P**	Cyclophosphamide Doxorubicin Oncovin® (vincristine) Prednisone	Lymphoma

	Agents	Clinical Uses
V **A** **C**	Vincristine Actinomycin D (dactinomycin) Cyclophosphamide	Rhabdomyosarcoma Wilms' Tumor
V **B** **C**	Vinblastine Bleomycin Cisplatin	Testicular carcinoma
V **B** **E**	Vinblastine Bleomycin Etoposide	Testicular carcinoma

Antimetabolites

Antimetabolites inhibit steps in DNA biosynthesis.
They exhibit cell cycle specific killing in **S phase**.

Drug	MOA & Pharmacokinetics	Clinical Uses	Side Effects
6-Mercaptopurine (Purinethol®) Azathioprine, a derivative of 6-mercaptopurine, is used as an immunosuppressant.	A purine antimetabolite which is converted by hypoxanthine-guanine phosphoryl transferase (**HGPRT**) to the active form 6-thioinosinic acid which inhibits key enzymes in the **purine synthetic pathway**. This results in inhibition of DNA synthesis. Cell cycle specific for **S-phase** Given PO	**Leukemias**: ALL, AML	**Bone marrow suppression**: anemia, leukopenia, thrombocytopenia Hepatotoxicity Immunosuppression
Methotrexate (Folex®, Mexate®) Note: Administered with **leucovorin**.	A **folic acid antagonist** which prevents the conversion of dihydrofolate to tetrahydrofolate by inhibiting dihydrofolate reductase (**DHFR**). Tetrahydrofolate is required for the synthesis of thymidylate, DNA, RNA and some amino acids (Ser, Met). Metabolized to polyglutamates which are also active but retained better within cells. Cell cycle specific for **S-phase** Given PO, IV, IM and intrathecal	Psoriasis Rheumatoid arthritis Choriocarcinoma Breast carcinoma Head and neck carcinomas Lung cancer Leukemias: ALL, meningeal Non-Hodgkin's lymphoma Mycosis fungoides Osteosarcoma Abortifacient	GI effects: bleeding, ulceration, intestinal perforation, mucositis Bone marrow suppression: leukopenia, thrombocytopenia Nausea and vomiting Loss of appetite Treatment of overdose: administration of **leucovorin** (folinic acid) which replenishes the folate pool; this is known as **leucovorin rescue**.

Drug	MOA & Pharmacokinetics	Clinical Uses	Side Effects
Cytarabine (Cytosine Arabinoside, Ara-C) (Cytosar®)	**Pyrimidine analog** which is activated to the monophosphate nucleotide (AraCMP) which can then form AraCDP and **AraCTP** the latter of which **inhibits DNA synthesis** by preventing DNA chain elongation. Cell-cycle specific for **S-phase** Given SC, IV, intrathecal	**Leukemia**: **DOC for AML** Other leukemias: ALL, CML, meningeal and erythroleukemia Non-Hodgkin's Lymphoma	Bone marrow suppression: leukopenia, anemia, thrombocytopenia Stomatitis Nausea and vomiting Loss of appetite
5-Fluorouracil (Adrucil®)	Requires ribosylation (by PRPP) or phosphorylation by uridine phosphorylase and uridine kinase to be converted to **5-F-UMP**. 5-F-UMP can **inhibit RNA synthesis**. It also prevents DNA synthesis by inhibiting **thymidylate synthetase** (depletion of thymidine stores). Cell cycle specific for **S-phase**	**Breast carcinomas** **GI carcinomas**: colorectal, gastric Ovarian cancer Pancreatic cancer	Diarrhea Esophagopharyngitis Leukopenia Infection Dermatitis Nausea and vomiting GI ulceration
Hydroxyurea (Hydrea®)	Urea analog which **prevents DNA synthesis** by inhibiting **ribonucleotide reductase**, the enzyme which converts ribonucleotides to deoxyribonucleotides. Cell cycle specific for **S-phase** Given PO, IV	**CML** Melanoma Polycythemia vera Sickle cell anemia	Bone marrow suppression: leukopenia, megaloblastic anemia, thrombocytopenia Nausea, vomiting Diarrhea

DNA Alkylating Agents

DNA alkylating agents are cell cycle non-specific (CCNS) agents that react with DNA. Specific DNA targets are the N-7 and O-6 positions of guanine. Interaction of these agents with DNA results in DNA cross-linking, base-pair mismatching or DNA breakage. These agents can be divided into three classes: the nitrogen mustards, nitrosoureas and miscellaneous alkylating agents.

Nitrogen Mustards

Drugs	MOA & Pharmacokinetics	Clinical Uses	Side Effects
Mechlorethamine (Mustargen®)	Bifunctional **alkylating agent** which forms an ethylenimmonium that cross links strands of DNA and RNA. Cell cycle **non-specific** Given IV (must be administered with care due to its tissue damaging properties)	**Hodgkin's disease**: component of MOPP **<u>M</u>** = Mechlorethamine **O** = (Oncovin®) Vincristine **P** = Procarbazine **P** = Prednisone	Nausea and vomiting Lacrimation Bone marrow suppression: leukopenia, thrombocytopenia Gonadal suppression Risk of phlebitis and necrosis at the site of injection
Cyclophosphamide (Cytoxan®)	**Prodrug** which is metabolized by the hepatic P_{450} system to many metabolites, the two most important of which are **phosphoramide mustard** (active metabolite) and **acrolein** (toxic metabolite). The **phosphoramide mustard** metabolite cross-links DNA and RNA. Cell cycle **non-specific** Given PO, IV	Ovarian and breast carcinoma Hodgkin's and Non-Hodgkin's lymphoma Leukemias: ALL, AML, CLL and CML Childhood malignancies: neuroblastoma, retinoblastoma Multiple myeloma	Nausea, vomiting and diarrhea Skin pigmentation Loss of hair (alopecia) Gonadal suppression Leukopenia High doses or long term use: cardiotoxicity, hemorrhagic cystitis (due to acrolein) and SIADH.
Melphalan (Alkeran®)	**Phenylalanine** derivative of nitrogen mustard that cross links strands of DNA and RNA. Cell cycle **non-specific** Given PO, IV	Ovarian carcinoma Multiple myeloma	Bone marrow suppression: leukopenia, thrombocytopenia

Nitrosoureas

These agents are lipophilic and are thus able to cross the blood brain barrier which makes them particularly useful in the treatment of meningeal leukemia and brain tumors.

Drugs	MOA & Pharmacokinetics	Clinical Uses	Side Effects
Lomustine (CeeNU®)	Inhibits DNA, RNA and protein synthesis via bifunctional alkylation and protein modification (carbamoylation of lysine residues). Crosses blood brain barrier due to high lipophilicity. Cell cycle **non-specific** Given **PO**	**Brain tumors**: primary Melanoma GI cancers	Nausea and vomiting Loss of appetite Bone marrow suppression: leukopenia, thrombocytopenia Immunosuppression
Carmustine (BiCNU®)	Inhibits DNA, RNA and protein synthesis via bifunctional alkylation and protein modification (carbamoylation of lysine residues). Crosses blood brain barrier due to high lipophilicity. Cell cycle **non-specific** Given **IV**	**Brain tumors**: astrocytomas and metastatic tumors to the brain Hodgkin's and Non-Hodgkin's lymphoma Multiple myeloma GI cancers	Nausea and vomiting Bone marrow suppression: leukopenia, thrombocytopenia Phlebitis at the site of injection Pulmonary fibrosis Renal toxicity
Streptozocin (Zanosar®) Note: streptozocin is a naturally occurring antibiotic derived from *Streptomyces acromogenes*.	Alkylating agent which inhibits DNA synthesis by cross linking strands of DNA. Diabetogenic agent in experimental animals due to high affinity for and toxicity to **pancreatic β cells**. Crosses blood brain barrier due to high lipophilicity. Cell cycle **non-specific** Given IV	Pancreatic carcinoma: islet cell (insulinomas)	Nausea and vomiting Bone marrow suppression: leukopenia, thrombocytopenia Renal failure

Miscellaneous Alkylating Agents

Drugs	MOA & Pharmacokinetics	Clinical Uses	Side Effects
Cisplatin (Platinol®)	**Platinum coordination complex** which enters cells by diffusion and is hydrolyzed to form an activated electrophile which alkylates DNA. Also interacts with proteins. Cell cycle **non-specific** Should be given to a well-hydrated patient. Given IV or intraperitoneally (for ovarian carcinoma)	**Testicular carcinoma**: component of VBC. The VBE regimen, in which etoposide replaces cisplatin, is equally effective. **V** = Vinblastine **B** = Bleomycin **C** = Cisplatin **Bladder carcinoma** Lung carcinoma Ovarian carcinoma	**Nephrotoxicity** **Ototoxicity** Nausea and vomiting Bone marrow suppression: anemia, leukopenia, thrombocytopenia Peripheral neuropathy Hyperuricemia
Carboplatin (Paraplatin®)	Same MOA as cisplatin. Cell cycle **non-specific** Given IV or intraperitoneally (for ovarian carcinoma)	Ovarian carcinoma	Bone marrow suppression: anemia, leukopenia, thrombocytopenia Less nephrotoxicity, neuropathy, nausea and ototoxicity than cisplatin
Busulfan (Myleran®)	An alkylsulfonate type bifunctional alkylating agent which alkylates and cross-links strands of DNA. Cell cycle **non-specific** Given PO	**Leukemia**: **DOC for CML**	Bone marrow suppression: anemia, leukopenia, thrombocytopenia Amenorrhea, ovarian suppression Skin pigmentation High doses: pulmonary fibrosis, seizures and hepatic veno-occlusive disease
Dacarbazine (DITC®)	Hepatically activated alkylating agent which is thought to inhibit DNA and RNA synthesis via formation of carbonium ions. Cell cycle **non-specific** Given IV	**Hodgkin's lymphoma**: component of ABVD **A** = Adriamycin **B** = Bleomycin **V** = Vinblastine **D** = Dacarbazine Malignant melanoma	Nausea and vomiting, loss of appetite Bone marrow suppression: anemia, leukopenia, thrombocytopenia Extravasation and damage in injected vein Hepatotoxicity (rare but fatal)

Antibiotics

Drugs	MOA & Pharmacokinetics	Clinical Uses	Side Effects
Dactinomycin (Actinomycin D) (Cosmegen®)	Antibiotic which binds double-stranded DNA and intercalates between adjacent G-C base pairs. This inhibits **DNA-dependent RNA polymerase**. Also causes single-stranded DNA breaks possibly through free radical intermediates or inhibition of **topoisomerase II**. Cell cycle **non-specific** Given IV	**Wilms' Tumor**: component of VAC **V** = Vincristine **A** = Actinomycin **C** = Cyclophosphamide **Rhabdomyosarcoma**: component of VAC Choriocarcinoma	Nausea and vomiting Anorexia Bone marrow suppression: anemia, leukopenia, thrombocytopenia GI problems: proctitis, diarrhea, ulcerative stomatitis Dermatologic effects
Doxorubicin (Adriamycin®)	**Anthracycline antibiotic** whose antitumor activity may result from any of several mechanisms including DNA intercalation, single-stranded DNA breaks and membrane disruption. Cell cycle specific: predominantly **S-phase** specific but at low doses cells may proceed through S-phase and die in G2. Metabolized by P_{450} system to a toxic metabolite which may cause **cardiomyopathy** by generating free radicals. Given IV	**Acute leukemia**: AML, ALL Hodgkin's disease: component of ABVD Non-Hodgkin's lymphoma Ovarian cancer Breast cancer Thyroid cancer: metastatic Soft tissue sarcomas	Nausea and vomiting Stomatitis or esophagitis Bone marrow suppression: leukopenia Alopecia Extravasation and tissue damage at the site of injection (vesicant) Cardiomyopathy
Daunorubicin (Cerubidine®)	Same MOA as doxorubicin. Cell cycle specific: predominantly **S-phase** specific but at low doses cells may proceed through S-phase and die in G2. Given IV	**Acute leukemias**: AML and ALL	

Drugs	MOA & Pharmacokinetics	Clinical Uses	Side Effects
Bleomycin (Blenoxane®)	Combines with iron and forms a complex which reacts with oxygen to produce free radicals. This cause strand scission and **DNA fragmentation**. Cell cycle specific for **G2 phase** Given IV, IM, SC	**Testicular carcinoma**: component of VBC or VBE **Hodgkin's disease**: component of ABVD Non-Hodgkin's lymphoma Head and neck carcinomas Ovarian carcinomas GU carcinomas Skin carcinomas	**Pulmonary toxicity**: pneumonitis which may progress to fibrosis. Fever and chills Mucocutaneous toxicity: "bleomycin blisters" Hypersensitivity Skin pigmentation
Mitomycin (Mutamycin®)	Reduced to a bi- or tri-functional **alkylating agent** which inhibits DNA synthesis. Reduction of mitomycin occurs preferentially in hypoxic environments. Cell cycle non-specific Given IV	Cervical carcinoma Bladder carcinoma GI carcinomas	Nausea and vomiting Loss of appetite Bone marrow suppression: leukopenia, thrombocytopenia Hemolytic-uremic syndrome (rare)

Plant Alkaloids

Plant alkaloids either interfere with tubulin function or **DNA topoisomerase II**. For the most part, they work in the M-phase of the cell cycle.

Drugs	MOA & Pharmacokinetics	Clinical Uses	Side Effects
Vinblastine (Velban®)	A **spindle poison** which binds **tubulin** and prevents assembly of **microtubules**. This inhibits formation of the mitotic spindle and blocks cells in mitosis. Cell-cycle phase specific for **M phase** Given IV	**Testicular carcinoma**: component of VBC and VBE **Hodgkin's Disease**: component of ABVD Non-Hodgkin's lymphoma Breast carcinoma	**Bone marrow suppression**: leukopenia Alopecia
Vincristine (Oncovin®)	Same MOA as vinblastine. Cell-cycle phase specific for **M phase** Given IV	**Hodgkin's lymphoma: component** of MOPP **Rhabdomyosarcoma**: component of VAC Non-Hodgkin's lymphoma Childhood tumors: Wilms' tumor, neuroblastoma and Ewing's sarcoma	**Neurotoxicity** Autonomic toxicity: constipation, stomach cramps Hyperuricemia Alopecia
Paclitaxel (Taxol®)	Binds tubulin promoting the **formation** and preventing the dissolution of microtubules. Cell-cycle phase specific for **M phase** Given IV	**Ovarian carcinoma** Breast carcinoma	Nausea, vomiting, diarrhea Bone marrow suppression: anemia, leukopenia, thrombocytopenia Arthralgias or myalgias Peripheral neuropathy Hypersensitivity reactions
Etoposide (VePesid®) Also called VP-16	Stabilizes the **DNA topoisomerase II-DNA complex** causing double strand DNA breaks during DNA replication. Cell cycle specific for **S** and **G2** phases Given PO, IV	**Testicular carcinoma**: component of **VBE** (equally effective as VBC, but less toxic). Lung carcinoma: oat cell	Nausea and vomiting Alopecia Bone marrow suppression: anemia, leukopenia, thrombocytopenia

Endocrine Agents

Drug	MOA & Pharmacokinetics	Clinical Uses	Side Effects
Glucocorticoids Prednisone Dexamethasone Hydrocortisone	Bind to intracellular glucocorticoid receptors in T cells and induce expression of glucocorticoid responsive genes. This results in suppression of cellular growth and proliferation as well as induction of apoptosis.	**Hodgkin's lymphoma**: part of the MOPP regimen. Non-Hodgkin's lymphomas Acute leukemias	Infection Hyperglycemia Gastric and duodenal ulcers Osteoporosis
Flutamide (Euflex®, Eulexin®)	**Nonsteroidal competitive antagonist** at androgen receptors.	**Prostatic carcinoma**: usually in combination with LHRH analogs such as **leuprolide**.	**Diarrhea**, **hot flashes**, **impotence**: due to combined flutamide and LHRH therapy Gynecomastia Hepatotoxic: mild, reversible
Tamoxifen (Nolvadex®)	**Nonsteroidal antiestrogen** which competitively inhibits estrogen at the estrogen receptor.	**Breast cancer**: **DOC** for endocrine management of estrogen receptor positive breast cancer. Metastatic breast cancer in men and women	**Hot flashes** **GI effects**: nausea, vomiting GU effects: menstrual irregularities, vulvar pruritus
Leuprolide (Lupron®)	Long acting **synthetic GnRH analog** which is used to **inhibit** the release of FSH and LH from the anterior pituitary when administered in a **continuous fashion**. Given SC, IM	**Prostatic carcinoma** **Endometriosis** Breast carcinoma Precocious puberty Infertility	Hot flashes Increased bone pain in patients with prostate cancer

Endocrine Drugs

Hypothalamic/Pituitary Hormones

Endocrinology is the study of hormones, the systems that regulate them and the glands that produce them. The body's endocrine glands include the hypothalamus, pituitary, thyroid, parathyroid, adrenal glands, gonads, liver, etc. This section focuses on hypothalamic and pituitary hormones as well as their analogs.

The hypothalamus controls the release of hormones from the pituitary. The pituitary gland consists of an anterior lobe (adenohypophysis), an intermediate lobe, and a posterior lobe (neurohypophysis). In response to hypothalamic releasing hormones, the anterior pituitary secretes growth hormone (GH), adrenocorticotropin (ACTH), follicle stimulating hormone (FSH), luteinizing hormone (LH) and prolactin. **The posterior pituitary** hormones (ADH, Oxytocin) are synthesized in the cell bodies of hypothalamic neurons and are delivered to the posterior lobe by neurosecretory fibers which release the hormones into the circulation directly. Secretion of posterior pituitary hormones is stimulated by osmotic and volume stimuli for ADH and by suckling of the breast for oxytocin.

Hypothalamic and anterior pituitary hormones and agonists can be functionally grouped into those which regulate growth, those which regulate gonadal function and those which regulate corticosteroid release. These drugs are used therapeutically for: **replacement therapy** for those with hormone deficiencies, **drug therapy** to elicit a hormonal effect not present at normal blood levels of the hormone and as **diagnostic tools** to evaluate hormone levels. Only the clinically used hypothalamic and pituitary hormones and their analogs are listed below:

Hormones that Regulate Growth	Hormones that Regulate Gonadal Function	Hormones that Regulate Corticosteroid Release
Growth hormone releasing hormone Somatostatin Octreotide Somatotropin Somatrem	Gonadorelin Goserelin acetate Histrelin acetate Leuprolide acetate Nafarelin acetate Human chorionic gonadotropin Menotropin Urofollitropin	Corticotropin releasing hormone Cosyntropin

Posterior Pituitary Hormones and Analogs
Oxytocin Vasopressin (ADH) Desmopressin acetate

Hormones that Regulate Growth

Drug	MOA & Pharmacokinetics	Clinical Uses	Side Effects
Growth-hormone-releasing hormone (GHRH, Somatocrinin®, Sermorelin®)	Stimulates the secretion of growth hormone from the anterior pituitary. Given IM or SC	**Diagnostic agent** to determine if a growth hormone deficiency is due to a hypothalamic or pituitary defect. Hypothalamic dwarfism: to promote normal growth rates in children with GHRH deficiency.	Few adverse effects, but may cause some facial flushing or injection site pain.
Somatostatin (Growth Hormone-Inhibiting Hormone, Somatotropin Release-Inhibiting Hormone)	**Inhibits growth hormone release** from the anterior pituitary. Also inhibits the release of gastrin from the GI tract, insulin and glucagon from the pancreas and TSH and prolactin from the pituitary. Short $t_{1/2}$ = 1-3 min	Not used clinically due to short half-life and non-specific inhibition of growth hormone.	Rebound hypersecretion of growth hormone when treatment stops.
Octreotide (Sandostatin®)	**Synthetic somatostatin analog** which selectively inhibits growth hormone release. More potent than somatostatin Long $t_{1/2}$ = 80 min Given PO, SC	**Acromegaly**: giantism secondary to growth hormone hypersecretion. **Endocrine tumors**: carcinoid, gastrinoma, glucagonoma	GI effects: malabsorption, loose stools, nausea, flatulence, abdominal cramps Gallstones commonly occur in patients treated for 6 months. Does not elicit rebound hypersecretion.

Drug	MOA & Pharmacokinetics	Clinical Uses	Side Effects
Somatotropin (Humatrope®) Somatrem (Protropin®) Growth hormone was originally isolated from human cadavers but due to the incidence of Creutzfeldt-Jacob disease only recombinant forms are now used.	**Synthetic growth hormone analogs** which stimulate the production of insulin-like growth factors (IGFs) in the liver resulting in increased cell number. IGFs share homology with insulin and have insulin-like effects. Somatrem is identical to somatotropin except that it possesses an additional methionine. Given IM or SC	**Hypopituitary dwarfism**: to promote normal growth rates in children with growth hormone deficiency.	Rapid growth may result in slipped capital femoral epiphyses, leading to a limp or lower extremity pain. ◆ Contraindications: Patients with closed epiphyses or an expanding intracranial mass.

Hormones that Regulate Gonadal Function

Drug	MOA & Pharmacokinetics	Clinical Uses	Side Effects
Gonadorelin (Factrel®, Lutrepulse®)	Synthetic **GnRH analog** which is used to **stimulate** the secretion of FSH and LH from the anterior pituitary when given in a **pulsatile fashion**. Given IV, SC	**Diagnosis** of gonadotropin deficiency. Stimulates LH and FSH secretion in patients with hypogonadotropic hypogonadism and delayed puberty.	Headache Abdominal discomfort Flushing
Goserelin acetate (Zoladex®) Histrelin acetate (Supprelin®) Leuprolide acetate (Lupron®) Nafarelin acetate (Synarel®)	Long acting **synthetic GnRH analogs** which are used to **inhibit** the release of FSH and LH from the anterior pituitary when administered in a **continuous fashion**. Given SC (goserelin, histrelin, leuprolide), IM (leuprolide) or nasally (nafarelin)	Treatment of children with gonadotropin dependent **precocious puberty**. Treatment of hormone sensitive tumors such as **prostate and breast cancer**. Infertility	Hot flashes Increased bone pain in patients with prostate cancer.
Human chorionic gonadotropin (APL®, Pregnyl®)	Produced by the placenta and extracted from the urine of pregnant women. Similar to **LH** in both structure and function. Given IM	Used to distinguish **cryptorchidism** from **pseudocryptorchism** **Prepubertal cryptorchidism** Infertility in men due to pituitary dysfunction. Stimulate ovulation: used in conjunction with menotropin or urofollitropin in patients refractory to clomiphene.	**Thromboembolic events** **Ovarian cysts, ovarian enlargement** Ovarian hyperstimulation syndrome Peripheral edema Headache, depression Precocious puberty may occur when treating cryptorchidism.

Drug	MOA & Pharmacokinetics	Clinical Uses	Side Effects
Menotropin (hMG) (Pergonal®)	**FSH** and **LH** containing extracts derived from the urine of postmenopausal women. Given IM	Infertility in men and women	Ovarian enlargement Ovarian hyperstimulation syndrome Thromboembolism Atelectasis, ARDS Gynecomastia in men
Urofollitropin (Metrodin®)	A substance with **FSH-like activity** isolated from human urine. Given IM	Infertility in women	Ovarian enlargement Ovarian hyperstimulation syndrome

Hormones that Regulate Corticosteroid Release

Drug	MOA & Pharmacokinetics	Clinical Uses	Side Effects
Corticotropin releasing hormone (CRH)	Stimulates the secretion of ACTH from the anterior pituitary. Given IV	Used diagnostically to differentiate Cushing's disease from ectopic ACTH production. The dexamethasone suppression test, however, is more frequently used clinically. ACTH response to CRH is usually used as an adjuvant test.	Transient facial flushing
Cosyntropin (Cortrosyn®)	A **synthetic ACTH derivative** (the first 24 amino acids only) which stimulates the release of adrenocorticosteroids. Given IM	Diagnosis of adrenal insufficiency	Similar to glucocorticoids

Bromocriptine

Drug	MOA & Pharmacokinetics	Clinical Uses	Side Effects
Bromocriptine (Parlodel®)	An **ergot-derived dopamine agonist** which decreases pituitary prolactin secretion. Growth hormone stimulant Given PO, IM	**Prolactinoma** **Amenorrhea, galactorrhea** and **infertility** secondary to hyperprolactinemia. **Acromegaly** due to its ability reduce serum growth hormone levels. Parkinsonism: usually in conjunction with L-dopa/carbidopa	In low doses: nausea, lightheadedness and confusion At high doses: cold-induced digital vasospasm, neuropsychiatric effects

Posterior Pituitary Hormones and Analogs

These hormones are synthesized in the hypothalamus and stored and released from the posterior pituitary.

Drug	MOA & Pharmacokinetics	Clinical Uses	Side Effects
Oxytocin (Pitocin®)	Stimulates the force and frequency of **uterine contractions**. The uterus becomes more sensitive to oxytocin as pregnancy evolves. It causes **milk ejection** by contracting myoepithelial cells surrounding mammary alveoli. Enhances dilation of the cervix. Exhibits weak antidiuretic and pressor activity. Given IV or intranasally	**Induces** and **reinforces labor** especially at term in patients with delivery problems. **Stimulates milk ejection** in patients with impaired lactation (administered nasally) Control of postpartum and postabortal uterine hemorrhage Used to diagnose fetal distress or utero-placental insufficiency in high risk pregnancies.	**Hypertensive episodes** **Uterine rupture** At high doses: • Long lasting contractions ("hard uterus") which may be detrimental to the fetus • Decreased blood pressure, flushing and reflex tachycardia due to vascular smooth muscle relaxation • Hyponatremia secondary to water retention due to its antidiuretic effects
Vasopressin (ADH) (Pitressin®, Pressyn®) ADH: Adds hydration to the body	Activates $\mathbf{V_2}$ receptors on the renal tubule cells to increase the number of water channels in the kidney collecting tubules. This results in the increased reabsorption of water and the formation of a concentrated urine. It interacts with $\mathbf{V_1}$ receptors on vascular smooth muscle cells to cause smooth muscle contraction. Increases the release of Factor VIII and von Willebrand factor. Given IV or intranasally	**Central diabetes insipidus** Variceal bleeding or colonic diverticular bleeding: causes the cessation of bleeding because of its vasoconstrictive properties.	Headache, nausea, abdominal cramps Hyponatremia due to antidiuretic effect Hypertension Bradycardia

Drug	MOA & Pharmacokinetics	Clinical Uses	Side Effects
Desmopressin acetate (DDAVP®)	Long acting **synthetic analog** of **vasopressin** which activates V_2 receptors on the renal tubule cells to increase the number of water channels in the kidney collecting tubules. This increases the reabsorption of water and the formation of a concentrated urine. Minimal activity at V_1 receptors. Increases the release of Factor VIII and von Willebrand factor. Given IV, SC or intranasally	**Central diabetes insipidus**: **DOC** Nocturnal enuresis Hemophilia A von Willebrand's disease	Headache, nausea, abdominal cramps Hyponatremia at high doses

Thyroid and Antithyroid Drugs

Thyroid diseases manifest in the gland's hypo- or hyperfunction. Control of **hypothyroidism** is achieved by replacing the absent hormones. Treatment of **hyperthyroidism** aims at decreasing excessive functioning of the gland. There are many agents available to treat hyperthyroidism; they act pharmacologically at various points in the synthesis of thyroid hormones. The modalities used in treating these various thyroid conditions are summarized below.

Treatment of Hypothyroidism	
T3	T4
Liothyronine sodium	Levothyroxine sodium

Treatment of Hyperthyroidism					
Antithyroid Drugs	Iodide	Radioiodine	Ionic Inhibitors	Miscellaneous	Symptomatic Therapy
Propylthiouracil Methimazole	Lugol's solution Potassium iodide	^{123}I ^{131}I	Thiocyanate Perchlorate	Iopanoic acid Sodium ipodate	β-blockers

Thyroid Hormone Synthesis

Before looking at the agents available for treating thyroid disorders, it is helpful to review some thyroid physiology. The thyroid gland secretes two types of hormones. The first type is the iodine-containing proteins, thyroxine (T4) and triiodothyronine (T3), which are important for growth, development and maintenance of metabolic homeostasis. The second type is calcitonin which helps maintain calcium homeostasis.
T3 and T4 are formed by the iodination of tyrosine residues of the protein thyroglobulin in a series of discrete steps. Below is a summary of the major processes involved in thyroid hormone synthesis.

Figure 7.1: Thyroid hormone synthesis

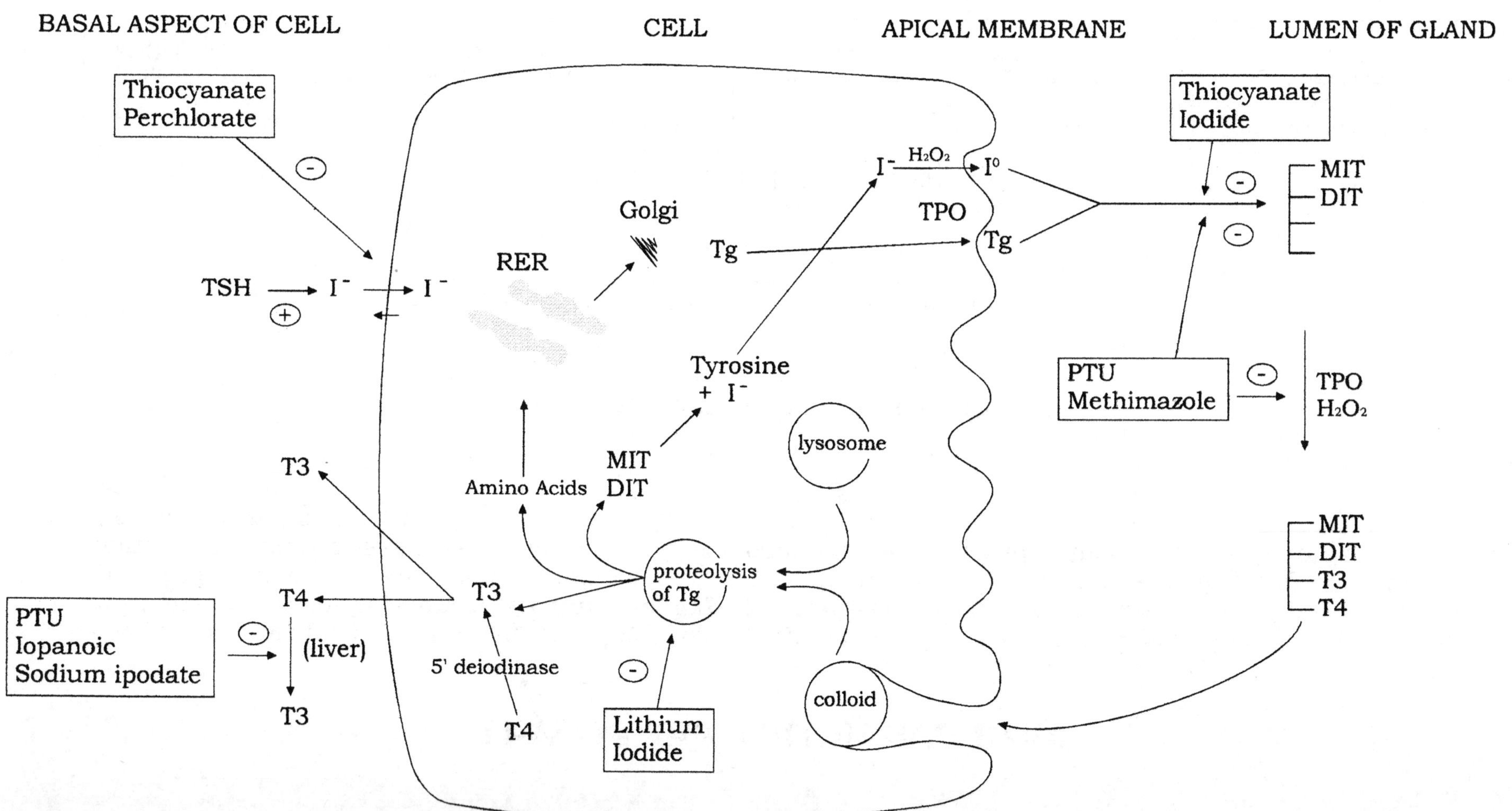

Process	Description
Iodide transport and oxidation	Iodide is transported into the thyroid gland by a facilitated sodium coupled transport system. Once in the cell, iodide is oxidized. The oxidized iodide then diffuses across the apical membrane of the cell and is concentrated in the follicular lumen.
Thyroglobulin (Tg) secretion	Thyroglobulin is a large 660 kD polypeptide composed of four subunits. Each subunit has a preferred tyrosine residue for iodination. Once thyroglobulin is formed, it is secreted into the follicular lumen.
Thyroglobulin iodination Coupling of iodotyrosine residues	At the apical surface of the follicular thyroid cell, tyrosine residues of thyroglobulin are iodinated by the enzyme thyroperoxidase (TPO) to form monoiodotyrosines (MIT) and diiodotyrosines (DIT). TPO is also responsible for facilitating the coupling of DIT to either another DIT or a MIT to form tetraiodothyronine (thyroxine, T4) or triiodothyronine (T3), respectively.
Secretion of thyroid hormones	Colloid droplets, reabsorbed by the thyroid follicular cell, fuse with lysosomes. Thyroglobulin is hydrolyzed into its constituent amino acids within the lysosomes. The liberated T3 and T4 diffuse into the circulation.
Recirculation of hydrolysis products	The monoiodotyrosines and diiodotyrosine of the hydrolyzed thyroglobulin are deiodinated by iodotyrosine deiodinase. The released iodide ions recirculate to participate again in the iodination of thyroglobulin. The amino acids released from the hydrolysis of thyroglobulin and MIT and DIT are also recirculated.
Circulating thyroid hormones	The majority of secreted T3 and T4 are not free in the circulation but are bound by several proteins such as thyroxine-binding globulin (TBG), albumin, and thyroxine-binding prealbumin (TBPA).
Regulation of thyroid hormone secretion	Thyroid function is under the control of the hypothalamic-pituitary-thyroid axis. Thyrotropin-releasing hormone (TRH), secreted by the hypothalamus, reaches the anterior pituitary and causes increased production of thyroid-stimulating hormone (TSH). TSH in turn acts on thyroid follicular cells to increase thyroid hormone synthesis and release. T3 and T4 provide negative feedback to both the anterior pituitary and hypothalamus.

Salient Features of Thyroid Hormones

Comparison of thyroid hormones:

T3 and T4 are the major forms of thyroid hormone released from the thyroid gland. After release into the bloodstream, the majority of T3 and T4 is bound to several serum proteins but only unbound (free) hormone is metabolically active. The major carrier for T3 and T4 is thyroxine-binding globulin (TBG). Although both T3 and T4 can also bind albumin, only T4 can bind thyroxine-binding prealbumin (TBP). The half life of these hormones is dependent on their affinity for the carrier proteins. Thyroxine, which binds serum proteins with a higher affinity, has a half-life of 8 days whereas triiodothyronine, which is less avidly bound, has a half life of 1 day.

	Concentration (μg/dL)			% Bound to Serum Proteins				
	Total	Free	% Free	TBG	Albumin	TBPA	$t_{1/2}$	Activity
Triiodothyronine (T3)	0.12	0.0004	0.3%	60	40	-	1 day	10
Thyroxine (T4)	8.5	0.002	0.03%	50	35	15	8 day	1

Peripheral metabolism of thyroid hormones:

Whereas T4 is produced only by the thyroid gland, the majority of T3 is produced by peripheral deiodination of T4 in many tissues. The major extra-thyroid site of conversion of T4 to T3 is the liver; other sites include the kidney, heart and anterior pituitary. T4 is metabolized to active T3 or reverse T3, which is an inactive metabolite.

Actions of thyroid hormones:

Thyroid hormones have many functions within the body. Thyroid hormones stimulate calorigenesis, increase cardiac output and promote growth and development including CNS development. Thyroid hormones also affect carbohydrate metabolism, lipid turnover and protein metabolism. The effects of T3 and T4 are mediated by **nuclear receptors** which increase the transcription of various genes. Although both T3 and T4 can bind to these receptors, the affinity of **T3 is about 10-fold greater**, and most consider **T4** to be a **prohormone**.

Treatment of Hypothyroidism

Drug	MOA & Pharmacokinetics	Clinical Uses	Side Effects
Levothyroxine sodium (T4) (Synthroid®, Levothroid®)	Absorbed in the small intestine. Cholestyramine resins and $Al(OH)_3$ decrease absorption. $t_{1/2}$ = 7 days	**Hypothyroidism**: most therapeutic uses involve administration of **thyroxine (T4)** due to its prolonged duration of action. One possible exception is myxedema coma in which T3 might be preferred due to its quicker onset of action. **Hormone replacement therapy** in hypothyroid patients **Prevention of cretinism** in hypothyroid newborns; therapy must be initiated at or shortly after birth to prevent detrimental consequences including mental retardation. Treatment after thyroid cancer in which the goal of therapy is suppression of TSH. Note: in pregnant hypothyroid women, dosage often needs to be increased (most likely due to increased production of TBG caused by estrogen).	Cardiac effects: palpitations, arrhythmias Thyrotoxicosis
Liothyronine sodium (T3) (Cytomel®, Triostat®)	Absorbed in the small intestine. Cholestyramine resins and $Al(OH)_3$ decrease absorption. $t_{1/2}$ = 2 days	**Myxedema coma**: this medical emergency is seen in cases of severe, long-standing hypothyroidism and is characterized by hypothermia, respiratory depression and unconsciousness.	Cardiac effects: palpitations, arrhythmias Thyrotoxicosis

Treatment of Hyperthyroidism

Antithyroid drugs

Drugs	MOA & Pharmacokinetics	Clinical Uses	Side Effects
Propylthiouracil (PTU) (Propyl-Thyracil®) Remember: only one antithyroid drug inhibits the peripheral conversion of T4 to T3: PTU.	**Inhibits thyroid peroxidase** thereby preventing iodination of tyrosyl residues of thyroglobulin and coupling of iodotyrosine residues. **Inhibits the peripheral deiodination** of T4 to T3. 80% is bound to serum proteins, primarily albumin. Because it is highly protein bound PTU has a lower concentration in breast milk and crosses the placenta to a **lesser degree** than methimazole. Shorter $t_{1/2}$ than methimazole (1-2 hours).	Graves' disease Radiation adjuvant: used in patients treated with ^{131}I while awaiting radiation effects. Conversion of a hyperthyroid patient to euthyroid prior to surgical treatment. This has been shown to reduce operative morbidity and mortality. Thyrotoxicosis in pregnant and nursing women.	**Transient leukopenia** Fever Skin rash Itching Joint pain Hypothyroidism Agranulocytosis in 0.44%
Methimazole (Tapazole®)	**Inhibits thyroid peroxidase** thereby preventing iodination of tyrosyl residues of thyroglobulin and coupling of iodotyrosine residues. Does NOT inhibit peripheral deiodination of T4 to T3. Because it is less protein bound, methimazole has a higher concentration in breast milk and crosses the placenta to a **greater degree** than PTU. Longer $t_{1/2}$ than PTU (5-6 hours).	Same as for PTU, except it is not indicated in treating pregnant women with thyrotoxicosis due to its higher transplacental and breast milk transfer.	Same as PTU except that the incidence of agranulocytosis is less than with PTU (0.12%).

Iodide based agents

Drugs	MOA & Pharmacokinetics	Clinical Uses	Side Effects
Lugol's solution (Strong iodine solution)	Inhibits release of T3 and T4 from the thyroid gland. Acutely inhibits the iodination of thyroglobulin (**Wolff-Chaikoff Effect**). Contains 5% iodine, 10% potassium iodide. The iodine component is reduced to iodide in the intestine prior to absorption.	Graves' disease Radiation adjuvant: used in patients treated with ^{131}I while awaiting radiation effects. Conversion of a hyperthyroid patient to euthyroid prior to surgical treatment. This has been shown to reduce operative morbidity and mortality.	Acute reaction: • **Angioedema** • Swelling of the larynx • Cutaneous hemorrhages • Symptoms of serum sickness such as fever, arthralgia, lymphadenopathy and eosinophilia Chronic reaction (**iodism**): • Brassy taste and burning in the mouth • Soreness of teeth and gums • Increased salivation • Coryza and sneezing • Swelling of the eyelids • Skin lesions • Respiratory problems
Potassium iodide (KI, Pima®, Thyro-Block®)	Inhibits release of T3 and T4 from the thyroid gland. Acutely inhibits the iodination of thyroglobulin (**Wolff-Chaikoff Effect**). Saturated solution of iodide.	Same as for Lugol's solution. Sporotrichosis	Iodine-induced hypothyroidism in euthyroid patients who have a history of various underlying thyroid disorders.

Radioactive iodide

^{123}I and ^{131}I are radioactive iodide species which are specifically taken up by the thyroid gland, incorporated into thyroglobulin and concentrated in colloid. These radioactive species are cytotoxic and eventually destroy the thyroid gland without causing damage to other cells in the body.

Drugs	MOA & Pharmacokinetics	Clinical Uses	Side Effects
^{131}I	Emits both β particles and γ rays. The β particles cause destruction of the thyroid parenchyma with little effect on surrounding structures. $t_{1/2}$ = 8 days Crosses the placenta and may cause severe and irreversible hypothyroidism in the fetus. Found in breast milk.	Hyperthyroidism Treatment of hyperthyroidism in older patients and those with cardiac diseases. Graves' disease: DOC for persistent or recurrent Graves' disease after subtotal thyroidectomy or antithyroid drugs have failed. Toxic nodular goiter	High incidence of delayed hypothyroidism. Delayed onset of therapeutic effects. Although there is no definitive evidence that radioactive iodine causes thyroid or other cancers, its use is primarily restricted to patients over the age of 30. ◆ Contraindications: Pregnancy Nursing mothers Coexisting severe ophthalmopathy (may exacerbate condition)
^{123}I	Emits γ and x-rays. $t_{1/2}$ = 13 hrs	^{123}I is used as a diagnostic tool for thyroid function (thyroid scanning).	

Ionic Inhibitors

Drugs	MOA & Pharmacokinetics	Clinical Uses	Side Effects
Thiocyanate	Competitively inhibits iodide transport mechanism in thyroid follicular cells. In high doses, inhibits thyroglobulin iodination.	Rarely used to treat hyperthyroidism; seldomly used diagnostically.	
Perchlorate	Same MOA as thiocyanate.	Same as thiocyanate.	Fatal aplastic anemia

Miscellaneous agents

Drugs	MOA & Pharmacokinetics	Clinical Uses	Side Effects
Iopanoic acid (Telepaque®) Sodium ipodate (Oragrafin®)	Inhibit the peripheral conversion of T4 to T3.	Short term treatment of hyperthyroid states	

Symptomatic therapy

Drugs	MOA & Pharmacokinetics	Clinical Uses	Side Effects
Propanolol	Blocks both β_1 and β_2 receptors on tissues. No effect on thyroid function.	Hyperthyroidism: used to alleviate the signs and symptoms of such as sweating, tremor, palpitations and tachycardia. Radiation adjuvant: used in patients treated with ^{131}I while awaiting radiation effects.	

Surgical treatment

Procedure	Clinical indication
Subtotal thyroidectomy	Graves' disease in young patients with very large goiters Children and pregnant women allergic to antithyroid drugs Patients who prefer surgery to drug treatment or radioactive iodine Toxic nodular goiter (since it is usually unresponsive to antithyroid drugs)

Figure 7.2: Steroid hormone synthesis

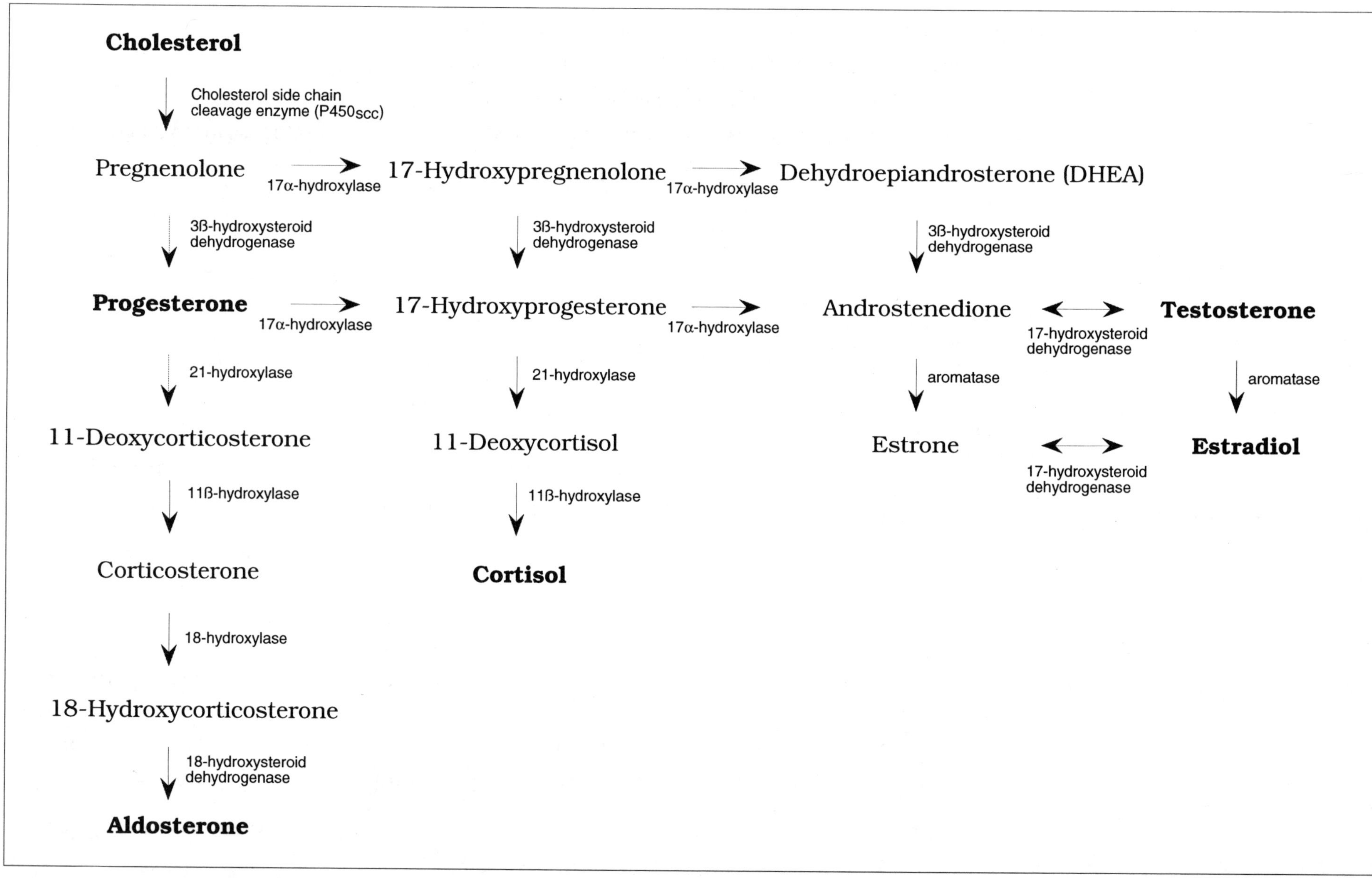

Adrenocorticosteroids and Antagonists

Adrenocorticosteroids are steroid hormones secreted from the adrenal cortex. They include glucocorticoids, mineralocorticoids and sex hormones. Analogs of these hormones are used in the diagnosis and treatment of adrenal, inflammatory and immunologic diseases.

Steroid hormones mediate their effects via transcriptional activation of target genes. These hormones are extremely lipophilic and are therefore able to diffuse through the lipid bilayer. Once inside the cell, they bind to either cytoplasmic or nuclear receptors. These complexes are then able to bind hormone responsive elements located in the promoter of genes and thus activate transcription. Once transcribed, the mRNAs are subsequently translated into proteins which mediate the observed physiological effects induced by these hormones.

Glucocorticoids	Glucocorticoid Antagonists	Mineralocorticoids
Cortisol Cortisone Corticosterone Prednisolone Prednisone Methylprednisolone Triamcinolone Dexamethasone Betamethasone Beclomethasone	Aminoglutethimide Metyrapone O.p'DDD RU486	Fludrocortisone Aldosterone

Secretion of adrenocorticosteroids is regulated by the hypothalamic-pituitary axis. In response to low levels of adrenocorticosteroids, the hypothalamus secretes corticotropin-releasing hormone (CRH) which stimulates the release of ACTH from the anterior pituitary. ACTH binds receptors on the adrenal cortex resulting in the secretion of adrenocorticosteroids. Mineralocorticoid secretion is also controlled by renin-angiotensin system.

The adrenal cortex has three components each of which secretes different hormones:

Region	Hormones Released	Effects
Zona glomerulosa	mineralocorticoids	salt retention
Zona fasciculata	glucocorticoids	anti-inflammatory immunosuppressive
Zona reticularis	sex hormones	sexual development fertility

Glucocorticoids

Cortisol is a potent endogenous glucocorticoid secreted by the adrenal cortex in response to ACTH. It is highly plasma protein bound: 75% to cortisol binding protein, 15% to albumin and 10% free. The actions of cortisol are listed below.

Actions	Mechanism
Anti-inflammatory	Suppresses cyclooxygenase expression. Increases expression of lipocortin, an inhibitor of phospholipase A2.
Immunosuppression	Prevents proliferation of activated T cells. Inhibits production of antibodies.
Increased blood glucose	↑ gluconeogenesis ↑ lipolysis ↑ muscle catabolism
Increased salt uptake	Stimulates the Na^{+}-H^{+} antiport system at the luminal epithelium of the kidney, gut and salivary glands.

Glucocorticoid Therapy

Among available glucocorticoids, there is variation in glucocorticoid activity (anti-inflammatory properties) and mineralocorticoid activity (Na^+ retention). In addition, glucocorticoids can be divided into different categories based on half-life: short-acting ($t_{1/2}$ = 8-12 hrs), intermediate-acting ($t_{1/2}$ = 12-36 hrs) and long-acting ($t_{1/2}$ = 36-72 hrs). Another glucocorticoid, **beclomethasone**, is noteworthy because it is available as an inhalant and is used in the treatment of asthma.

<table>
<tr><th>Drug</th><th>Anti-inflammatory activity</th><th>Na^+-retaining activity</th><th>$t_{1/2}$ (hrs)</th><th>Clinical Uses</th><th>Side Effects</th></tr>
<tr><td>Cortisol</td><td>1</td><td>1</td><td rowspan="3">8-12</td><td rowspan="3">Replacement therapy: DOC
Anti-inflammatory</td><td rowspan="9">Adrenal suppression: muscle wasting, striae, truncal obesity, moon facies, buffalo hump
Salt retention
Hyperglycemia
Psychological disturbances
Osteoporosis
Growth defects
Immunosuppression</td></tr>
<tr><td>Cortisone</td><td>0.8</td><td>0.8</td></tr>
<tr><td>Corticosterone</td><td>0.85</td><td>15</td></tr>
<tr><td>Prednisolone</td><td>4</td><td>0.8</td><td rowspan="3">12-36</td><td rowspan="3">Prednisone is the inactive precursor of prednisolone.
Anti-inflammatory
Immunosuppressive
Chemotherapy: prednisone is part of the MOPP regimen</td></tr>
<tr><td>Prednisone (Delta-cortef®, Deltasone®)</td><td></td><td></td></tr>
<tr><td>Methylprednisolone (Depro-medrol®, Medrol®)</td><td>5</td><td>0.5</td></tr>
<tr><td>Triamcinolone (Aristocort®, Kenacort®)</td><td>5</td><td>0</td><td>12-36</td><td>Anti-inflammatory
Immunosuppressive</td></tr>
<tr><td>Dexamethasone (Decadron®, Decaderm®, Gammacorten®, Hexadrol®, Maxidex®)</td><td>30</td><td>0</td><td>36-72</td><td>Diagnosis of Cushing's disease
Anti-inflammatory
Immunosuppressive
ACTH suppression
Cerebral edema</td></tr>
<tr><td>Betamethasone (Benisone®, Celestone®)</td><td>30</td><td>0</td><td>36-72</td><td>Anti-inflammatory
Immunosuppressive
ACTH suppression
Induction of surfactant synthesis in fetal lung for preterm labor</td></tr>
</table>

Adrenocorticosteroid Antagonists

Adrenocorticosteroid antagonists are used to treat adrenal gland hypersecretion. They either prevent the synthesis of adrenal corticosteroids or block corticosteroid receptors.

Drug	MOA & Pharmacokinetics	Clinical Uses	Side Effects
Aminoglutethimide (Cytadren®)	Prevents the synthesis of cortisol by inhibiting **desmolase**.	Breast cancer: used in conjunction with dexamethasone Cushing's syndrome: secondary to adrenocortical cancer	Lethargy at high doses
Metyrapone (Metopirone®)	Prevents cortisol production by inhibiting 11 β-hydroxylase.	Diagnostic tests of adrenal function	Edema Hirsutism
O.p'DDD (Mitotane®, Lysodren®)	Destroys cells of the zona fasciculata and zona reticularis.	Adrenocortical carcinoma	
RU486 (Mifepristone®)	Inhibits glucocorticoid and progesterone receptors.	Cushing's syndrome Abortifacient	

Mineralocorticoid Therapy

Mineralocorticoids increase the excretion of K^+ and H^+ and the reabsorption of Na^+ and water in the distal tubule of the kidney. The most important endogenous mineralocorticoid is aldosterone. Like cortisol, its synthesis and secretion are stimulated by ACTH from the pituitary. However, the most important stimuli for aldosterone release are a decrease in blood volume (via renin-angiotensin) and an increase in plasma K^+.

Drug	Anti-inflammatory activity	Na^+-retaining activity	$t_{1/2}$ (hrs)	Clinical Uses	Side Effects
Aldosterone	0	500			
Fludrocortisone (Florinef®)	15	150	8-12	**Addison's disease**	Anaphylaxis Congestive heart failure Hypokalemia Drug Interactions: Digitalis Phenytoin Rifampin Hypokalemic drugs

Notes

Sex Hormones

The sex hormones **progestins**, **estrogens** and **androgens**, are part of the steroid family. They are all derived from cholesterol and confer activity by a similar mechanism. Analogs of these hormones are used for hormone replacement therapy, oral contraception and treatment of hormone-responsive cancers. Conversely, antagonists of sex hormones are used to treat disorders characterized by the overproduction of hormones. The following table lists the drugs that will be discussed in this section

Estrogens	Antiestrogens
Estradiol Estrone Ethinyl estradiol Mestranol	Clomiphene Tamoxifen

Progestins	Antiprogestins
Medroxyprogesterone Norethindrone Norethindrone acetate	Mifepristone Danazol

Androgens	Antiandrogens
Testosterone Methyltestosterone Fluoxymesterone	Finasteride Spironolactone Cyproterone Flutamide

Steroid Hormone Synthesis

Progesterone, the most important progestin, is an early derivative of cholesterol and is the compound from which estrogens, androgens and adrenocorticosteroids are ultimately derived.

Figure 7.3: Sex hormone synthesis

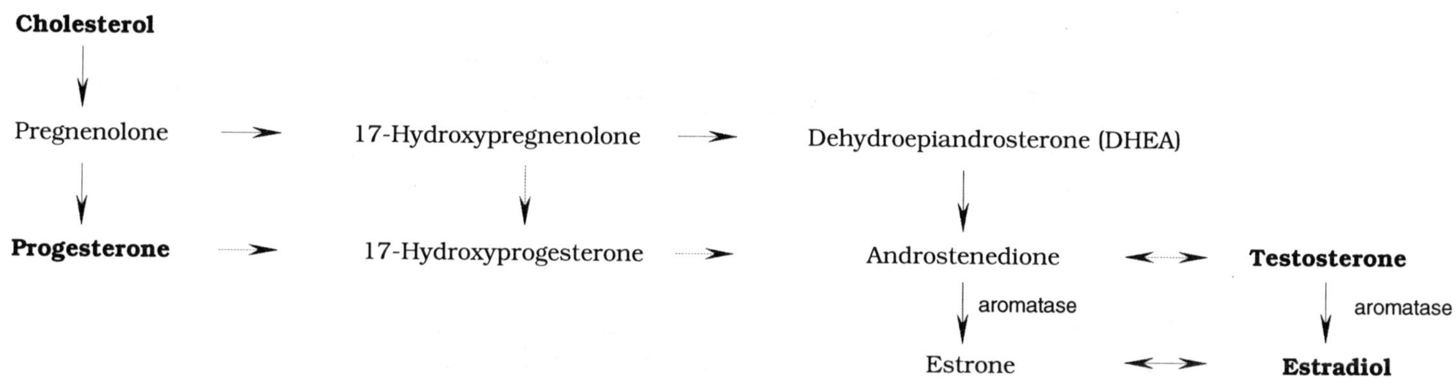

Estrogens

The estrogens are cholesterol derivatives which are involved in female development and regulation of the menstrual cycle. They are 18-carbon steroids which are directly converted from androstenedione or testosterone by **aromatase**. In premenopausal women, the granulosa cells of the ovaries are the major site of estrogen synthesis. In men and postmenopausal women, the major site of estrogen production is adipose tissue. Of the endogenous estrogens, estradiol is the most potent.

Action	
Development in females	Important in the development of female secondary sexual characteristics.
Neuroendocrine effects	Regulation of the menstrual cycle and pregnancy. Provides negative feedback to the pituitary and down regulates LH and FSH release.
Metabolic effects	1) ↑ in bone mass by promoting Ca^{2+} retention 2) ↑ HDL while ↓ LDL and triglycerides 3) ↑ production of sex hormone binding globulin, corticosteroid binding globulin and clotting factors II, VII, IX and X 4) Promotes fat mobilization and subcutaneous deposition 5) ↑ in protein formation (anabolic effect)

Estrogens

Although estrogen itself cannot be administered orally, several synthetic estrogens are available for oral administration. Therapeutic uses of **estrogens** include oral contraception and treatment of conditions which decrease estrogen production, such as menopause. **Antiestrogens** are used to treat infertility and breast cancer.

Drug	MOA & Pharmacokinetics	Clinical Uses	Side Effects
Estradiol Estrone Ethinyl estradiol (Estinyl®, Feminone®) Mestranol (Enovid®, Norinyl®)	Bind the estrogen receptor and form a complex which stimulates transcription of target genes. Exogenous administration inhibits FSH secretion and prevents ovulation. Mestranol is the methyl derivative of ethinyl estradiol. Given PO, transdermally	**Oral contraceptives**: in combination with progestins **Postmenopausal hormone therapy**: in combination with progestin. Can be given alone in women who have had a hysterectomy. **Hypogonadism in females** Osteoporosis: prevention and treatment Infertility Dysmenorrhea Prostate cancer	Hypertension Breast tenderness Endometrial hyperplasia Breakthrough bleeding Edema ◆ Contraindications: Pregnancy Breast cancer

Antiestrogen

Drug	MOA & Pharmacokinetics	Clinical Uses	Side Effects
Clomiphene (Clomid®, Serophene®)	A **partial agonist** at estrogen receptors in the pituitary which imparts antiestrogen activity via **competitive inhibition** in the presence of estrogen. This prevents feedback inhibition, increases LH and FSH and stimulates ovulation. Given PO	**Female infertility**: to stimulate ovulation. Male infertility: has been used to induce spermatogenesis.	**Hot flashes** Ovarian enlargement, ovarian cysts Multiple births Ovarian hyperstimulation
Tamoxifen (Nolvadex®)	**Nonsteroidal antiestrogen** which competitively inhibits estrogen at the estrogen receptor. Given PO	**Breast cancer**: drug of choice for endocrine management of estrogen receptor positive breast cancer.	**Hot flashes** **GI effects**: nausea, vomiting GU effects: menstrual irregularities, vulvar pruritus

Progestins

Progesterone is the prototypical progestin in the body. It is produced in various tissues including the ovary, testis, adrenal cortex and placenta. In the ovary, progesterone is secreted from the corpus luteum during the second half of the menstrual cycle. In cases where the ovum is successfully fertilized, the resulting trophoblast secretes human chorionic gonadotropin (hCG) into the maternal circulation. hCG maintains the corpus luteum resulting in high plasma progesterone levels. The presence of urinary hCG is evaluated as a positive pregnancy test.

The hormonal effects of progestins are outlined below:

Effects of Progestins	
Neuroendocrine effects	Progestins produced in the luteal phase decrease the frequency of the hypothalamic pulse.
Reproductive tract	1. Development of secretory endometrium. 2. Modification of the vaginal epithelium to a pregnancy epithelium (maintains pregnancy). 3. Alteration in cervical gland secretion from watery to viscous.
Mammary glands	Proliferation of mammary glands during pregnancy.
CNS	1. ↑ in body temperature (1°C) corresponding to the time of ovulation. 2. ↑ ventilatory response to CO_2 during the luteal phase and pregnancy.
Metabolic effects	1. ↑ insulin secretion. 2. Stimulation of lipoprotein lipase activity resulting in fat deposition. 3. ↓ in Na^+ reabsorption by inhibiting aldosterone receptors at the renal tubule resulting in increased aldosterone release. 4. ↓ HDL, ↑ LDL

Progestins

Due to its high first-pass effect, progesterone is not used therapeutically. However, several synthetic progestins have been developed which are maintained more effectively in the body. These synthetic **progestins** are used for replacement therapy and in contraceptives. **Antiprogestins** are used as abortifacients or for postcoital contraception.

Drug	MOA & Pharmacokinetics	Clinical Uses	Side Effects
Medroxyprogesterone (Provera®) Norethindrone (Norlutin®) Norethindrone acetate (Norlutate®, Aygestin®)	Binds to progestin receptors and stimulates transcription of target genes. Given IM, PO (medroxyprogesterone) Given PO (norethindrone and norethindrone acetate)	**Contraception**: alone or with estradiol. **Postmenopausal hormone therapy**: in combination with estrogens. Dysmenorrhea and endometriosis	Weight gain Edema Depression Thrombophlebitis

Antiprogestins

Drug	MOA & Pharmacokinetics	Clinical Uses	Side Effects
Mifepristone (RU486®)	A **competitive inhibitor** of progestins at progesterone receptors in the presence of progestin. In the absence of progestin, mifepristone acts as a **partial agonist**. Mifepristone is also a competitive inhibitor of glucocorticoids at the glucocorticoid receptor. $t_{1/2}$ = 20-40 hrs Given PO	**Abortifacient**: usually given concomitantly with PGE or PGF to increase myometrial contractions. Postcoital contraception Cushing's syndrome	Infrequent but include: Heavy bleeding GI effects: nausea, vomiting, anorexia and abdominal pain
Danazol (Cyclomen®, Danocrine®)	Exhibits agonist effects at progesterone, androgen and glucocorticoid receptors.	**Endometriosis** Fibrocystic disease of the breast	Weight gain Edema Acne

Androgens

Androgens are 19-carbon steroids which are fundamental to male development. In males, 95% of androgen production occurs in the Leydig cells of the testes and 5% in the adrenal cortex. In females, the ovary is the major site of androgen production. Four androgens are produced by the testes: testosterone, dihydrotestosterone (DHT), dehydroepiandrosterone (DHEA) and androstenedione. Of these, testosterone is the most important.

Leydig cells produce testosterone in response to LH secretion by the anterior pituitary. Meanwhile, FSH induces the synthesis of androgen-binding protein by the Sertoli cells of the testes. Testosterone is responsible for the negative feedback which inhibits secretion of LH from the pituitary. Testosterone is converted to DHT by 5α-reductase in the skin, epididymis, seminal vesicles and prostate.

Testosterone exhibits both androgenic and anabolic activities. Synthetic androgens which maintain anabolic effects while minimizing androgenic effects have been used (abused) in order to enhance athletic performance. Since the anabolic effects of these drugs cannot be completely separated from the androgenic effects, use of these drugs to increase muscle strength is accompanied by androgenic side effects.

Testosterone and dihydrotestosterone	
Male development	1. Stimulate development and maturation of sperm. 2. Stimulate development of the epididymis, vas deferens and seminal vesicles. 3. Provide negative feedback to gonadotropin secretion. 4. Stimulate development of the scrotum, penis and prostate. 5. Stimulate development of secondary sexual characteristics in males.
Others	1. Anabolic effects on muscle and bone mass. 2. Increase erythrocyte production. 3. Masculinization in females.

Androgens

Synthetic **androgens** are used to treat pituitary or hypothalamic diseases which result in the loss of gonadotropins. A less common use is the treatment of anemia. **Antiandrogens** are used to treat androgen excess in females and prostate disease in males.

Drug	MOA & Pharmacokinetics	Clinical Uses	Side Effects
Methyltestosterone (Android®) Fluoxymesterone (Halotestin®)	Bind the androgen receptor and stimulate transcription from genes containing androgen responsive elements. Given PO	**Hormone replacement therapy**: for hypogonadism in men and hypopituitarism in women. Anemia: testosterone can enhance erythropoietin secretion in some refractory anemias. Breast cancer: due to testosterone's antiestrogenic activity. Osteoporosis	Masculinizing effects in women: hirsutism, acne, clitoral enlargement. Alteration in serum lipid profiles. Hepatocellular carcinoma ◆ Contraindications: Pregnant women Patients with prostate cancer

Antiandrogens

Drug	MOA & Pharmacokinetics	Clinical Uses	Side Effects
Finasteride (Proscar®)	Prevents the synthesis of dihydrotestosterone by **inhibiting** the activity of **5 α-reductase**. Given PO	**Benign prostatic hyperplasia**	
Spironolactone (Aldactone®)	Competitive inhibitor at androgen and aldosterone receptors. Decreases androgen levels by reducing 17α-hydroxylase activity.	Potassium sparing diuretic Hirsutism	Hyperkalemia GI disturbances
Cyproterone (Androcur®)	Steroid inhibitor at androgen receptors.	Hirsutism Prostatic carcinoma	
Flutamide (Eulexin®)	A **nonsteroidal competitive antagonist** at androgen receptors.	Prostatic carcinoma	Gynecomastia Hepatotoxic: mild, reversible

Notes

Hormonal Contraceptives

Hormonal contraceptives prevent the fertilization of an ovum. They utilize the negative feedback effects of estrogen and progesterone on the pituitary. The suppression of the LH and FSH surges prevents ovulation. While progesterone and estrogen can individually achieve this effect, they are more effective when combined. Presently, available contraceptives include oral combination pills and progestin only contraceptives. Oral combination contraceptives are approximately 98% effective; progestin only contraceptives are marginally less effective (approximately 97%). Additionally, some of these agents can be used as postcoital contraceptives.

Combination Oral Contraceptives		
Monophasic	Biphasic	Triphasic
Ethinyl estradiol/norethindrone Ethinyl estradiol/levonorgestrel Ethinyl estradiol/norgestrel Ethinyl estradiol/ethynodiol diacetate Mestranol/norethindrone Ethinyl estradiol/desogestrel Ethinyl estradiol/norgestimate	Ethinyl estradiol/norethindrone	Ethinyl estradiol/norethindrone Ethinyl estradiol/norgestimate Ethinyl estradiol/levonorgestrel

Progestin Only Contraceptives		
Oral (mini-pill)	Subdermal Implants	Injectable
Norethindrone Norgestrel	Levonorgestrel	Medroxyprogesterone acetate

Combination Oral Contraceptives

Combination oral contraceptives are available in three formulations: monophasic, biphasic and triphasic. Oral contraceptives are given 21 of a 28 day cycle which allows menses to occur in the remaining 7 days. For a complete listing of the different preparations available refer to the appendix. The side effects of these drugs can be decreased by altering the relative amounts of estrogen and progestin in the preparations. A **lower incidence** of **endometrial** and **ovarian cancer** has been observed in women taking oral contraceptives.

Drug	MOA & Pharmacokinetics	Side Effects
Monophasic: Ethinyl estradiol/norethindrone Ethinyl estradiol/levonorgestrel Ethinyl estradiol/norgestrel Ethinyl estradiol/ethynodiol diacetate Mestranol/norethindrone Ethinyl estradiol/desogestrel Ethinyl estradiol/norgestimate	Provide negative feedback on the pituitary which prevents LH and FSH release. This results in: • Depression of ovarian function and follicular development • Increased viscosity of cervical mucus • Production of stromal deciduation at the end of the cycle Provide a constant dose of estrogen and progestin throughout the 21 day cycle.	**Cardiovascular disease**: there is an increased of myocardial infarction especially for women over the age of 35 who smoke. Weight gain GI disturbances: nausea, bloating Acne and hirsutism Edema Breast tenderness Skin pigmentation CNS effects: dizziness, headaches Thromboembolism
Biphasic: Ethinyl estradiol/norethindrone	Same as for monophasic pills. Provides varying amounts of progestin while maintaining a constant dose of estrogen.	
Triphasic: Ethinyl estradiol/norethindrone Ethinyl estradiol/norgestimate Ethinyl estradiol/levonorgestrel	Same as for monophasic pills. Provide varying amount of progestin and estrogen.	

Progestin Only Contraceptives

In addition to the combination pills, single hormone contraceptive therapy is available. Progestin only contraception is appealing to patients who should not be given exogenous estrogens. Although these preparations prevent pregnancy by blocking ovulation, they are less effective than combination therapy.

Drug	Description	Side Effects
Oral Formulation: Norethindrone (Micronor®, Nor-QD®) Norgestrel (Ovrette®)	The "minipill". This formulation does not always inhibit ovulation and has been shown to be less effective than the combination pills.	**Bleeding irregularities**: especially spotting and breakthrough bleeding Weight gain Headaches GI disturbances: nausea, bloating Edema Thromboembolism Thromboembolic disorders
Subdermal: Levonorgestrel (Norplant®)	Delivered via 6 silastic tubes implanted in the upper arm. These implants deliver the hormone for up to 5 yrs.	
Injectable: Medroxyprogesterone acetate (Depo-provera®)	A single injection is given once every 3 months.	

Postcoital Contraception

Various agents can be used as postcoital contraceptives. These include high doses of estrogen (e.g. ethinyl estradiol) or estrogen progestin combination (e.g. ethinyl estradiol and norgestrel). In addition, RU486, an antagonist at glucocorticoid and progesterone receptors, is also used as a postcoital contraceptive.

Notes

Agents Influencing Bone Mineral Homeostasis

Calcium and phosphorous are important in maintaining adequate cellular function and are the two primary elements of bone. The body uses bone as its resource to maintain a constant serum concentration of calcium and phosphorous. The major regulators of serum calcium and phosphorous are parathyroid hormone (PTH) and vitamin D; minor regulators include calcitonin, glucocorticoids and estrogen.

This chapter focuses on the treatment of hypocalcemia and hypercalcemia. The major causes of hypocalcemia are **hypoparathyroidism**, **chronic renal failure** and **vitamin D deficiency**. The major symptoms of hypocalcemic states are **neuromuscular excitability** (tetany), **neurological complications** and **cataracts**. Calcium supplements and vitamin D agents are the two major forms of treatment for hypocalcemia.

Agents used in the Treatment of Hypocalcemia	
Calcium Salt Preparations	Vitamin D preparations
Calcium carbonate Calcium chloride Calcium gluceptate Calcium gluconate	Calcifediol Calcitriol Dihydrotachysterol Ergocalciferol

The major causes of hypercalcemia include **hyperparathyroidism**, **neoplasms** and **milk-alkali syndrome**. The major symptoms of hypercalcemic states are related to **nervous system depression** (muscle weakness, constipation and coma). The goal in treatment of hypercalcemic disorders is to normalize the serum calcium levels. Agents clinically used include bisphosphonates, calcitonin and others.

Agents used to Treat Hypercalcemic States		
Bisphosphonates	Calcitonin (CT)	Others
Etidronate Pamidronate Others	Human calcitonin Salmon calcitonin	Gallium nitrate Plicamycin Glucocorticoids Diuretics

The effects of the major endogenous regulators of serum calcium and phosphate levels are summarized below (Note: absorption occurs in the gut, reabsorption in the kidney and resorption in bone).

	Serum Ca^{2+} & PO_4^{2-}	Effect on Bone	Effect on Intestine	Effect on Kidney
Calcitonin	↓ Ca^{2+} ↓ PO_4^{2-}	↓ resorption	↓ Ca^{2+} absorption	
PTH	↑ Ca^{2+} ↓ PO_4^{2-}	↑ resorption	↑ Ca^{2+} and PO_4^{2-} absorption (secondary to ↑ Vitamin D)	↑ renal tubular Ca^{2+} reabsorption ↓ renal tubular PO_4^{2-} reabsorption ↑ conversion of vitamin D to calcitriol
Vitamin D	↑ Ca^{2+} ↑ PO_4^{2-}	↑ Ca^{2+} resorption	↑ Ca^{2+} and PO_4^{2-} absorption	↓ renal clearance of Ca^{2+} and PO_4^{2-}

Figure 7.4: Biosynthesis of Vitamin D

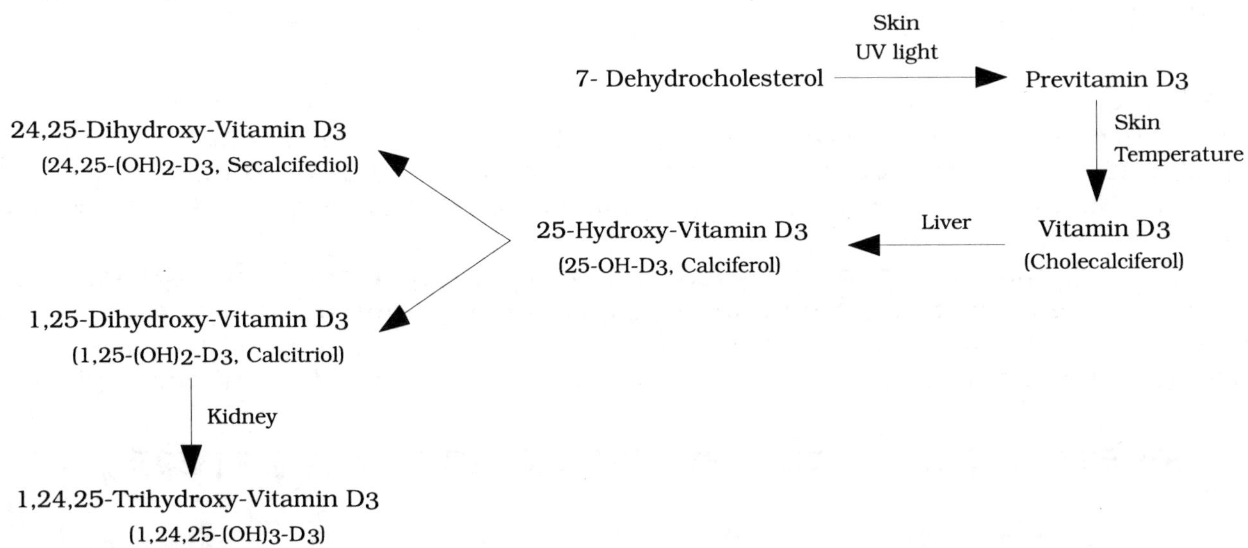

Treatment of Hypocalcemia

The treatment of hypocalcemia includes calcium salts and vitamin D agents. Calcium salts are used for the immediate treatment of **hypocalcemic tetany** (IV forms) as well as for **dietary supplementation** (oral forms). There are many different calcium salt preparations which have additional indications to those discussed here. For a more comprehensive list of available agents as well as additional properties, see Appendix.

Calcium Salt Preparations

Drug	IV	Oral	IM	Clinical Uses	Side Effects
Calcium carbonate (Tums®, Os-Cal®)		✓		Mild hypocalcemic symptoms	
Calcium chloride	✓			Hypocalcemic tetany Laryngospasm	Peripheral vasodilation which may lead to a fall in blood pressure Cutaneous burning sensation
Calcium gluceptate	✓		✓	Severe hypocalcemic tetany	Transient tingling sensation
Calcium gluconate	✓	✓	✓	**Severe hypocalcemic tetany**: IV form is DOC. Mild hypocalcemic symptoms: oral	

Vitamin D Agents

Drug	MOA & Pharmacokinetics	Clinical Uses	Side Effects
Calcifediol (Calderol®) Calcitriol (Calcijex®, Rocaltrol®) Dihydrotachysterol (DHT®, Hytakerol®) Ergocalciferol (Calciferol®, Drisdol®)	Increase Ca^{2+} and PO_4^{2-} absorption from the intestine Decrease renal excretion of Ca^{2+} Increase renal excretion of PO_4^{2-} Given PO	Nutritional rickets Metabolic rickets and osteomalacia Hypoparathyroidism Osteoporosis Chronic renal failure Vitamin D deficient states Chronic forms of tetany	Vascular calcification Nephrocalcinosis Soft tissue calcification Growth arrest in children Vitamin D toxicity can cause renal failure and death (rare).

Treatment of Hypercalcemia

Bisphosphonates

Drug	MOA & Pharmacokinetics	Clinical Uses	Side Effects
Etidronate (Didronel®, EHDP®)	Adsorbed to bone, where it is taken up by osteoclasts and inhibits their activity. This slows the formation and dissolution of hydroxyapatite crystals (anti-resorptive effect). Etidronate is the most potent mineralization inhibitor of the bisphosphonates and can lead to **osteomalacia** over time. Only 0.5-3% of an oral dose is adsorbed to bone. Must be taken on an empty stomach with water, not milk or antacids, both of which prevent absorption. Given PO, IV	Paget's disease of bone Heterotopic ossification (myositis ossificans): especially in patients with total hip replacement or with spinal cord injuries due to its antimineralizing effect. **Malignancy-associated hypercalcemia** usually in conjunction with saline hydration and diuretics to increase the urine output and rate of calcium excretion. Osteoporosis	Bone pain in patients with Paget's disease usually around the pagetic lesion (more common in patients receiving long term high doses). Osteomalacia and bone fractures (more common in patients receiving long term high doses). Diarrhea Nausea
Pamidronate (Aredia®, APD®) Less toxic than Etidronate	Same MOA as for etidronate. About 50% of an IV dose is adsorbed to bone. Given IV	Paget's disease of bone Malignancy-associated hypercalcemia usually in conjunction with saline hydration and a loop diuretic.	Hypocalcemia leading to abdominal cramps, confusion and muscle spasms. Leukopenia or lymphopenia Pain and swelling at the site of injection

Alendronate Teludronate	These newer bisphosphonates are currently in development and do not inhibit mineralization like etidronate. These agents may clinically replace etidronate in the future.

Calcitonin Agents

Drugs	MOA & Pharmacokinetics	Clinical Uses	Side Effects
Human calcitonin (Cibacalcin®) Another alternatively spliced product of the calcitonin gene, calcitonin gene-related peptide (CGRP), is produced in the brain. There is little or no CGRP produced by the thyroid gland.	A 32 amino acid peptide synthesized and secreted by the parafollicular C cells of the thyroid which lowers serum Ca^{2+} and PO_4^{2-} by acting on bone and kidney. Interacts with receptors on **osteoclasts** producing a decrease in the ruffled membrane surface area resulting in a decrease in resorptive activity. Reduces Ca^{2+} and PO_4^{2-} reabsorption in the kidney. Serum $t_{1/2}$ after a single dose = 60 min	Paget's disease of bone Used in patients who have developed resistance to salmon-calcitonin.	Allergic reactions: skin rash and urticaria Flushing, redness, or tingling of the face, ears, hands and feet GI effects: diarrhea, nausea and vomiting
Salmon calcitonin (Calcimar®, Miacalcin®)	Same MOA as human calcitonin. More potent than human calcitonin due to its longer half-life (80 min) and reduced metabolic clearance.	Paget's disease of bone Postmenopausal osteoporosis in conjunction with an adequate intake of calcium Hypercalcemia: given with saline hydration and a loop diuretic	

Miscellaneous Agents

Drugs	MOA & Pharmacokinetics	Clinical Uses	Side Effects
Gallium nitrate (Ganite®)	Decreases serum calcium by inhibiting abnormal bone resorption associated with neoplastic tissue.	**Malignancy associated hypercalcemia** in patients with normal kidney function. Usually given in conjunction with saline hydration and diuretics to increase the urine output and rate of calcium excretion.	**Nephrotoxicity**: observed as hematuria, changes in the frequency of urination, nausea and vomiting Hypophosphatemia: resulting in bone pain and muscle weakness ◆ Contraindication: Patients with impaired renal function
Plicamycin (formerly called Mithramycin) (Mithracin®)	A cytotoxic antibiotic which also lowers serum calcium concentration. The MOA for plicamycin's antineoplastic action and effect on serum calcium are unknown. The antineoplastic action is thought to involve inhibition of DNA-directed RNA synthesis. Thought to lower serum calcium by blocking the hypercalcemic effect of vitamin D or by inhibiting the effect of PTH on osteoclasts. Reduction in Ca^{2+} occurs within 24-48 hours following administration. Duration of a single dose is 7-10 days. The dose used in hypercalcemia is about 1/10th the cytotoxic dose.	Malignancy associated hypercalcemia and hypercalciuria: (NOT the drug of first choice due to its toxicity). Paget's disease of bone refractory to other agents. Testicular cancer refractory to other treatments.	Loss of appetite, nausea, and vomiting (most common) **Hemorrhagic diathesis** (most significant): • GI bleeding • Nosebleeds • Petechial bleeding • Thrombocytopenia Hepatic and renal toxicity Hypocalcemia

Drugs	MOA & Pharmacokinetics	Clinical Uses	Side Effects
Glucocorticoids	Reduce plasma Ca^{2+} by: • Decreasing GI absorption of Ca^{2+} • Increasing renal excretion of Ca^{2+} • Decreasing sarcoid tissue High doses of **prednisone** are usually required. Response to therapy is slow (1-2 weeks).	Hypercalcemia secondary to sarcoidosis, lymphoma and hypervitaminosis D.	There are many side effects of long term glucocorticoid therapy including osteoporosis in adults and poor skeletal development in children.
Loop diuretics	Hypocalcemic effect is due to an increase in the urinary excretion of calcium. This occurs by inhibiting the absorption of calcium in the ascending loop of Henle.	Hypercalcemia: must be given concurrently with saline because loop diuretics administered by themselves can cause volume contraction (which results in increased calcium reabsorption in the proximal tubule).	Hypercalcemia if not administered with hydration. Orthostatic hypotension Hypokalemic metabolic alkalosis Hyponatremia Hypochloremia Hyperuricemia Ototoxicity Hypomagnesemia Allergic reactions: eosinophilia and rash

Notes

Hypoglycemics

Hypoglycemic drugs are used to lower elevated serum glucose levels as seen in patients with diabetes mellitus. **Diabetes mellitus**, diagnosed by a fasting blood glucose of ≥140 mg/dl, is due to a deficiency in insulin.

There are 2 classifications of diabetes based on the patient's requirement for insulin. **Type I**, also known as insulin-dependent diabetes mellitus (IDDM) or juvenile-onset diabetes, is due to an absence of insulin. These patients require insulin. **Type II** diabetes, also known as non-insulin dependent (NIDDM) diabetes mellitus or adult-onset diabetes, is the more common of the two, affecting 5% of adult Americans. NIDDM is secondary to insulin resistance and the goal of therapy is to reduce glucose and utilize existing insulin. NIDDM patients, however, may eventually require insulin.

Several hypoglycemic drugs are available in injectable and oral forms. For most IDDM patients, injectable insulin is necessary due the to short life of ingested insulin. Oral hypoglycemic preparations are used for NIDDM patients as adjuvant therapy to dietary modifications.

Injectable hypoglycemics (Insulin preparations)	Oral hypoglycemics (Sulfonylureas & biguanides)
Ultrashort Acting: Zinc insulin ("regular insulin," crystalline) Prompt insulin zinc (semilente) Short Acting: Isophane insulin suspension (NPH) Insulin zinc suspension (lente) Long Acting: Protamine zinc insulin (PZI) Extended insulin zinc suspension (ultralente)	Sulfonylureas: Tolbutamide Acetohexamide Tolazamide Chlorpropamide Glyburide Glipizide Biguanides: Metformin

Glucagon
Glucagon Emergency Kit

Some of the major differences in Type I and Type II diabetes are summarized below:

	Type I (IDDM)	Type II (NIDDM)
Level of insulin secretion	Low or absent	Normal or increased
β-cell function	Absent	Decreased
Age at Onset	Under 20 yrs	After 30 yrs
Body Weight	Normal	Overweight
Genetic factors (parents or siblings with diabetes)	<20%	>60%
Management	Insulin and diet	Diet, oral hypoglycemics and insulin, if necessary
Insulin resistance	None	Mild to severe

Clinically, diabetes presents as the classic triad of **polydipsia**, **polyuria** and **polyphagia**. The pathognomonic finding, thickening of the capillary basement membranes, is seen in both types of diabetes. This change may ultimately result in other complications of diabetes, such as microvascular disease, nephropathy, retinopathy and peripheral neuropathies. Another complication is a predisposition to atherosclerosis which may compromise the blood supply to the extremities and result in the need for amputation. Diabetes is a common cause of nontraumatic amputations in the U.S. However, recent studies indicate that control of blood sugar reduces the risk of cardiovascular complications as well as renal and retinal pathologies.

Most hypoglycemic drugs are designed to prevent the clinical complications of diabetes by supplying the body with insulin. Insulin is comprised of two polypeptide chains connected by disulfide bridges. It is synthesized by the **β-cells** of the pancreas as preproinsulin and cleaved to form proinsulin. Cleavage of preproinsulin liberates A, B and C peptides. The A and B peptides are joined by disulfide bridges to form an active insulin monomer which binds to insulin receptors and initiates a cellular signalling cascade which results in increased glucose uptake by cells.

The drugs presently available fall into two categories: injectable forms of insulin (usually precipitates of insulin which are degraded more slowly than pure insulin) and oral hypoglycemics which stimulate the secretion of insulin from the remaining functional β cells of the pancreas.

Injectable Hypoglycemics

The **injectable** forms of insulin are used for Type I diabetics and are divided into ultrashort, short and long acting insulin preparations. These drugs are **precipitates** of insulin (derived from porcine or bovine pancreas, or recombinant human insulin) and zinc.

	Drug	MOA & Pharmacokinetics	Activity (hrs) Peak	Activity (hrs) Duration	Side Effects
Ultrashort Acting	Crystalline zinc insulin (CZI, regular insulin)	A **crystalline** mixture of insulin and zinc to form an injectable precipitate. Given SC normally Given IV in emergencies	2-4	5-7	**Hypoglycemia**: **insulin shock**[1], sweating, tachycardia, hunger Antigenic response to animal insulins. Weight gain Local sensitivity reactions at the site of injection.
Ultrashort Acting	Prompt zinc insulin suspension (semilente insulin)	**An amorphous** insulin and zinc suspension. Given SC. Usually used as a supplement to intermediate or long acting insulin preparations.	1-4	12-16	
Short Acting	Isophane insulin suspension (neutral protamine Hagedorn, NPH)	A **suspension** of CZI and protamine (a positively charged peptide). Protamine decreases the solubility of CZI thereby increasing its duration of action. Given SC	8-12	18-24	
Short Acting	Insulin zinc suspension (lente insulin)	Composed of 30% semilente and 70% ultralente insulins. Given SC	8-12	18-24	
Long Acting	Protamine zinc insulin (PZI)	A precipitate of CZI and protamine. Given SC	8-16	24-36	
Long Acting	Extended insulin zinc suspension (ultralente insulin)	A poorly soluble CZI.	8-16	24-36	

[1] Insulin shock: hypoglycemia may result in CNS effects such as brain damage and convulsions. Treatment includes immediate administration of glucose or glucagon.

Oral Hypoglycemics

Oral hypoglycemics are used to treat patients with NIDDM. The two classes of oral hypoglycemics are sulfonylurea derivatives and biguanides. **Sulfonylurea derivatives** stimulate secretion of insulin by β-cells of the pancreas. These agents are ineffective in patients who lack functional β-cells. The **second generation sulfonylureas** (glyburide and glipizide) are more potent than their first generation counterparts. Sulfonylureas block K^+ channels causing depolarization. This triggers insulin release from the β-cells of the pancreas. In addition, the sulfonylureas decrease glucagon levels and increase the binding of insulin to its receptors.

Sulfonylurea derivatives

Drug	Pharmacokinetics	Clinical Uses	Side Effects
Tolbutamide (Orinase®)	Onset is 30 min. Duration = 6-12 hrs. Tolbutamide is the least potent, shortest-acting sulfonylurea. Given PO	**Type II diabetics** (NIDDM) refractory to dietary modifications alone.	**Hypoglycemia**: in elderly patients and those with hepatic or renal insufficiency. GI effects: nausea, vomiting Cutaneous reactions Hematologic effects: leukopenia, agranulocytosis, thrombocytopenia
Acetohexamide (Dymelor®)	Peak effect at 3 hrs. Duration = 12-18 hrs. Given PO. Its metabolite, **hydroxyhexamide**, possess much of the drug's activity.		
Tolazamide (Tolinase®)	Peak effect at 6 hrs. Duration = 24 hrs. Given PO. Hepatic metabolism to products with weaker hypoglycemic effects than parent.		
Chlorpropamide (Diabinese®)	Duration = 24-60 hrs. Given PO		
Glyburide (Micronase®) Glipizide (Glucotrol®)	**Second generation** sulfonylureas. The most potent sulfonylurea agents. Duration = 24 hrs. Given PO		

Biguanides

Drug	Pharmacokinetics	Clinical Uses	Side Effects
Metformin (Glucophage®)	Thought to decrease hepatic glucose production and improve insulin sensitivity by increasing peripheral glucose uptake and utilization. Does **not** stimulate the β cells of the pancreas to secrete insulin. Not metabolized Renally excreted Given PO	**Type II diabetics** (NIDDM) refractory to dietary modifications alone.	GI effects: anorexia, diarrhea, nausea, vomiting, flatulence Lactic acidosis

Glucagon

Glucagon is produced by α cells of the pancreas in response to hypoglycemia. It binds to glucagon receptors on hepatocytes and stimulates gluconeogenesis, ketogenesis, and metabolism of stored glucagon. Other physiological effects include relaxation of smooth muscle, especially in the GI tract, and a positive inotropic effect.

Drug	MOA & Pharmacokinetics	Clinical Uses	Side Effects
Glucagon (Glucagon Emergency Kit)	Binds glucagon receptors on the liver, activates adenyl cyclase and increases intracellular cAMP. In hepatocytes, this causes glycogenolysis and gluconeogenesis. Given IV, IM	**Severe hypoglycemia**: only if liver glycogen stores are available. GI radiography: glucagon decreases the tonicity of smooth muscle	Allergic reactions: dizziness, skin rash, dyspnea Symptoms of overdose include continuous nausea and vomiting and hypokalemic syndrome.

Notes

Anti-inflammatory Drugs

Non-Steroidal Anti-Inflammatory Drugs (NSAIDs)

NSAIDs are a class of drugs which exhibits antiplatelet, analgesic, antipyretic and anti-inflammatory effects. NSAIDs are most effective in treating pain associated with inflammation but are also useful for treating neurogenic, myogenic and headache pain. Listed below are the NSAIDs discussed in this section:

Salicylate Derivatives	Propionic Acid Derivatives	Oxicam Derivative	Acetic Acid Derivatives
Aspirin Salicylic acid Salsalate Diflunisal	Ibuprofen Naproxen	Piroxicam	Indomethacin Sulindac Ketorolac

All NSAIDs have a common mechanism of action; they inhibit cyclooxygenase, an enzyme which converts arachidonic acid to prostaglandins (PG) and thromboxane (TxA_2). Shown below is the point at which NSAIDs act on the cyclooxygenase pathway.

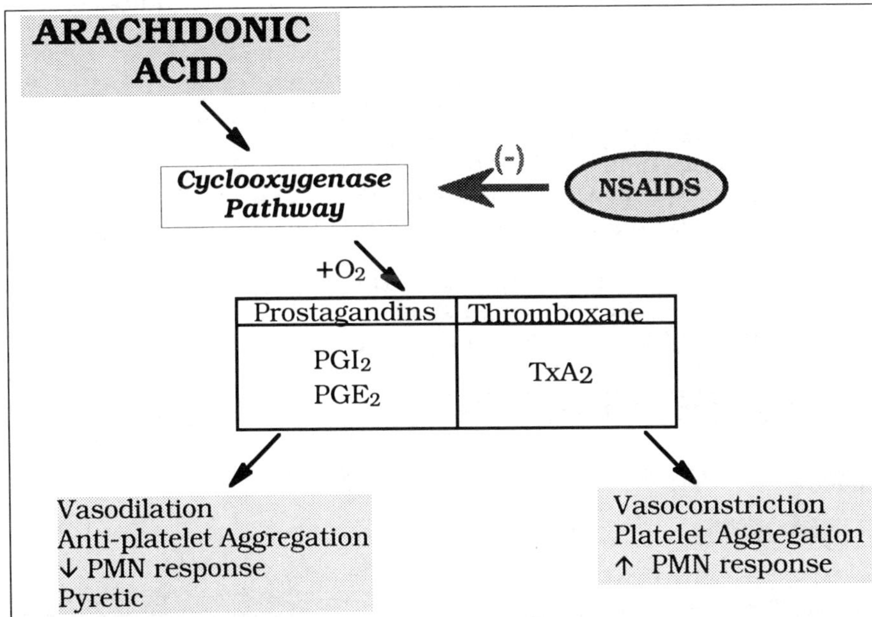

Antiplatelet activity is due to the decreased production of thromboxane, a key mediator of platelet function which normally influences platelets to change shape, release granules and aggregate.

Analgesic effects are due to the inhibition of prostaglandin synthesis. Prostaglandins, such as PGE_2, are thought to mediate hyperalgesia by sensitizing nerve endings to the action of bradykinin, histamine and other chemical mediators released during inflammation.

Antipyretic effects are due to decreased production of PGE_2. PGE_2 acts on the thermoregulatory center in the hypothalamus to elevate body temperature. Antipyretic effects are observed in febrile patients only.

Anti-inflammatory activity is due to several mechanisms which may include decreased prostaglandin synthesis in inflamed tissue, inhibition of other inflammatory mediators and inhibition of leukocyte migration.

Salicylate Derivatives

Aspirin, an acetylated salicylic acid, is the prototype of NSAIDs.

Drug	MOA & Pharmacokinetics	Clinical Uses	Side Effects
Aspirin (Acetylsalicylic acid, ASA) (Bayer®, Bufferin®) Note: Other salicylate derivatives such as **salicylic acid**, **salsalate** and **diflunisal** reversibly inhibit cyclooxygenase.	**Irreversibly** inhibits cyclooxygenase decreasing the production of prostaglandins and thromboxane. Due to its irreversibility, the antiplatelet activity of aspirin lasts for the life-span of the platelet (7-10 days). Patients undergoing elective surgery should stop administration 1 week prior to their procedure. **Salicylic acid**, a metabolite of aspirin, also contributes to the drug's activity by **reversibly** inhibiting cyclooxygenase. Exhibits a uricosuric effect at high doses (5000 mg/day). Given PO; $t_{1/2}$ = 2-3 hrs Hepatic metabolism Renal excretion; alkalinization of the urine significantly increases the rate of excretion.	Myocardial infarction: DOC Antiplatelet (<300 mg/day) Analgesia: low to moderate pain (300-2400 mg/day) Antipyretic: only in febrile patients (300-2400 mg/day) Anti-inflammatory (2400-4000 mg/day)	Bleeding complications Gastric intolerance Hypersensitivity reactions Renal toxicity Hepatotoxicity **Reye's Syndrome**: a fatal, fulminating hepatitis and cerebral edema seen in children with fever caused by viral illness who are given aspirin. Children with fever should be given acetaminophen. **Salicylate poisoning**: characterized by hyperventilation (respiratory alkalosis), metabolic acidosis, hyperpyrexia, coma, renal, vasomotor and respiratory failure, tinnitus and vertigo. Treatment of overdose includes induction of emesis, correction of electrolyte imbalance, alkalinization of the urine and dialysis. ◆ Contraindications: Pregnancy Peptic ulcer disease Hemophilia Children with fever caused by viral illnesses (associated with **Reye's Syndrome**)

Propionic Acid Derivatives

The propionic acid derivatives exhibit analgesic, antipyretic and anti-inflammatory activities but possess only mild antiplatelet activity. In contrast to aspirin, these drugs inhibit cyclooxygenase in a **reversible** manner.

<table>
<tr><th>Drug</th><th>MOA & Pharmacokinetics</th><th>Clinical Uses</th><th>Side Effects</th></tr>
<tr><td>Ibuprofen
(Advil®, Motrin®, Nuprin®)</td><td>Reversibly inhibits cyclooxygenase decreasing the production of prostaglandins and thromboxane.

Given PO; $t_{1/2}$ = 2 hrs</td><td rowspan="2">Analgesia

Rheumatoid arthritis

Osteoarthritis</td><td rowspan="2">GI disturbances

◆ Contraindication: Pregnancy</td></tr>
<tr><td>Naproxen
(Naprosyn®, Aleve®)</td><td>Same as ibuprofen except:

$t_{1/2}$ = 12-15 hrs</td></tr>
</table>

Oxicam Derivative

Piroxicam, an oxicam derivative, exhibits analgesic, antipyretic and anti-inflammatory activities. Due to its long half-life, piroxicam can be administered once a day.

Drug	MOA & Pharmacokinetics	Clinical Uses	Side Effects
Piroxicam (Feldene®)	**Reversibly** inhibits cyclooxygenase decreasing the production of prostaglandins and thromboxane. Given PO; $t_{1/2}$ = 50 hrs	Rheumatoid arthritis Osteoarthritis Ankylosing spondylitis Acute gout	GI effects: abdominal pain and discomfort, nausea, pancreatitis CNS effects: headache, vertigo

Acetic Acid Derivatives

These drugs, like propionic acid derivatives, confer analgesic, antipyretic, anti-inflammatory and mild antiplatelet activities by **reversibly** inhibiting cyclooxygenase. Ketorolac is notable for 2 reasons: analgesic potency is morphine-like and it is one of the few injectable NSAIDs.

Drug	MOA & Pharmacokinetics	Clinical Uses	Side Effects
Indomethacin (Indocin®)	**Reversibly** inhibits cyclooxygenase decreasing the production of prostaglandins and thromboxane. Given PO; $t_{1/2}$ = 4 hrs	**Acute gout**: DOC **Ankylosing spondylitis:** DOC Barter's syndrome: juxtaglomerular cell hyperplasia with secondary hyperaldosteronism. Rheumatoid arthritis Osteoarthritis Induce closure of patent ductus arteriosus (PDA): the only indication in children	CNS effects: headache, vertigo, mental confusion GI effects: abdominal pain, diarrhea, pancreatitis Hypersensitivity reactions: rash, urticaria Hematopoietic reactions: thrombocytopenia, neutropenia Renal toxicity: less pronounced with sulindac
Sulindac (Clinoril®)	Same MOA as indomethacin but is less potent. **Prodrug** which is metabolized by the liver to its active form, sulindac sulfide. Given PO; $t_{1/2}$ = 18 hrs (sulindac sulfide)	Rheumatoid arthritis Osteoarthritis Ankylosing spondylitis Acute gout	
Ketorolac (Toradol®) Note: An ophthalmic preparation (Acular®) is used to treat seasonal allergic conjunctivitis.	Same MOA as indomethacin. Analgesic properties are greater than anti-inflammatory effects. Potency is **morphine-like**. Given PO, IM or IV; $t_{1/2}$ = 5 hrs	**Analgesia** (moderate to severe): for short term management of pain; commonly used postoperatively instead of opioid analgesics.	GI effects: abdominal pain, dyspepsia, nausea CNS effects: somnolence, dizziness, headache Pain at injection site

Acetaminophen

Acetaminophen has analgesic and antipyretic effects but, unlike NSAIDs, it does not have antiplatelet or anti-inflammatory activity. It is most useful as an alternative analgesic and antipyretic when NSAIDs are contraindicated. Acetaminophen is derived from phenacetin, a relatively toxic non-narcotic analgesic which is not available in the U.S.

Drug	MOA & Pharmacokinetics	Clinical Uses	Side Effects
Acetaminophen (Tylenol®)	Inhibits prostaglandin synthesis, primarily in the CNS, through an unclear mechanism. This activity is thought to account for its analgesic and antipyretic effects. It is a weak inhibitor of cyclooxygenase in the periphery which accounts for its lack of anti-inflammatory activity. Approximately 95% is hepatically metabolized to non-toxic species. A minor route of metabolism is via the P_{450} system which produces toxic species. Given PO; $t_{1/2} = 2$ hrs Hepatic metabolism Renal excretion	Analgesic (mild to moderate pain): especially useful for patients in whom aspirin is contraindicated. Antipyretic: especially useful for patients in whom aspirin is contraindicated, including children with febrile viral illnesses.	Allergic reactions (rare): skin rash Symptoms of overdose: nausea, vomiting, anorexia, abdominal cramps and ultimately, fatal **hepatic necrosis**. In overdose, saturation of the major route of acetaminophen metabolism results in increased production of toxic metabolites through the P_{450} system. An abundance of these metabolites, which are normally scavenged by glutathione, exhaust hepatic glutathione stores. The toxic metabolites are then free to react with sulfhydryl groups of hepatic proteins ultimately leading to hepatic necrosis. Antidote for overdose: **acetylcysteine** (Mucomyst®) should be initiated within 24 hrs. Acetylcysteine protects against acetaminophen-induced hepatotoxicity by restoring hepatic concentrations of **glutathione**.

Notes

Antigout Drugs

Gout is a disorder characterized by increased serum uric acid (hyperuricemia) and the deposition of urate crystals in the joints and kidneys. Uric acid is a product of purine catabolism and is eliminated by renal excretion. Therefore, gout can be the result of several metabolic disturbances such as:

1) ↑ production of purines
2) ↑ catabolism of nucleic acids
3) ↓ salvage of free purine bases
4) ↓ excretion of uric acid

Physiologically, the hyperuricemic state results in the deposition of urate crystals in tissues, usually joints but also in soft tissue. These precipitates absorb fibronectin and complement and elicit an inflammatory reaction mediated by phagocytes. Clinically, gout presents as the sudden onset of severe pain in a single joint, usually in the foot or ankle. Treatment is geared towards limiting the inflammatory response to urate crystal deposits (acute gout) or controlling hyperuricemia (chronic gout). The drugs used to treat gout are divided into two categories:

Acute Gout	Chronic Gout
Colchicine Indomethacin Phenylbutazone	Probenecid Sulfinpyrazone Allopurinol Colchicine

Acute Gout

The drugs used to treat acute gout are anti-inflammatory agents and include colchicine and NSAIDs (indomethacin and phenylbutazone).

Drug	MOA & Pharmacokinetics	Clinical Uses	Side Effects
Colchicine	**Inhibits microtubule formation** in leukocytes causing a decrease in motility, phagocytosis and release of chemotactic factors. This is responsible for its anti-inflammatory activity. Given PO, IV	**Acute gout** **Chronic gout**: prophylaxis against gouty flares.	GI effects: diarrhea, nausea, vomiting, abdominal pain Bone marrow depression: aplastic anemia and agranulocytosis have been associated with long term use Alopecia: with long term use
Indomethacin (Indocin®)	**Reversibly** inhibits **cyclooxygenase** decreasing the production of prostaglandins and thromboxane. This is responsible for its anti-inflammatory activity. Given PO	**Acute gout:** DOC **Ankylosing spondylitis:** DOC Barter's syndrome: juxtaglomerular cell hyperplasia with secondary hyperaldosteronism. Rheumatoid arthritis Osteoarthritis **Induce closure of patent ductus arteriosus** (PDA)	CNS effects: headache, vertigo, mental confusion GI effects: abdominal pain, diarrhea, pancreatitis Hypersensitivity reactions: rash, urticaria Hematopoietic reactions: thrombocytopenia, neutropenia Renal toxicity
Phenylbutazone (Butazolidin®, Azolid®)	Same MOA as indomethacin Given PO; $t_{1/2}$ = 65 hrs	Acute gout: for short term use only when other drugs have failed.	GI effects: nausea, vomiting, abdominal pain Edema Skin rash Hematopoietic reactions: aplastic anemia and agranulocytosis

Chronic Gout

The drugs used to treat chronic gout are geared at controlling hyperuricemia and include uricosuric agents (probenecid and sulfinpyrazone) and allopurinol.

Drug	MOA & Pharmacokinetics	Clinical Uses	Side Effects
Probenecid (Benemid®)	**Inhibits tubular reabsorption** of uric acid in the proximal convoluted tubule thereby increasing its excretion (uricosuric). Competitively inhibits the renal tubular secretion of weak organic acids such as penicillin, methotrexate and some NSAIDs. Given PO	**Chronic gout** Adjuvant in antibiotic therapy: potentiates the effects of penicillin G	**Acute gouty attacks**: at low doses, uricosuric agents may decrease the secretion of uric acid. Other side effects are uncommon but include headache, nausea, GI irritation and hypersensitivity reactions.
Sulfinpyrazone (Anturane®)	**Inhibits tubular reabsorption** of uric acid in the proximal convoluted tubule thereby increasing its excretion (uricosuric). Given PO	Chronic gout	**Acute gouty attacks**: at low doses, uricosuric agents may decrease the secretion of uric acid. GI irritation: stomach pain Hypersensitivity reactions (rare)
Allopurinol (Lopurin®, Zyloprim®)	Allopurinol and its metabolite, **alloxanthine** (oxypurinol), **inhibit xanthine oxidase (XO)**, the enzyme which catalyzes the formation of uric acid from hypoxanthine. Allopurinol is metabolized by xanthine oxidase to alloxanthine. Given PO	**Chronic gout** Hyperuricemia secondary to blood dyscrasias or antineoplastic therapy Renal calculi Hyperuricemia of Lesch-Nyhan syndrome: does not improve neurological and behavioral abnormalities or alter the course of the disease.	Hypersensitivity reactions: allergic dermatitis, fever, malaise Acute gouty attacks: seen early in treatment due to mobilization of tissue stores of uric acid. GI upset Inhibits P_{450} system thus decreases the metabolism and inactivation of other drugs such as anticoagulants.

Notes

Histamine Antagonists

Histamine is an autocoid which mediates inflammation, allergic reactions, anaphylaxis and digestion. The physiological effects of histamine release include smooth muscle contraction, capillary dilation and gastric acid secretion. Histamine is used clinically as a diagnostic agent to assess gastric function, nonspecific bronchial hyperreactivity and allergic skin reactions. Histamine antagonists are used for the treatment of allergies, motion sickness, gastric acid hypersecretion and asthma.

Histamine antagonists work by two mechanisms: 1) inhibiting binding of histamine to histamine receptors (H_1- and H_2-blockers) and 2) preventing the release of histamine (cromolyn sulfate). Although there are three types of histamine receptors (H_1, H_2 and H_3), only H_1 blockers and H_2 blockers are used therapeutically. Presently there are no clinical applications for H_3-receptor blocking agents.

H_1-Receptor Antagonists	H_2-Receptor Antagonists	Inhibitor of Histamine Release
Diphenhydramine Dimenhydrinate Chlorpheniramine Meclizine Terfenadine Loratadine Astemizole	Cimetidine Ranitidine Nizatidine Famotidine	Cromolyn sulfate

Properties of histamine receptors

Receptor	2nd Messenger	Actions
H_1	↑ IP_3/DAG	Vasodilation Increases vascular permeability Bronchoconstriction
H_2	↑ cAMP	Gastric acid hypersecretion by parietal cells Vasodilation Positive inotropic and chronotropic effects

H_1- Receptor Antagonists

H_1-receptor blockers reversibly inhibit the effect of histamine at H_1-receptors. Second generation drugs (terfenadine, loratadine and astemizole) have the least CNS effects and are non-sedating. In general, H_1-blockers are chosen for the side effect profile rather than their H_1- blocking properties.

First Generation H_1-Blockers

Drug	MOA & Pharmacokinetics	Clinical Uses	Side Effects
Diphenhydramine (Benadryl®) Dimenhydrinate (Dramamine®) Chlorpheniramine (Chlor-Trimeton®) Meclizine (Antivert®)	**Reversible**, competitive inhibitors of histamine at H_1-receptors. Given PO; $t_{1/2}$ = 4-6 hrs except meclizine (12-24 hrs)	**Allergies**: hayfever, rhinitis, urticaria and pruritus Motion sickness Sedative Vestibular disturbances including Menière's disease and vertigo Drug-induced extrapyramidal effects	**Sedation** Anticholinergic effects: dry mouth, urinary retention, blurred vision GI disturbances: nausea, vomiting Loss of appetite Drug Interactions: Potentiate the effects of **CNS depressants** (i.e. alcohol, benzodiazepines).

Second Generation H_1-Blockers: Non-sedating

Drug	MOA & Pharmacokinetics	Clinical Uses	Side Effects
Terfenadine (Seldane®) Loratadine (Claritin®) Astemizole (Hismanal®)	Same MOA as above Do not cross the blood-brain barrier therefore are **non-sedating**. $t_{1/2}$ = 12-24 hrs terfenadine 24 hrs loratadine >24 hrs astemizole	**Allergies**: hayfever, rhinitis, urticaria and pruritus	Arrhythmias: ventricular tachycardia (torsades de pointes) can be precipitated by high dose of terfenadine or astemizole or concurrent use of these agents with inhibitors of the P_{450} system. Loratadine has not been associated with arrhythmias. Drug Interactions: Potentiation of the effects of **CNS depressants** (i.e. alcohol, benzodiazepines).

H_2-Receptor Antagonists

H_2-receptor blockers competitively inhibit histamine binding at H_2-receptors. Their primary effect is on parietal cells of the stomach which produce acid in response to histamine. They have little, if any, effect on H_1-receptors.

Drug	MOA & Pharmacokinetics	Clinical Uses	Side Effects
Cimetidine (Tagamet®)	Competitively inhibits histamine at H_2-receptors.	Duodenal and gastric ulcers Zollinger-Ellison syndrome Gastroesophageal reflux disease	Cimetidine has a **high incidence** of side effects. Most commonly: sedation, headache, dizziness, GI distress, muscle pain (arthralgia). CNS effects in elderly patients: slurred speech, delirium, confusional states. Endocrine effects: galactorrhea in women, gynecomastia and low sperm count in men. Drug Interactions: Increases blood levels of several other drugs by inhibiting P_{450}.
Ranitidine (Zantac®) Nizatidine (Axid®) Famotidine (Pepcid®)	Same MOA as cimetidine. $t_{1/2}$ = 2-3 hrs Given PO	Duodenal and gastric ulcers Zollinger-Ellison syndrome Gastroesophageal reflux disease	Ranitidine has less CNS effects, endocrine effects and inhibitory effects on the P_{450} system than cimetidine. Nizatidine and famotidine appear to be **free** of CNS, endocrine effects and inhibitory effects on the P_{450} system.

Cromolyn Sulfate

Drug	MOA & Pharmacokinetics	Clinical Uses	Side Effects
Cromolyn sulfate (Intal®, Nasalcrom®)	Inhibits the release of histamine from mast cells.	**Asthma** (prophylaxis): the drug has no benefit during an acute asthmatic attack.	Infrequent but include bronchospasm, cough or wheezing.

Notes

Special Topics

Drugs Affecting the Immune System

This section describes agents used to suppress the immune system (immunosuppressors) as well as drugs used to bolster the immune system (immunomodulators). The major clinical indication for immunosuppressive agents is organ transplantation. Immunomodulators are mainly used as an adjuvant to chemotherapy.

Immunosuppressive Agents	Immunomodulators
Cyclosporine Tacrolimus Azathioprine Glucocorticoids Antibody reagents Muromonab-CD3 Rh_0(D) Immune Globulin Antilymphocytic Globulin	G-CSF (Filgrastim®) GM-CSF (Sargramostim®) Levamisole BCG Aldesleukin

Immunosuppressive Agents

Drug	MOA & Pharmacokinetics	Clinical Uses	Side Effects
Cyclosporine (Sandimmune®) A peptide elaborated by the fungus *Tolypocladium inflatum Gams.*	**Blocks T cell activation** by binding cyclophilin (an intracellular receptor) and decreasing the activity of **calcineurin** (a protein phosphatase). This ultimately prevents production of **IL-2**, IL-3 and IFN-γ. Given PO	**Organ transplantation**: DOC for kidney, liver, heart and pancreas transplantation. Graft-vs-host disease subsequent to bone marrow transplantation.	**Nephrotoxicity** Hepatotoxicity Neurotoxicity Hypertension Hyperglycemia GI effects: vomiting, diarrhea Increased incidence of lymphoma Hirsutism: *cyclosporine* Gingival hyperplasia: *cyclosporine*
Tacrolimus (FK 506)	**Inhibits T cell activation** by binding the FK506 binding protein. This complex decreases **calcineurin** activity ultimately preventing production of **IL-2**, IL-3 and IFN-γ. 100 times more potent than cyclosporine but has equivalent toxicity. Given PO, IV	**Organ transplantation**: **hepatic**, renal, cardiac	
Azathioprine (Imuran®)	**Pro-drug** activated to **mercaptopurine**, an **antimetabolite** which inhibits purine synthesis preventing T cell proliferation.	**Organ transplant rejection**: renal Rheumatoid arthritis	Bone marrow suppression Leukopenia, infection Megaloblastic anemia GI distress: nausea, vomiting Increase incidence of skin cancer and lymphomas with prolonged use.
Glucocorticoids Dexamethasone Hydrocortisone Prednisone Prednisolone	Suppress cell-mediated immune reactions, decrease T cells, decrease interactions of immunoglobulins with cell surface receptors and inhibit the synthesis of interleukins such as IL-1, **IL-2** and IL-6.	Anti-inflammatory Organ transplantation, particularly in preventing transplant rejection. Adrenal insufficiency	Infections Hyperglycemia Muscle wasting Osteoporosis Capillary fragility Cataracts Central obesity

Antibody Reagents

Drug	MOA & Pharmacokinetics	Clinical Uses	Side Effects
Muromonab CD3(OKT-3) (Orthoclone OKT3®)	Murine monoclonal antibody directed against the **CD3** molecule of the **T-cell antigen** receptor complex. This interaction initially causes cytokine release (first-dose) but ultimately blocks the actions of T-cells. Specifically blocks **T-cell** function. Given IV	Acute renal transplant rejection Steroid-resistant acute rejection of cardiac or hepatic transplants	**Cytokine-release syndrome**: due to the initial activation of lymphocytes. Observed as diarrhea, dizziness and fever. Anaphylaxis Hypersensitivity
Rh_0(D) Immune Globulin (Rhogam®, MICRhoGAM®)	Human IgG globulin preparation containing antibodies against **Rh(D) erythrocytic antigens**. Prevents maternal antibody response to Rh_0(D)-positive cells which may enter Rh-negative mother's bloodstream.	**Rh-hemolytic disease** of newborn (erythroblastosis fetalis): prophylaxis. Administered to **Rh_0(D)-negative mothers** within 72 hours after the birth of a Rh_0(D)-positive baby to prevent hemolytic disease of the newborn during subsequent pregnancies.	Pain and erythema at injection site Slight temperature elevation
Antilymphocytic globulin (Antithymocyte globulin) (ALG) (Atgam®)	Binds to and induces complement-mediated destruction of **T-lymphocytes**. A purified Ig prepared from hyperimmune serum of horses, rabbits, sheep or goats which have been immunized with human thymic lymphocytes. No effect on humoral immunity.	Organ transplant: acute rejection episodes in solid organ and bone marrow transplantation.	Pain and erythema at injection site Serum sickness Nephritis Anaphylaxis Histiocytic lymphoma at the site of injection

Immunomodulators

Drug	MOA & Pharmacokinetics	Clinical Uses	Side Effects
Granulocyte colony stimulating factor (G-CSF) (Filgrastim®) Granulocyte-macrophage colony stimulating factor (GM-CSF) (Sargramostim®)	Recombinant proteins which stimulate the proliferation and activation of **neutrophils** (G-CSF) or **macrophages/granulocytes** (GM-CSF).	Recovery from chemotherapy: accelerate the recovery of neutrophils or macrophages and granulocytes following chemotherapy or other marrow suppressing therapies.	Excessive leukocytosis Fever Allergic reactions Capillary leak syndrome (*sargramostim*): due to an increase in capillary permeability. Can lead to hypotension and pulmonary edema or respiratory failure.
Levamisole (Ergamisol®)	Stimulates delayed hypersensitivity and T-cell mediated immunity. Also increases monocyte, macrophage and neutrophil activity.	**Colorectal cancer**: adjuvant to chemotherapy. Hodgkin's disease Rheumatoid arthritis	Blood dyscrasias: agranulocytosis, leukopenia, thrombocytopenia Ataxia
BCG (Theracys®) Bacillus Calmette-Guerin	An attenuated strain of *Mycobacterium bovis* which activates T-cells and may also stimulate natural killer cells. Active metabolite is muramyl dipeptide.	**Bladder cancer**: intravesicular injection	Hypersensitivity Shock, chills, fever Immune complex disease
Aldesleukin (Proleukin®)	Recombinant preparation of **IL-2** which promotes the proliferation and differentiation of lymphocytes into cytotoxic cells and natural killer cells.	**Renal cell carcinoma**	**Capillary leak syndrome** due to increased capillary permeability. Can lead to hypotension and pulmonary edema or respiratory failure. Renal failure, cardiac arrest, stroke Severe anemia

Treatment of Migraine Headaches

Migraines are episodic unilateral, throbbing headaches associated with nausea, vomiting and photophobia. They are thought to be due to alterations in cerebral blood flow. Specifically, the migraine phase results from excessive vasoconstriction of cerebral vessels while the headache phase is due to vasodilation of extracranial and other arteries. Studies implicate aberrations in serotonergic pathways as the underlying cause of this disorder. The following drugs are currently available.

Drug	MOA & Pharmacokinetics	Clinical Uses	Side Effects
Sumatriptan (Imitrex®)	**Serotonin agonist** which selectively stimulates **5-HT$_{1D}$** receptors and causes vasoconstriction of cerebral vessels. Given PO, SC	**Acute migraine headaches**: in patients refractory to acetaminophen or NSAIDs.	Mild and transient effects include: dizziness, tingling, muscle weakness and neck pain.
Ergotamine Cafergot® is a mixture of ergotamine and caffeine.	An ergot alkaloid which stimulates **5-HT$_{1D}$** and α-adrenergic receptors providing relief of acute headaches by causing vasoconstriction of cerebral vessels. Antagonist activity at **5-HT$_2$** receptors provides headache prophylaxis. Given PO, PR (per rectal)	**Acute migraine attacks**: most effective when administered during the prodrome of an acute attack. Cluster headaches	**GI effects**: nausea, vomiting, diarrhea Vasospasm Muscle weakness in the extremities **Overdose**: can result in ischemia and gangrene.
Methysergide (Sansert®)	An ergot alkaloid with partial agonist activity at 5-HT receptors.	**Migraine headache** prophylaxis Cluster headaches	**GI effects**: nausea, vomiting, diarrhea Vasospasm Retroperitoneal fibrosis **Overdose**: can result in ischemia and gangrene.
Propranolol (Inderal®) See section IV	A nonselective β-adrenergic blocker whose antimigraine action is mediated through an undefined mechanism unrelated to β-blockade.	**Migraine headache** prophylaxis	Side effects are due to β-blockade

Treatment of Gastrointestinal Disorders

Common disorders of the GI tract are acid-peptic disease, decreased upper GI motility, vomiting and constipation. **Acid-peptic diseases** include peptic ulcer disease (PUD), hypersecretory states and gastroesophageal reflux, all of which involve gastric acid hypersecretion. Treatments for gastric acid hypersecretion include antacids and a proton pump inhibitor (omeprazole). H_2-blockers are commonly used for peptic ulcers and are described in the histamine antagonists section. Decreased **upper GI motility** may be a symptom of diabetes and treatment includes agents with prokinetic activity. **Antiemetic** therapy is usually employed as an adjuvant to chemotherapy. **Constipation** is often treated with laxatives.

Acid-Peptic Disease Agents	Prokinetic agents and Antiemetics	Laxatives
Antacids Calcium carbonate Aluminum hydroxide Magnesium hydroxide Proton pump inhibitor Omeprazole Miscellaneous Sucralfate Bismuth, Tetracycline and Metronidazole Misoprostol	Cisapride Metoclopramide Dronabinol Ondansetron Granisetron Hydroxyzine Prochlorperazine	Bulk-forming Saline and Osmotics Stimulant Surfactants

Antidiarrheals are described in the CNS chapter.

Antidiarrheals
Loperamide Diphenoxylate

Treatment of Acid-Peptic Disease

Antacids are weak bases which are used to neutralize gastric acid.
These compounds are a combinations of hydroxide and metallic cations.

Antacids

Drug	MOA & Pharmacokinetics	Clinical Uses	Side Effects
Calcium carbonate (Tums®)	Reacts chemically to buffer stomach acid with little effect on acid secretion.	Hyperacidity Duodenal/gastric ulcer Gastroesophageal reflux Hypocalcemia	Metabolic alkalosis Belching Fecal impaction Abdominal distension Drug Interaction: Prevent absorption of tetracyclines
Aluminum hydroxide	Buffers stomach acid.	Hyperacidity Duodenal/gastric ulcer Gastroesophageal reflux	**Constipation** Hypophosphatemia Drug Interaction: Prevent absorption of tetracyclines
Magnesium hydroxide (Milk of Magnesia®)	Buffers stomach acid.	Hyperacidity Duodenal/gastric ulcer Gastroesophageal reflux	**Diarrhea** Drug Interaction: Prevent absorption of tetracyclines

Proton pump inhibitor

Drug	MOA & Pharmacokinetics	Clinical Uses	Side Effects
Omeprazole (Losec®, Prilosec®)	A **prodrug** which is activated at an acidic pH to a sulfenamide derivative that binds **irreversibly** to the **H^+-K^+ ATPase** proton pump on the luminal surface of stomach parietal cells. This results in decreased H^+ secretion.	**Gastroesophageal reflux** Hypersecretory conditions: Zollinger-Ellison disease, multiple endocrine adenoma, mastocytosis Duodenal ulcer	GI effects: nausea, diarrhea, abdominal colic

Miscellaneous

Drug	MOA & Pharmacokinetics	Clinical Uses	Side Effects
Sucralfate (Carafate®, Sulcrate®)	Forms a polymer in acidic environments which binds to and protects damaged tissue (ulcers) from further acid attack.	Duodenal ulcer Stress ulcer: prophylaxis	Drowsiness Constipation
Bismuth subsalicylate (Pepto-Bismol®), Tetracycline and Metronidazole	Treatment regimen to eradicate *Helicobacter pylori*, a putative etiologic agent in peptic ulcer disease and gastric carcinoma, from the GI tract.	Peptic ulcer disease Gastroesophageal reflux: *bismuth* Diarrhea: *bismuth*	GI effects: nausea, diarrhea Dizziness
Misoprostol (Cytotec®)	A PGE_1 analog which inhibits gastric acid secretion. Also stimulates the secretion of bicarbonate and mucus which can prevent ulcer development or progression.	Duodenal/gastric ulcers: NSAID induced.	Diarrhea ◆ Contraindication: Pregnancy due to its stimulatory effects on the uterus (potential abortifacient).

Treatment of GI Motility Disorders and Emesis

Delayed gastric emptying and severe bloating may result from destruction of neurons innervating upper GI viscera. Metoclopramide and cisapride are prokinetic agents used to stimulate upper GI motility.

Prokinetic Agents

Drug	MOA & Pharmacokinetics	Clinical Uses	Side Effects
Cisapride (Propulsid®)	Enhances esophageal sphincter tone and esophageal clearance by increasing the release of acetylcholine in the **myenteric plexus** (prokinetic activity). Given PO	**Gastroesophageal reflux** Gastroparesis Chronic constipation Colonic hypomotility	Abdominal cramping Constipation Diarrhea Note: does not cause extrapyramidal side effects.
Metoclopramide (Apo-Metoclop®, Clopra®)	**Antagonist** at $\mathbf{D_2}$ and $\mathbf{5\text{-}HT_3}$ receptors in gastric smooth muscle resulting in acceleration of GI emptying and intestinal transit time (prokinetic activity). **Antagonist** at $\mathbf{D_2}$ receptors in the chemoreceptor trigger zone (antiemetic effect). Given PO	**Diagnostic procedures**: GI radiography and intestinal intubation. **Gastroparesis**: resulting from diabetes. **Gastroesophageal reflux** Antiemetic: postoperative and cancer chemotherapy induced.	**Extrapyramidal side effects** **Diarrhea** Drowsiness, dizziness, anxiety Agranulocytosis Methemoglobinemia has been reported in neonates receiving metoclopramide.

Antiemetic Drugs

Drug	MOA & Pharmacokinetics	Clinical Uses	Side Effects
Dronabinol (Marinol®) Schedule II Drug	Dronabinol (∂-9THC) is the active ingredient in **marijuana**. The MOA of this drug, although unclear, appears to involve inhibition of the chemoreceptor trigger zone in the medulla. Given PO	**Antiemetic**: Chemotherapy-induced **Anorexia**: AIDS-associated	Unsteadiness Dizziness Drowsiness Nausea

Drug	MOA & Pharmacokinetics	Clinical Uses	Side Effects
Ondansetron (Zofran®) Granisetron (Kytril®) Note: Granisetron is more efficacious when used in conjunction with dexamethasone.	Selectively and **competitively inhibits serotonin** at **5-HT$_3$** receptors in the periphery (vagal nerve terminals) and CNS (area postrema). It is not yet established which of these 2 effects is responsible for antiemesis. Given PO, IV	**Antiemetic**: chemotherapy (cisplatin) induced, post-operative and radiation therapy induced emesis.	Headache Constipation Diarrhea Dizziness Somnolence: *Granisetron* Note: Do not produce extrapyramidal side effects.
Hydroxyzine (Vistaril®)	Mechanism is unclear, however, its effects may be related to its anticholinergic effects or action on the chemoreceptor trigger zone. Given **IM**	Antiemetic Antihistaminic Antianxiety Sedative-hypnotic	Drowsiness Anticholinergic effects Blood dyscrasias
Prochlorperazine (Compazine®)	An antipsychotic agent that blocks **D$_2$** receptors in the medullary chemoreceptor trigger zone as well as the vagus nerve in the GI tract. Given PO, PR, IM	**Antiemetic**	Drowsiness Hypotension Extrapyramidal effects

Note: **Apomorphine** is a dopamine agonist used in the diagnosis of idiopathic Parkinsonism syndrome. It also stimulates **D$_2$** receptors in the chemoreceptor trigger zone and is used as a potent emetic agent to treat overdose in patients who are found within ~ 30 minutes after drug ingestion. This drug is often abused by those who suffer from **bulimia**.

Laxatives

Laxatives are used to accelerate the movement of food through the gastrointestinal tract. These agents work by a variety of mechanisms. **Bulk forming** laxatives attract water and ions into the intestinal lumen which reflexively causes contraction of the bowel. **Saline** and **osmotic** laxatives retain water and allow the stool to pass easier through the bowel. **Stimulant** laxatives increase the secretion of water and ions into the lumen and stimulate the bowel wall to contract. **Surfactants** soften the stool and increase the amount of water and electrolytes secreted into the intestinal lumen.

Bulk-Forming	Saline and Osmotic	Stimulants	Surfactants
Dietary fiber (bran) Methylcellulose Psyllium	Saline Magnesium hydroxide Magnesium citrate Osmotic Glycerin Lactulose Polyethylene glycol	Phenolphthalein Bisacodyl Senna Casarca sagrada	Docusate sodium Poloxamers Castor oil

Bulk Forming Laxatives

These are among the most satisfactory preventative and therapeutic agents used for common constipation.

Drug	MOA & Pharmacokinetics	Clinical Uses	Side Effects
Dietary fiber (bran) Methylcellulose Psyllium (Metamucil®, Serutan®)	Undigestible plant, fruit and vegetable parts which form gels within the large intestine causing water retention and distention leading to an increase in GI peristaltic activity. Work in 1-3 days Given PO	Constipation	Flatulence Drug Interactions: Reduced drug absorption (e.g. cardiac glycosides) ◆ Contraindications: GI ulcers, stenosis and adhesions

Saline and Osmotic Laxatives

Saline Laxatives

Drug	MOA & Pharmacokinetics	Clinical Uses	Side Effects
Magnesium hydroxide (Milk of Magnesia®) Magnesium citrate	Hypertonic solutions of non-absorbable salts that retain water within the colonic lumen by osmotic forces leading to distention and increased peristaltic activity. Effective in 1-3 hours Given PO, PR	Constipation Colonic lavage: prior to surgery, radiologic and colonoscopic procedures. Elimination of parasites Poisoning	Dehydration Electrolyte imbalance ◆ Contraindications: Congestive heart failure Impaired renal function

Osmotic Laxatives

Drug	MOA & Pharmacokinetics	Clinical Uses	Side Effects
Glycerin	Softens the stool and lubricates the bowel by increasing water retention (osmotic properties) in the intestinal lumen. May also stimulate rectal contractions. Given PR. Poorly absorbed.	Constipation	
Lactulose (Chronulac®, Cephulac®)	Synthetic disaccharide which is not absorbed and acts as an osmotic laxative to attract water into the intestinal lumen.	Constipation Chronic hepatic encephalopathy by reducing absorption of ammonia.	Flatulence Abdominal cramps Nausea, vomiting, diarrhea ◆ Contraindication: Patients on galactose-free diet.
Polyethylene glycol (GoLYTELY®, CoLyte®)	An isotonic electrolyte solution containing a large amount of an nonabsorbable polymer (polyethylene glycol, PEG). This solution flushes the colon of its contents and causes water diarrhea.	**Colonic lavage** used in preparation for colonoscopy. Patients must drink 3-4 liters of the solution.	Diarrhea ◆ Contraindications: GI obstruction or perforation Toxic megacolon

Stimulant Laxatives

Drug	MOA & Pharmacokinetics	Clinical Uses	Side Effects
Phenolphthalein (Modane®, Ex-Lax®) Bisacodyl (Dulcolax®) Senna (Senokot®) Casarca sagrada ("sacred bark")	Reduces the net absorption of fluid and electrolytes and induces GI motility by stimulating Auerbach's plexus. May inhibit Na^{+}-K^{+}-ATPase causing an increase in secretion of fluid and electrolytes within the colon. Effective in 6-8 hours Given: PO, PR	Constipation Evacuation of the bowel prior to surgery or diagnostic exams. Note: *phenolphthalein* is one of the most abused laxatives.	Fluid and electrolyte deficiencies Abdominal cramps Pink coloration of urine and feces: *phenolphthalein* Nephritis and melanotic pigmentation in large doses: *senna, cascara*

Surfactants

Drug	MOA & Pharmacokinetics	Clinical Uses	Side Effects
Docusate sodium (Colace®) Poloxamers	Anionic surfactants which emulsify and soften the stool facilitating the passage of feces. Increase net water and electrolyte secretion into the intestine. Effective in 1-3 days Given PO, PR	Constipation Note: These agents soften the stool but do not stimulate GI motility.	Diarrhea, nausea Abdominal cramps Rash Drug interactions: Increases absorption of other drugs.
Castor oil Note: Castor oil is too strong to use for common constipation and long-term use should be avoided.	An extremely strong and distasteful oil which is hydrolyzed to glycerol and ricinoleate. Ricinoleate, an anionic surfactant, decreases fluid and electrolytes absorption and increases peristalsis in the small intestine causing rapid accumulation and evacuation. May cause uterine contractions. Effective in 1-6 hours Given PO	Preparation for radiographic examinations Severe constipation	Dehydration Electrolyte imbalance Colic ◆ Contraindication: Pregnant women

Antitussives

Antitussive agents are used to relieve cough. The **cough reflex** is a means by which the passageway of the lungs are maintained free of foreign matter. Irritation of the trachea, larynx, pharynx, or bronchi stimulate sensory stretch receptors which have afferent nerve fibers going to the cough center in the **medulla**. There are two types of drugs employed in treating cough: anodynes and peripheral acting antitussives. **Anodynes** are CNS agents which reduce the excitability of the cough center ; they are described in the narcotic analgesics section. Dextromethorphan, an opioid derivative, is a non-narcotic antitussive. **Peripheral acting** antitussives diminish input to the cough center by inhibiting afferent signals from the vagus and glossopharyngeal nerves.

Anodynes	Peripheral Acting Antitussives
Morphine Methadone Hydromorphone Hydrocodone Codeine Dextromethorphan	Benzonatate Guaifenesin Demulcents

Peripheral Acting Antitussives

Drug	MOA & Pharmacokinetics	Clinical Uses	Side Effects
Benzonatate (Tessalon®)	A **local anesthetic** which suppresses stretch or cough receptors of vagal afferents located in respiratory passages, lungs and pleura. Also may inhibit transmission of the cough reflex to the medulla.	**Antitussive**	Constipation Dizziness Drowsiness Skin rash
Guaifenesin (Anti-Tuss®)	Acts as an **expectorant** to increase the volume and decrease the viscosity of tracheal and bronchial secretions.	**Antitussive**	Rare but include diarrhea, dizziness, headache, nausea, rash
Demulcents (honey, olive oil, glycerin)	Substances which soothe esophageal-pharyngeal membranes.	**Antitussive**	

Notes

Toxicology

Toxicology is the study of adverse effects of chemicals on biological systems. Toxic agents exist in gas, liquid and solid forms. This section includes clinically relevant air pollutants, insecticides, herbicides and heavy metals.

Air Pollutants	Insecticides	Herbicides
Carbon Monoxide Sulfur dioxide Nitrogen dioxide Ozone Hydrocarbons	Chlorinated hydrocarbons Cholinesterase inhibitors Botanicals	Chlorophenoxy compounds Bipyridyls

Heavy Metals	Chelators
Lead Arsenic Mercury	Dimercaprol Succimer Penicillamine EDTA (Edetate) Deferoxamine

Air Pollutants

Chemical	Description	Effects
Carbon monoxide (CO)	Accounts for ~50% of air pollutants in industrialized countries. Colorless, odorless and non-irritating gas. Causes **tissue hypoxia** by competing with oxygen for hemoglobin binding (forms carboxy-Hb). Its affinity for hemoglobin is 200 times greater than that of oxygen.	Headaches, confusion, decreased visual acuity, tachycardia, tachypnea and syncope. Ultimately, it can cause coma, respiratory failure, convulsions and death. **Treatment** includes removal of the carbon monoxide source and administration of pure oxygen gas.
Sulfur dioxide (SO_2)	Colorless, irritating gas Forms **sulfurous acid** upon contact with moist mucous membranes. Affects the **upper respiratory tract**.	Bronchoconstriction and irritation of eyes, nose and throat. May cause pulmonary edema.
Nitrogen dioxide (NO_2)	Brown, irritating gas Less water soluble than SO_2, accesses the **lower respiratory tract**.	Irritation of lungs, eyes, nose and throat and pulmonary edema. At high concentrations acute pulmonary edema may be fatal. Exposure to high levels of NO_2 leads to **Silo-Fillers disease** which is characterized by cough and dyspnea presenting ≤ 30 hrs after exposure.
Ozone (O_3)	Blue, irritating gas Affects the **upper** (low dose) and **lower** (high dose) **respiratory tract**.	Dryness of mucosal membrane and irritation. At higher concentrations, pulmonary function may be impaired. Chronic effects include bronchitis, bronchiolitis, fibrosis and edema.
Hydrocarbons: Carbon tetrachloride Benzene Toluene Chloroform		Potent CNS depression, nausea, vertigo, headache, motor disturbances and coma. **Benzene** may cause **hematologic** disturbances (aplastic anemia, leukopenia, pancytopenia, thrombocytopenia).

Insecticides

Chemical	Description	Effects
Chlorinated hydrocarbons	Includes **DDT** and its analogs: benzene hexachloride, cyclodienes, toxaphene. Lipophilic and long-lived. Inhibit the physiologic **inactivation** of neuronal **sodium channels** resulting in continuous firing of action potentials.	Tremors, convulsions
Cholinesterase inhibitors	**Organophosphates** and **carbamates** which inhibit acetylcholinesterase. Much shorter $t_{1/2}$ than chlorinated hydrocarbons.	Miosis, sweating, salivation, bronchoconstriction, diarrhea, vomiting, muscle fasciculation, paralysis and respiratory failure. **Treatment**: atropine and pralidoxime (2-PAM)
Botanicals	Includes **pyrethrum** and **rotenone**.	**Pyrethrum** causes paresthesia, tremors and convulsions **Rotenone** causes GI distress (when ingested), conjunctivitis and dermatitis (topical).

Herbicides

Chemical	Description	Effects
Chlorophenoxy compounds	Includes **2,4-D** (2,4-dichlorophenoxyacetic acid) and **2,4,5-T** (2,4,5-trichlorophenoxyacetic acid). The manufacture of these compound produces the **dioxin** contaminant: **TCDD** (2,3,7,8-tetrachlorodibenzo-p-dioxin, **Agent orange**).	**Acute effects of TCDD**: muscle weakness and coma **Chemical worker's chloracne** **Chronic effects**: infertility and ma be implicated in the development of cancer.
Bipyridyls	Includes **paraquat**. Results in the formation of O_2 radicals. Toxic only when ingested.	GI irritation which initially presents as hematemesis or blood in the stools; progressive pulmonary impairment and death.

Heavy Metals

The following principles regarding heavy metal toxicity and availability

1. Toxicity is caused by the **unbound** form of the metal.
2. Heavy metals **bioaccumulate** and target specific **organs**.
3. Therapy involves metal **chelators**.

Metal	Description	Effects	Treatment
Lead (Pb)	**Most common** cause of heavy metal poisoning. Exposure by ingestion (70%) and by inhalation. A common means of exposure in children is by ingestion of lead-containing paint (pica).	Acute effects: abdominal colic and CNS alterations Chronic effects: GI distress, weight loss, peripheral neuropathy (including **wrist-drop** and foot-drop), lead lines on long bones in X-ray, anemia (microcytic, hypochromic), and infertility Childhood encephalopathy: behavioral effects, ataxia, stupor, coma	Edetate Dimercaprol Penicillamine Succimer (children)
Arsenic	Exposure: skin, lungs, GI	Acute effects: GI distress (vomiting, rice water stools), garlic breath, capillary transudation and hypotension. Chronic effects: skin discoloration, malaise, fatigue and neurological symptoms	Dimercaprol Succimer
Mercury (Hg) There are 3 forms: Hg^0, Hg^+, Hg^{2+}	Exposure: **Inhalation**: **elemental** mercury (Hg^0) is oxidized to Hg^{2+} in the kidney and CNS. $t_{1/2}$ = 35-90 days. **Oral**: **inorganic** mercury (Hg^+, Hg^{2+}) accumulates in the kidneys. $t_{1/2}$ = 40 days. **Oral**: **organic** mercury (alkyl mercury): exposure via food; accumulates in the brain. $t_{1/2}$ = 70 days.	**Elemental mercury**: Acute effects include bronchitis, pneumonitis, tremor and excitability. Chronic effects include neurasthenic symptoms, tremor and personality changes. **Inorganic mercury**: Acute effects include GI ulceration, bleeding and necrosis and renal failure. Chronic effects include renal tubular toxicity and neurological alterations. **Organic mercury**: Chronic effects include visual field and hearing changes and ataxic gait. Also, impaired intelligence and speech abnormalities.	Dimercaprol

Chelators

Chelators are useful for the treatment of metal ion overload or poisoning.
Most chelators can form multiple bonds with metal ions (polydentate).
The most clinically relevant chelators are listed below.

Chelator	Uses	Comments
Dimercaprol (BAL)	**Arsenic** **Mercury** Lead Cadmium	Forms 2 bonds (bidentate chelator) with metal ions, which prevents the metal from binding to tissue proteins. Must be given **parenterally**. **Toxicities**: **hypertension**, nausea, vomiting, headache and pain at injection site.
Succimer	**Lead** (in children) Arsenic	**Oral** congener of dimercaprol. Less toxic than BAL.
Penicillamine	Copper poisoning Wilson's disease Lead	A derivative of penicillin. A bidentate chelator of copper. Toxicities: acute allergic reactions, nephrotoxicity, aplastic anemia, SLE and hemolytic anemia
Edetate (EDTA)	Divalent and trivalent cations, especially **lead**	A polydentate chelator. Given with calcium disodium to prevent severe hypocalcemia. Nephrotoxic at high doses.
Deferoxamine	Iron	Polydentate bacterial compound which has a high affinity for iron. Toxicities: dermatologic reactions, neurotoxicities, hepatic and renal dysfunction.

Notes

Vitamins

Vitamins are a group of unrelated organic substances essential for normal biochemical and physiological processes. They are either obtained from the diet or are synthesized in the body. They are necessary in small quantities for nutritional purposes and in higher doses for therapeutic purposes in deficient states. Higher doses have been suggested to prevent cardiovascular diseases, cancer, emphysema and aging.

The Recommended Dietary Allowance (RDA) are recommended levels of intake to satisfy the nutritional needs of healthy individuals and are higher than levels which prevent vitamin deficiency diseases. A well balanced diet offers all vitamins in sufficient quantities and healthy individuals consuming a well-balanced diet do not need supplementation for nutritional well-being.

Vitamins are generally classified as fat soluble or water soluble. Water soluble vitamins are excreted in the urine and rarely cause toxicities at high doses. Fat soluble vitamins are stored and more likely to cause toxicities at high doses.

Water Soluble	Fat Soluble
B-complex Folic acid C	A D E K

Water Soluble Vitamins

Vitamin	Deficiency	Clinical Uses	Toxicology
B1 (thiamine) Found in meats and whole grains	**Dry beri-beri**: peripheral neuropathy with muscle atrophy; **wet beri-beri**: characterized by high cardiac output failure. Commonly observed in chronic alcoholics as **Wernicke syndrome** (dementia, ataxia and ophthalmoplegia) and **Korsakoff's psychosis**.	Thiamine deficiency	Relatively non-toxic
B2 (riboflavin) Found in milk products, meats, green leafy vegetables and grains.	**Sore throat** and **stomatitis** **Cheilosis**: fissures in the skin at the angles of the mouth, **seborrheic dermatitis**, **glossitis**, interstitial keratitis and vascularization of the cornea, anemia	Riboflavin deficiency	Relatively non-toxic
B3 (niacin, nicotinic acid) Found in meat, eggs, and milk and grains.	**Pellagra**: **dermatitis, diarrhea** and **dementia** (3 D's); glossitis, degeneration of posterior and lateral columns, death.	**Pellagra** **Hyperlipidemia**, especially type IIb	Flushing, pruritus, cramps, nausea, vomiting Hepatotoxicity, arrhythmias
B6 (pyridoxine, pyridoxal) Found in meats, grains, and vegetables	Rash, sores on lips, anemia, sensory neuritis and confusion. Rarely due to diet, usually drug-induced (especially isoniazid and penicillamine).	B6-deficient states Prophylaxis in isoniazid treated patients.	Low toxicity, but some neurologic symptoms have been reported at high doses.
B12 (cobalamin) Found in meats, eggs and cheese. Absorption requires **intrinsic factor**.	Hematologic: megaloblastic anemia CNS: degeneration of the posterior columns of the spinal cord. Vitamin B12 deficiency takes years to develop because body stores are used up slowly.	**Megaloblastic anemia**	Low toxicity

Vitamin	Deficiency	Clinical Uses	Toxicology
Folic acid Found in meats, eggs and vegetables.	Megaloblastic anemia and growth failure. Folic acid deficiency can develop within months.	Megaloblastic anemia **Pregnant** or **lactating women**	Low toxicity
C **(ascorbic acid)** An antioxidant found in citrus fruits, green vegetables, potatoes and tomatoes.	**Scurvy**: subperiosteal, skin, subungual, and joint hemorrhages due to inadequate collagenous support of capillaries. Observed as tooth loss, gingivitis, inability to limit infections, poor wound healing and arrested skeletal development (children).	Scurvy Supplementation during pregnancy	Low toxicity, however megadoses can lead to kidney stones.

Fat Soluble Vitamins

Vitamin	Deficiency	Clinical Uses	Toxicology
A Occurs naturally as **retinoids** (liver) or as a precursor, β-**carotene** in green, leafy vegetables.	Keratomalacia, xerophthalmia, bronchopneumonia, kidney stones (due to squamous metaplasia) **Diminished vision in dim light**: Vitamin A is a component of rods and is active in light transduction.	Vitamin A deficient states Acne Supplementation in pregnant and lactating women	Drowsiness, irritability, dizziness, headache, vomiting Dry and pruritic skin, skin desquamation, fissures of the lips Joint pain, hepatosplenomegaly, Papilledema, increased intracranial pressure (may mimic a brain tumor)
D Found in milk products and fish Formed naturally from sterols in the skin by UV light.	**Rickets** (children), **osteomalacia** (adults)	Rickets Osteomalacia Hypocalcemia Hypophosphatemia Osteodystrophy Tetany	Constipation, diarrhea, dryness of mouth, increased thirst, increased frequency of urination, loss of appetite, nausea and vomiting Vascular calcification, nephrocalcinosis, soft tissue calcification
E (tocopherols) An **antioxidant** found in vegetable oils.	Hemolytic anemia Peripheral neuropathy, decreased proprioception and necrotizing myopathy	Vitamin E deficient states	Very low toxicity In high doses, diarrhea, dizziness, headache, nausea, stomach cramps
K (quinones) Vitamin K1 is found in green leafy vegetables. Vitamin K2 is synthesized by normal intestinal bacteria.	Usually seen in newborns because vitamin K does not cross the placenta and the gut of the newborn is sterile. In anticoagulant and antibiotic therapy increased bleeding in gut, eyes and gums Necessary for the activity of the clotting factors: II (prothrombin) and factors VII, IX, and X.	Hypoprothrombinemia may occur during anticoagulant or certain antibiotic therapy. Hemorrhagic disease of the newborn. Coumadin overdose	Low toxicity In high doses, hemolytic anemia and jaundice can occur: toxicity occurs most often in newborns.

Drug Interactions

In most cases, the concurrent use of two or more drugs results in the independent action of each drug. In some cases, however, the simultaneous use of two or more drugs can result in altered therapeutic and/or adverse effects. This may be due to changes in pharmacokinetics, pharmacodynamics and/or toxicities of the individual agents.

Possible outcomes of drug interactions		
Additivity	The outcome is **equal** to the combined effects of the individual drugs.	$1 + 1 = 2$
Synergism	The outcome is **greater** than the combined effects of the individual drugs.	$1 + 1 > 2$
Antagonism	A drug with no inherent activity **decreases** the effect of another drug.	$0 + 1 < 1$
Potentiation	A drug with no inherent activity yet **enhances** the effect of another drug.	$0 + 1 > 1$

Listed below are selected drug interactions:

Drug 1	Drug 2	Outcome of Interaction
Alcohol	CNS depressants	Additive CNS depression
	Disulfiram Some cephalosporins	**Disulfiram-like reaction** due to the inhibition of alcohol dehydrogenase by disulfiram.
Alcohol (chronic) Barbiturates Carbamazepine Phenytoin Rifampin	Drugs metabolized by the liver including: Oral Anticoagulants Lidocaine, quinidine Theophylline Some benzodiazepines	These five drugs **induce hepatic metabolic enzymes** (P_{450}) and thus increase clearance of hepatically metabolized agents.
Antacids	Tetracyclines	Antacids complex with drugs in the GI tract **reducing absorption** of tetracyclines.

Drug 1	Drug 2	Outcome of Interaction
Anticholinergic drugs	Drugs absorbed in the small intestine	Anticholinergic drugs **decrease gastric motility** and will thus decrease the onset of action of orally administered drugs which are absorbed from the gut.
Cimetidine	Drugs metabolized by the liver including: Oral Anticoagulants Lidocaine, quinidine Theophylline Some benzodiazepines	Cimetidine **inhibits hepatic metabolic enzymes** (P_{450}) and thus increases the plasma levels and drug action.
Digitalis glycosides	Amiodarone Diltiazem Quinidine	Increase digitalis levels by decreasing clearance.
	Erythromycin	Increases digitalis levels by increasing absorption from the gut.
	Thiazide diuretics	The **loss of K^+** due to thiazide diuretics results in an increased cardiac toxicity of digoxin.
MAO-inhibitors	Sympathomimetic amines (tyramine)	**Hypertensive crisis** due to release of stored norepinephrine.
	Tricyclic antidepressants Serotonin reuptake inhibitors	A combination of MAO-inhibitors with these other antidepressant agents may result in a hyperserotonergic state (serotonin syndrome).
Probenecid	Penicillin	Probenecid **reduces renal excretion** of penicillin resulting in higher levels of the antibiotic. This is an example of **potentiation**.
Bile-acid binding resins	Thiazide diuretics Thyroid hormones	Resins can bind to orally administered drugs in the small intestine resulting in a **decreased absorption**.
Thiazide diuretics	Lithium	Thiazides **interfere with lithium excretion** and subsequently increase lithium levels and toxicity.

Antidotes for Drug Overdose and Poisoning

Drug Overdose or Poisoning	Antidote
Acetaminophen	Acetylcysteine
Anticholinergics (including atropine)	Physostigmine
Anticholinesterases (including organophosphate pesticides)	Atropine Pralidoxime (PAM)
Arsenic Gold Mercury	Dimercaprol (BAL)
Benzodiazepines	Flumazenil
Carbon monoxide	Oxygen
Cyanide	Sodium thiosulfate Amyl nitrite
Digoxin	Digoxin-specific antibodies (F'ab)
Heparin	Protamine sulfate
Iron salts	Deferoxamine
Lead	EDTA Dimercaprol
Methanol Ethylene glycol (antifreeze)	Ethanol
Neuromuscular blocking drugs	Neostigmine Physostigmine
Opioid analgesics	Naloxone
Warfarin	Vitamin K

Notes

Perinatal, Pediatric and Geriatric Pharmacology

Very young (fetal and neonatal) and elderly (geriatric) patients have an increased susceptibility to the pharmacologic and/or toxic effects of many drugs when compared to healthy young and adult populations. This poses many health concerns for these two age groups and precautions must be taken to avoid the accumulation of toxic levels of drugs due to their altered capabilities to absorb, metabolize, distribute and excrete certain drugs.

Physiologic and pharmacokinetic differences between fetal, newborn and geriatric patients:

Parameters	Fetus	Newborn (< 1 month)	Elderly Adult (> 75)
Lean body mass	↓	↓	↓
Muscle mass	Low	Low	↓
% body fat	Less than newborn	15%	↑
Total body H_2O	Highest	Very high (~75%)	Low (~50%)
Metabolic rate	↓	↓	↓
Hepatic mass	↓	↓	↓
Hepatic blood flow	–	↓	Low (~60% of normal)
Renal function	↓	↓	↓
Serum albumin (g/dL)	↓	↓	↓
Absorption	Most drugs can cross the placenta especially those that are lipid-soluble, and have a low molecular weight.	Elevated GI pH and lowered GI enzymes may ↑ concentrations of certain drugs inactivated by low gastric pH and enzymes. Gastric emptying is prolonged	Normal (may be affected by decreased gastric emptying and various drug interactions)
Distribution Protein Binding	↓ (more free drug due to ↓ albumin levels)	↓ (more free drug due to ↓ albumin levels)	↓ (more free drug due to ↓ albumin levels)
Metabolism	Placenta and maternal liver	↓ (due to ↓ P_{450} enzymes)	↓ (due to ↓ in phase I reactions and ↓ in hepatic blood flow)
Elimination		↓ renal elimination due to ↓ GFR	↓ renal elimination due to ↓ GFR

Drug Therapy During Pregnancy

There are many drugs taken by pregnant women that cross the placenta and expose the fetus to their pharmacological and possibly teratogenic effects. Lipid-soluble drugs and those of small molecular size cross the placenta easily.

Teratogens

Drug	Trimester	Effect on Fetus
Aminoglycosides	All	Ototoxicity, nephrotoxicity
Antidepressants (tricyclic)	1st & 3rd	Congenital anomalies Neonatal withdrawal symptoms
Chloramphenicol	3rd	Gray Baby syndrome
Diethylstilbestrol	All	Reproductive abnormalities: including vaginal adenosis and carcinoma
Ethanol	All	Fetal alcohol syndrome
Lithium	1st	Cardiovascular anomalies (especially Ebstein malformation) and goiter
Phenytoin	All	Fetal Hydantoin Syndrome: characterized by heart defects, hypoplastic nails and digits and craniofacial abnormalities
Tetracycline	All	Tooth discoloration and bone alterations
Thalidomide	1st	Phocomelia, microtia

Drug Therapy During Lactation

Although drugs taken postpartum have less of an impact on the newborn, conservative measures should be continued in women who are breast feeding. A large number of drugs can be found in breast milk.

Drugs contraindicated during lactation

Drug	Effect on Infant
Chloral Hydrate	Sedation
Chloramphenicol	Bone marrow depression (concentrations too low to cause Gray Baby Syndrome)
Diazepam	Sedation and weight loss
Heroin	Narcotic dependence
Iodine (radioactive)	Thyroid suppression and skin rash
Lithium	Hypotonia, hypothermia, cyanosis and ECG changes
Methadone	Physical dependence
Methimazole	Suppression of thyroid function, agranulocytosis
Phenobarbital	Sedation at hypnotic doses
Sulfonamides	Kernicterus Hemolytic anemia in G-6-PD deficient infants
Tetracycline	Permanent staining of teeth, photosensitivity, bone alterations

Pediatric Drug Dosage

There is much variation in drug dosages for infants and children due to differences in pharmacokinetics. Drug therapy for pediatric patients must be tailored to their age, weight and body composition. Keep in mind that the pediatric dose should never exceed the adult dose. Listed below are selected examples of drugs whose adverse effects are more pronounced in pediatric populations.

Drugs adversely affecting infants and children

Drug	Effects
Aspirin	Reye Syndrome following viral illness
Antihistamine	Paradoxical hyperactivity
Benzodiazepines	Prolonged CNS depression
Fluoroquinolones	Not clinically tested in children due to abnormal development of cartilage and joints observed in experimental animals.
Phenobarbital	Sedation at hypnotic doses.
Phenytoin	Coarsening of facial features, excessive body hair and increased susceptibility to gingival hyperplasia.
Sulfonamides	Kernicterus in neonates
Tetracycline	Permanent staining of teeth, enamel hypoplasia and decrease in skeletal growth rate.

Geriatric Drug Dosage

There is much variation in drug dosages among the adult population due to differences in the pharmacokinetic properties of elderly individuals. Drug therapy for geriatric patients must be tailored to their age, weight and body composition. Listed below are selected examples of drugs whose adverse effects are more pronounced in geriatric populations.

Selected drugs affecting geriatric patients

Drug	Effects
Anticoagulants	Increased risk of hemorrhage
Cimetidine	Confusion
Aminoglycosides	Nephrotoxicity, ototoxicity
Isoniazid	Hepatitis (drug induced)

Pharmacogenetics

Pharmacogenetics is the study of the effects that genetic differences have on the metabolism of certain drugs. The major mechanisms of pharmacogenetic actions and specific examples are listed below:

Type	Genetic Alteration	Selected Examples	Clinical Manifestations
Slow vs. rapid acetylation	N-acetyltransferase	Isoniazid, hydralazine, procainamide	Increased toxicity
Slow vs. rapid hydrolysis	Pseudocholinesterase	Succinylcholine	Increased toxicity
Glucose-6-phosphate dehydrogenase (G-6-PD)	G-6-PD	Primaquine, aspirin, fava beans	Hemolysis
Uncontrolled calcium release	Heterogeneous	General anesthetics Neuromuscular blocking agents	Malignant hyperthermia

Example	Mechanism/Genetics	Notes
Slow vs. rapid acetylation **Isoniazid** **Hydralazine** **Procainamide**	**N-acetyltransferase**: enzyme activity varies in the population **Autosomal recessive**	These drugs are inactivated by **N-acetyltransferase** **Half of the population** metabolizes these drugs slower than the other half; there is a **bimodal distribution** of metabolizers **Slow metabolizers** are more likely to develop toxic side effects and thus require lower doses **Rapid metabolizers** are less likely to achieve therapeutic responses to a usual dose and thus require higher doses. There is an *in vivo* test which measures the blood level 6 hours after administration of a standard dose. It is thus recommended to test susceptible individuals and adjust dose accordingly

Example	Mechanism/Genetics	Notes
Slow vs. rapid hydrolysis **Succinylcholine**	**Pseudocholinesterase**: enzyme activity varies in the population **Autosomal recessive**	Succinylcholine is inactivated by **plasma pseudocholinesterase** Plasma pseudocholinesterase activity is normally high so excess drug must be given to compensate for the expected rapid loss in the plasma About 1/3,000 individuals have **atypical pseudocholinesterase** which is much less active A normal dose would be a serious overdose for those with deficient enzyme activity resulting in **respiratory failure**. Thus, it is recommended to test pseudocholinesterase activity before administering succinylcholine and always have respiratory support available There is an *in vitro* test available which indirectly characterizes the patient's esterase. This test utilizes **dibucaine** which inhibits atypical esterase **less** than it inhibits normal esterase. Thus measuring plasma pseudocholinesterase activity in the presence and absence of dibucaine will determine the phenotype of the patient.
Glucose-6-phosphate dehydrogenase deficiency **Primaquine** **Aspirin** **Fava beans**	Tissue metabolism disorder **Sex linked** G-6-PD deficiency is most prevalent in populations genetically derived from Africa and the Mediterranean basin. Observed in **15% of American black males.**	The enzyme deficiency is **glucose-6-phosphate dehydrogenase (G-6-PD)**. Although not the metabolic enzyme for primaquine and other compounds, G-6-PD, an enzyme in the **pentose-phosphate-shunt pathway**, generates NADPH which maintains **glutathione in a reduced state** (GSH) which in turn maintains the integrity of the RBC membranes. Patients with G-6-PD deficiency have marginal stores of NADPH. The administration of oxidant drugs such as primaquine depletes these stores and subsequently result in **hemolysis** There is an *in vitro* test for G-6-PD deficiency which measures GSH in the blood before and after the administration of an oxidant drug. GSH levels remains constant in normal individuals but decrease in G-6-PD deficient patients
Uncontrolled Ca^{2+} release **General anesthetics** **Neuromuscular blocking agents**	Various causes but many are due to mutated Ca^{2+} release channel (ryanodine receptor) in skeletal muscle. Autosomal dominant	Administration of general anesthetics or neuromuscular blocking drugs may cause uncontrolled **calcium release** leading to **uncoupled oxidative phosphorylation**. This can result in muscle rigidity and **malignant hyperthermia**. **Dantrolene** is used to treat malignant hyperthermia because it is a muscle relaxant which decreases calcium release

Prescription Writing

The following items are necessary when filling out a prescription:

- Full name of patient
- Address of patient
- Name & address of prescribing MD
- Signature of prescribing MD
- Date of issuance
- Name, strength and dosage of drug
- Quantity of drug prescribed
- Indication for use
- Number of refills
- Physician's licence number
- DEA registration number of MD (if controlled substance is prescribed)

Sample Prescription

Patient name　　　　Physician name

Address　　　　Address

Date________________

DOB___________

Rx

Marinol 5 mg PO tid ac
 # 90

Refill ___ times　　　　Indication_______________________________

( ) Place indication on prescription label

_______________________ Physician's Signature

_______________________ Physician's Name(print)

_______________________ Physician's Extension (pager#)

Physician's Lic. #_____________________　　DEA #_____________________

Abbreviations	Explanations
ac	before meals
bid	twice a day
hs	at bedtime
pc	after meals
PO	by mouth
PR	per rectum
prn	when needed
q	every
qd	every day
qh	every hour
qhs	every night at bedtime
qid	four times a day
qod	every other day
stat	at once
tid	three times a day

The **Controlled Substance Act** requires all prescribers and dispensers to register with the DEA and keep a record of all controlled substances that are prescribed and dispensed. A physician's **DEA registration number** is required for a prescription for any controlled substance to be filled (schedule I - schedule V).

Schedule	Example	Notes
I	Heroin Marihuana	High abuse and addictive potential. **Not available for prescription**; no therapeutic use.
II	Morphine Codeine Amphetamines	High abuse and addictive potential. These drugs are used clinically. Order must be in writing (no verbal orders). **No refills**
III	Tylenol with codeine	Less abuse and addictive potential than schedule I or II. May be submitted in writing or verbally. Limited to 5 refills or 6 months usage whichever is first.
IV	Valium	Even less abuse and addictive potential than schedule III. May be submitted in writing or verbally. Limited to 5 refills or 6 months usage whichever is first.
V	Lomotil	Low abuse and addictive potential. May be submitted in writing or verbally. Limited to 5 refills or 6 months usage whichever is first.

Principles of Drug Development

The time span between the discovery of an investigational drug and its FDA approval averages **12 years**. Approximately 1 in 8,000 compounds tested in animals reaches the drug market; one in 40,000 ultimately provides a significant contribution to medicine. The stages of the drug development process include:

Preclinical Studies (1-5 yrs)

Most new drugs are created by modification of known drugs, random testing of natural products, chemicals, peptides or nucleic acids or rational drug design based on knowledge of chemical structure. These drugs are screened and initially developed using **in vitro studies**. Once the drug has shown efficacy in vitro, **animal studies** may be initiated to assess acute, subacute and chronic toxicity as well as carcinogenic, mutagenic and reproductive effects. These studies may also address pharmacokinetic parameters.

Clinical Studies (2-10 yrs)

Once animal data indicate that a drug is relatively safe and has the potential for clinical use, the chemical and biological data must be submitted to the FDA as a **Notice of Claimed Investigational Exemption for a New Drug** (IND) which requests permission to begin human trials. If denial is NOT received within 30 days, human studies may be initiated. Clinical research involves three phases prior to approval for marketing and a fourth phase which follows the marketing of the product.

Phase	General Notes	Main Emphasis	Size of Study
I	First introduction into humans to evaluate if the effects seen in animal studies are reproducible in humans.	**Safety** Is it safe?	< 50 **healthy volunteers**
II	Usually involves single-blind or double-blind evaluation against placebo and currently marketed drugs in patients with the disease the drug is designed to treat.	**Efficacy** Does it work?	< 300 patients with the target disease
III	Usually involves a double-blind **multicenter** trial against placebo and currently marketed drugs in patients with the disease the drug is designed to treat.	**Safety** and **Efficacy**	> 1,000 patients with target disease
Data from Phases I, II, and III are combined and submitted to the FDA for review and approval of a **New Drug Application** (NDA). Once a NDA has been approved, the drug may be manufactured, labeled, and marketed for the indications approved by the FDA. This process usually takes 2 months to 7 years (average 2.6 years).			
IV	These are studies conducted by pharmaceutical companies to gain approval for additional indications.	Post-marketing surveillance	Available to public

Note: The time required before human tests are started depends on the urgency and importance of the agent in question. For example, anti-cancer and HIV medications are accelerated through preclinical and clinical phases which makes them available sooner, however the safety of some of these agents may still be in question.

Appendix

Page	Topic
323	Appendix I. Glossary
326	Appendix II. Contraceptive Formulations
328	Appendix III. Calcium Salt Preparations and Uses

Acute intermittent porphyria: clinically manifested as intermittent abdominal pain, peripheral neuropathy, seizures and psychosis. Laboratory findings include hyponatremia and an increased amount of porphobilinogen in the urine. The underlying cause of this disorder is a deficiency of porphobilinogen deaminase, an enzyme involved in heme biosynthesis.

Afterload: describes the force that the ventricle must overcome during systolic ejection. Afterload is directly related to arterial pressure.

Anaphylaxis: an immediate, transient allergic reaction characterized by smooth muscle contraction and capillary dilation.

Capillary leak syndrome: due to an increase in capillary permeability. Can lead to hypotension and pulmonary edema or respiratory failure.

Chloracne: acne-like eruptions due to exposure to some chlorinated compounds.

Chorea: observed as involuntary, spastic movements of the extremities or facial muscles.

Chronotropic effects: an alteration in heart rate.

Conn's Syndrome (primary hyperaldosteronism): characterized by elevated aldosterone levels, muscular weakness, polyuria, hypertension, hypokalemic alkalosis and decreased plasma renin activity. Conn's syndrome is due to excessive aldosterone secretion. The two primary causes are adrenocortical adenoma and cortical hyperplasia.

Coomb's test: a hematologic test to determine autoantibody status. A positive Coomb's test indicates the presence of autoantibodies and may predispose the patient to hemolytic anemia. There are two types of Coomb's tests, indirect and direct.

Cretinism: characterized by stunted growth and mental development usually presenting during infancy. May result from endocrine disorders or insufficient iodine intake during pregnancy.

Cytokine: proteins released by cells which act as intercellular mediators.

Diabetes insipidus: characterized by polyuria and polydipsia. There are two types: central and nephrogenic. Central diabetes insipidus results from a deficiency in vasopressin. Nephrogenic diabetes insipidus results from an inability of the kidney to reabsorb water.

Diabetes mellitus: characterized by the classic triad of polydipsia, polyuria and polyphagia and a fasting blood glucose $\geq$ 140 mg/dL. The underlying cause of this disorder is a deficiency of insulin.

Disulfiram reaction: characterized by flushing, tachycardia, nausea and hyperventilation. This reaction is due to the accumulation of acetaldehyde.

Dyskinesias: disorders of voluntary movement control.

Erythema multiforme: an acute eruption of multiple dermatologic lesions over the dorsal aspect of the upper extremities. Stevens-Johnson syndrome occurs when erythema multiforme runs a severe course with a fatal outcome.

Extrapyramidal effects: observed as parkinsonism (rigidity, tremor), akathisia (inability to remain in a seated posture) and acute dystonic reactions. Long term effects include tardive dyskinesia (choreoathetoid movements and lip smacking). These effects occur secondary to dopamine blockade in the CNS which can disturb the dopamine:acetylcholine balance.

Familial periodic paralysis: represents a group of disorders characterized by episodes of muscular weakness. There are three types of this disorder: hypokalemic, hyperkalemic and normokalemic.

Fanconi's syndrome: a hematologic disorder characterized by pancytopenia, hypoplasia of the bone marrow and congenital abnormalities.

Gilles de la Tourette syndrome: observed as multiple motor and phonic tics which usually present before the age of 21.

Hemophilia A: an X-linked disorder characterized by a deficiency of clotting factor VII. Hemophilia A is manifested as a severe bleeding tendency, most frequently into joint capsules.

Hypertensive crisis: characterized by headache, nausea, tachycardia, hypertension, cardiac arrhythmias and possibly stroke. May be induced by concomitant ingestion of tyramine-containing foods and administration of MAO-inhibitors.

Inotropic effect: an alteration in the force of contractility.

Iodism: iodine overdose characterized by acne-like eruptions, weakness, salivation and halitosis.

Lupus-like syndrome: characterized by photosensitivity, polyarthralgia, myalgia and fever. Less severe than systemic lupus erythematosus and may be induced by a variety of agents.

Malignant hyperthermia: is an autosomal dominant disorder which can result from administration of fluorinated hydrocarbons or depolarizing muscle relaxants such as succinylcholine. Malignant hyperthermia results from an excessive release of Ca^{2+} from the sarcoplasmic reticulum and presents as hyperthermia, metabolic acidosis, tachycardia and accelerated muscle contractions. **Treatment** includes rapid cooling, 100% O_2, control of the acidosis and IV administration of **dantrolene** which blocks the release of Ca^{2+} from the sarcoplasmic reticulum.

Meniere's disease: observed as the triad of vertigo, tinnitus and sensorineural hearing loss.

Methemoglobinemia: characterized by the presence of methemoglobin in the blood. Methemoglobin is a combination of oxyhemoglobin with ferric rather than ferrous iron. This form of oxyhemoglobin is useless in respiration.

Monoclonal antibody: a specific antibody directed against a single epitope of its target molecule.

Myxedema: presents as edema of the extremities, tongue and eyelids. This state is caused by an accumulation of proteoglycans in the extracellular matrix and is seen in hypothyroidism. May also present with neurologic effects such as paranoid ideation, depression or agitation (myxedema madness).

Nephrotic syndrome: characterized by proteinuria, peripheral edema and hyperlipidemia and is caused by non-inflammatory glomerulonephropathies.

Neuroleptic malignant syndrome: a serious complication of neuroleptic treatment characterized by a catatonic state, extrapyramidal signs, fever, changes in blood pressure and alterations in consciousness.

Papilledema: optic disk swelling due to increased intracranial pressure.

Preload: defined as the passive tension/unit cross-sectional area in ventricular muscle. Preload describes the pressure in the ventricle at the onset of ventricular contraction and is directly related to the end-diastolic pressure.

Prodrug: an inactive drug which must be metabolized to its active form.

Prophylaxis: prevention of a disease or the process which leads to disease.

Red man syndrome: rapid IV infusion of vancomycin can cause histamine release which leads to hypotension and a red pruritic rash on the patient's torso. Patients may be pre-treated with H_1-receptor antagonists and aspirin to avoid this uncomfortable but not life-threatening side effect.

Reye's syndrome: a fatal, fulminating hepatitis and cerebral edema seen in children with fever caused by viral illness who are given aspirin.

Serotonin syndrome: observed as rigidity, hyperthermia, myoclonus, confusion and coma. May be caused by concomitant administration of various antidepressants.

Serum sickness: characterized by fever, arthralgia, vasculitis and glomerulonephritis observed within one week of injection of a foreign protein.

Stevens-Johnson syndrome: a severe, possibly fatal form of erythema multiform which involves mucosal membranes and internal organs.

Torsades de pointes: a spontaneous or drug-induced ventricular tachycardia with varying QRS morphology.

von Willebrand's disease: an autosomal dominant disorder due to a deficiency in von Willebrand factor. This disorder commonly presents as bleeding on mucosal surfaces.

Wernicke-Korsakoff Syndrome: a combination of Wernicke encephalopathy and Korsakoff syndrome both of which are observed in the setting of chronic alcoholism. Wernicke's encephalopathy presents as nystagmus, truncal ataxia and confusion. Korsakoff's syndrome is observed as amnesia and confabulation.

Appendix II. Available Oral Contraceptives:

Type	**Trade Name**	**Progestin** (mg)	**Estrogen** (μg)
Monophasic Ethinyl estradiol/norethindrone	Loestrin 1/20	1	20
	Loestrin 1.5/30	1.5	30
	Brevicon	0.5	35
	Modicon	0.5	35
	Genora 0.5/35	0.5	35
	Nelona 0.5/35	0.5	35
	Norinyl 1+35	1	35
	Ortho-Novum 1/35	1	35
	Ovcon-35	0.4	35
	Ovcon-50	1	50
Ethinyl estradiol/levonorgestrel	Levlen	0.15	30
	Nordette	0.15	30
Ethinyl estradiol/norgestrel	Lo-Ovral	0.3	30
	Ovral	0.5	50
Ethinyl estradiol/ethynodiol diacetate	Demulen 1/35	1	35
	Demulen 1/50	1	50
Mestranol/norethindrone	Norinyl 1+50	1	50
	Ortho-novum 1/50	1	50
	Norethin1/50 M	1	50
	Genora 1/50	1	50
	Nelova 1/50M	1	50
Ethinyl estradiol/desogestrel	Desogen	0.15	30
	Ortho-cept	0.15	30
Ethinyl estradiol/norgestimate	Ortho-cyclen	0.25	35

Type	Trade Name	Progestin (mg)	Estrogen (μg)
Biphasic Ethinyl estradiol/norethindrone	Ortho-novum 10/11	0.5	35
		1	35
	Nelova 10/11	5	35
		1	35
	Jenest-28	0.5	35
		1	35
Triphasic Ethinyl estradiol/norethindrone	Ortho-novum 7/7/7	0.5	35
		0.75	35
		1	35
	Tri-norinyl	0.05	35
		1	35
		0.5	35
Ethinyl estradiol/norgestimate	Ortho Tri-cyclen	0.18	35
		0.215	35
		0.25	35
Ethinyl estradiol/levonorgestrel	Tri-levlen	0.05	30
		0.075	40
		0.125	30
	Triphasil-21	0.05	30
		0.075	40
		0.125	30

Appendix III. Use and administration of various systemic calcium supplements.

Since the multitude of calcium supplements are varied in both clinical indiciation as well as administration, this appendix serves to expand on the calcium supplements already mentioned in the previous chapters. This chart **SHOULD NOT** be memorizied, but rather serve as a reference for the interested reader as well as provide an appreciation of the numerous calcium supplements and their various clinical uses.

	% Ca^{2+}	IV	Oral	IM	Antihypocalcemic	Antacid	Antihyperkalemic	Antihypermagnesemic	Antihyperphosphatemic	Cardiotonic	Nutrient Supplement	Electrolyte Replenisher
Calcium Acetate	25	✓			✓							✓
Calcium Carbonate	40		✓		✓	✓			✓		✓	
Calcium Chloride	27	✓			✓		✓	✓		✓		✓
Calcium Citrate	21		✓		✓				✓		✓	
Calcium Glubionate	7		✓		✓						✓	
Calcium Gluceptate	8		✓	✓	✓			✓			✓	✓
Calcium Gluconate	9	✓	✓		✓		✓ (IV)	✓ (IV)		✓ (IV)	✓	✓ (IV)
Calcium Lactate	13		✓		✓						✓	
Calcium Phosphate, Dibasic	23		✓		✓						✓	
Calcium Phosphate, Tribasic	38		✓		✓						✓	

Benzodiazepines

Flumazenil

Barbiturates

MAO Inhibitors

Isocarboxazid
Phenelzine
Tranylcypromine

TCA Antidepressants

Imipramine
Desipramine
Amitriptyline
Nortriptyline
Clominpramine

Fluoxetine

Chlorpromazine

Haloperidol

Clozapine

MOA: Enhance GABA binding to the $GABA_A$ receptor resulting in **prolonged duration** of **chloride channel opening**. This causes membrane hyperpolarization and a decrease in neuronal excitability.

Clinical Uses: status epilepticus, partial and generalized tonic-clonic seizures, narco-analysis

Side Effects: clumsiness, dizziness, drowsiness, induction of the P_{450} system

Page 36

MOA: **Competitive antagonist** of benzodiazepines at the $GABA_A$ receptor in the CNS.

Clinical Uses: reversal of benzodiazepine-induced sedation following anesthesia, zolpidem overdose, suspected **acute benzodiazepine overdose**.

Side Effects: few effects in benzodiazepine-free individuals; effects are mainly due to reversal of benzodiazepine activity.

Page 35

MOA: Enhance GABA binding to the $GABA_A$ receptor resulting in **increased frequency** of **chloride channel opening**. This causes membrane hyperpolarization and a decrease in neuronal excitability.

Clinical Uses: **anxiety**: diazepam, **panic disorders**: alprazolam, **insomnia**: flurazepam, triazolam, temazepam

Side Effects: drowsiness, decreased cognitive function, ataxia, dizziness

Page 34

MOA: Selectively inhibits serotonin reuptake. A **pro-drug** which is converted to its active metabolite, **norfluoxetine**.

Clinical Uses: depression: DOC, Obsessive compulsive disorder

Side Effects: nervousness, restlessness, irritability, sleep disturbances, nausea, diarrhea

Others: Sertraline and Paroxetine

Page 41

MOA: Block the active uptake of norepinephrine and serotonin at the cell membrane of presynaptic neurons causing desensitization of postsynaptic adrenergic and serotonergic receptors.

Clinical Uses: depression, enuresis in childhood, obsessive-compulsive disorder

Side Effects: orthostatic hypotension, sedation, anticholinergic effects

Page 40

MOA: Inhibit the activity of intraneuronal MAO which increases the release of **norepinephrine** and/or **serotonin** from the presynaptic neuron.

Clinical Uses: **depression**

Side Effects: orthostatic hypotension, hypertensive crisis with tyramine

Page 39

MOA: Blocks D_4 and D_2 receptors. Clozapine exhibits lesser affinity for blocking D_2 than chlorpromazine.

Clinical Uses: schizophrenia

Side Effects: agranulocytosis, convulsions, sedation, hypotension, tachycardia

Page 47

MOA: Competitively blocks postsynaptic dopamine (D_2) receptors in the CNS.

Clinical Uses: psychotic disorders, Gilles de la Tourette's Syndrome, Huntington's disease

Side Effects: extrapyramidal effects

Page 46

MOA: Blocks postsynaptic dopaminergic receptors (D_2) in the brain, medullary chemoreceptor trigger zone. Also blocks the vagus nerve in the GI tract.

Clinical Uses: **schizophrenia, antiemetic**, intractable hiccups

Side Effects: hypotensive effects, sedation

Others: Fluphenazine, trifluoperazine, thioridazine

Page 45

Lithium Carbonate

Phenytoin

Ethosuximide

Valproic Acid

Levodopa

Selegiline

Bromocriptine

Halothane

Droperidol

plus

Fentanyl

MOA: **Inhibits Ca^{2+} influx** through low threshold T-type channels in thalamic neurons.

Clinical Use: absences seizures

Side Effects: GI disturbances, CNS effects

Page 53

MOA: Binds to and prolongs the inactivated state of Na^+ channels (prevents high frequency firing of action potentials).

Clinical Uses: generalized tonic-clonic seizures, partial seizures, status epilepticus

Side Effects: **gingival hyperplasia,** CNS toxicity, hirsutism, induction of P_{450} enzymes, hypersensitivity reactions

Page 51

MOA: The mechanism is unclear but involves the inhibition of inositol phosphate recycling.

Clinical Uses: bipolar disorder, mania

Side Effects: CNS effects, nephrogenic diabetes insipidus, teratogenic

Drug Interactions: Thiazide diuretics may enhance lithium toxicity.

Page 48

MOA: Increases dopamine concentrations by **selectively inhibiting MAO-B**.

Clinical Uses: Parkinson's disease

Side Effects: dyskinesias, mood alterations

Page 56

MOA: Levodopa is rapidly converted to dopamine by dopa decarboxylase in the periphery and nervous system. Levodopa crosses the blood brain barrier.

Clinical Use: Parkinson's disease

Side Effects: GI disturbances, dyskinesia, cardiovascular effects, CNS effects

Note: Levodopa if often given alone. Carbidopa increase the concentration of dopamine in the CNS by inhibiting dop decarboxylase in the periphery.

Page 56

MOA: Inhibits high-frequency repetitive firing of neurons by **inhibiting Na^+ influx** through specific voltage-gated ion channels.

Clinical Uses: absence seizures, generalized tonic-clonic seizures, myoclonic seizures

Side Effects: GI disturbances, hepatotoxicity, CNS effects, teratogenic

Page 53

MOA: When a neuroleptic drug is combined with a narcotic, a state of **neurolept analgesia** is produced; most often produced by combining droperidol with fentanyl

Clinical Uses: analgesia, general anesthesia

Side Effects: nausea, vomiting, confusion and mental depression

Page 64

MOA: Inhalational anesthetic

Clinical Use: general anesthesia

Side Effects: malignant hyperthermia, hepatic necrosis with enflurane

Others: Enflurane, isoflurane, desflurane

Page 61

MOA: Ergot alkaloid which acts as a strong agonist at D_2 receptors and a partial antagonist at D_1 receptors.

Clinical Uses: Parkinson's disease, hyperprolactinemia, acromegaly

Side Effects: hypotension, CNS effects

Page 57

Ketamine

Local Anesthetics

Esters
Cocaine, Benzocaine
Procaine, Tetracaine

Amides
Lidocaine, Mepivacaine
Bupivacaine, Prilocaine

Morphine

Fentanyl

Codeine

Diphenoxylate HCl

Dextromethorphan

Pentazocine

Naloxone

MOA: Naturally occurring opioid agonist at μ receptors. Has an active metabolite, morphine 6-glucuronide.

Clinical Uses: analgesia, acute pulmonary edema, antitussive

Side Effects: constipation, histamine release, convulsions

Others: Methadone. meperidine, fentanyl is a synthetic opioid agonist.

MOA: Weak bases which block nerve transmission by inhibiting **Na^+ channels**.

Clinical Uses: surface anesthesia, nerve block anesthesia, spinal anesthesia, epidural anesthesia, arrhythmias

Side Effects: CNS effects, cardiovascular effects, allergic reactions (due to the formation of p-amino benzoic acid)

MOA: A **dissociative anesthetic** which blocks **NMDA** receptors. Ketamine is structurally similar to PCP (the original dissociative anesthetic).

Clinical Uses: trauma and emergency surgical procedures, radiological procedures in children

Side Effects: **hallucinations**, unpleasant dreams

MOA: A meperidine analog which acts at opioid receptors in the enteric nervous system to decrease intestinal motility

Clinical Uses: **antidiarrheal**, analgesia

Side Effects: anticholinergic effects

Others: Loperamide

MOA: A naturally occurring opioid agonist with low affinity at μ receptors. Twelve times less potent than morphine.

Clinical Uses: analgesia, **antitussive**

Side Effects: constipation

MOA: A synthetic opioid agonist at μ receptors. Eighty times more potent than morphine

Clinical Uses: **analgesia**, anesthesia (used in combination with droperidol)

Side Effects: apnea, CNS depression, hypoventilation

MOA: Antagonist at opioid receptors

Clinical Uses: **opioid toxicity**, **respiratory depression**

Side Effects: tachycardia, arrhythmias

Other: Naltrexone

MOA: An opioid agonist at κ and σ receptors and an antagonist at μ receptors.

Clinical Use: Analgesia

Side Effects: Subjective/psychotomimetic effects, respiratory depression which exhibits a "**ceiling effect**."

Other: Nalbuphine

MOA: A synthetic derivative of morphine which acts directly on the medullary cough center to suppress the cough reflex. Does not have any activity at opioid receptors.

Clinical Use: Antitussive

Reserpine

Guanethidine

α-Adrenergic Blockers

Prazosin
Terazosin

Propanolol

Metoprolol

Methyldopa

Hydralalazine

Minoxidil

ACE Inhibitors

MOA: Potent selective α_1-adrenergic receptor antagonists in arterioles and veins causing a decrease in peripheral vascular resistance (PVR) and venous return to the heart. Relax smooth muscle in the bladder neck and prostate by blocking α_1-adrenergic receptors.

Clinical Uses: hypertension, benign prostatic hyperplasia

Side Effects: First-dose phenomenon, dizziness, headache

Page 89

MOA: Enters neuron by norepinephrine reuptake transporter and slowly displaces norepinephrine in the synaptic vesicles. ("substitute neurotransmitter") and thereby blocks the release of norepinephrine normally produced by nerve stimulation

Clinical Use: hypertension

Side Effects: orthostatic hypotension, impotence

Page 88

MOA: **Irreversibly** binds to storage vesicles in adrenergic neurons causing a reduced uptake and storage of norepinephrine, dopamine and serotonin both centrally and peripherally

Clinical Uses: hypertension, Huntington's disease

Side Effects: sedation, inability to concentrate, dizziness

Page 88

MOA: **Prodrug** converted in the brain to its active metabolite methyl-norepinephrine which activates α_2-adrenergic receptors to inhibit sympathetic outflow.

Clinical Uses: hypertension

Side Effects: Edema, drowsiness, dry mouth, headache, development of a (+) Coombs test

Others: Clonidine

Page 92

MOA: Selective β_1-adrenergic receptor antagonist (cardioselective) with antianginal, antiarrhythmic (Class II) and antihypertensive effects.

Clinical Uses: hypertension, angina, arrhythmias, myocardial infarction

Side Effects: bradycardia, sedation, fatigue, bronchospasm, hypoglycemia, congestive heart failure

Page 91

MOA: Nonselective β_1, β_2-adrenergic receptor antagonist with antianginal, antiarrhythmic (Class II) and antihypertensive effects.

Clinical Uses: hypertension, angina, arrhythmias, myocardial infarction, pheochromocytoma

Side Effects: impotence, sedation, fatigue, bronchoconstriction, hypoglycemia

Others: Timolol

Page 90

MOA: Reversibly inhibit ACE (kininase II) preventing the conversion of angiotensin I into the vasoconstrictor **angiotensin II**.

Clinical Uses: hypertension and congestive heart failure. Captopril is also used for Scleroderma renal crisis

Side Effects: dry cough, headache, fatigue, hypotension (with first dose)

Page 94

MOA: **Prodrug** metabolized to minoxidil N-O sulfate which is an **arteriolar** smooth muscle vasodilator. Minoxidil sulfate increases K^+ efflux by opening K^+ channels causing hyperpolarization and relaxation of smooth muscle.

Clinical Use: **hypertension**: refractory to other antihypertensive medications.

Side Effects: edema, reflex tachycardia, hypertrichosis

Page 93

MOA: Direct vasodilator of **arteriolar** smooth muscle resulting in a significant ↓PVR. This action elicits a compensatory sympathetic response including ↑ HR and stroke volume (↑ cardiac output) and fluid retention.

Clinical Use: hypertension

Side Effects: headache, nausea, Lupus-like syndrome

Page 93

Losartan

Nifedipine

Diltiazem

Diazoxide

Sodium Nitroprusside

Nitrates

Nitroglycerin
Isosorbide nitrate
Amyl nitrate

Cardiac Glycosides

Digoxin
Digitoxin

PDE Inhibitors

Amrinone
Milrinone

Class IA Drugs

Quinidine
Procainamide
Disopyramide

MOA: Binds cardiac L-type Ca^{2+} channels and decreases **SA node** automaticity and **AV nodal conduction** with some negative inotropic effects on the heart.

Clinical Uses: hypertension (mild to moderate), angina, supraventricular arrhythmias

Side Effects: rare

Other: Verapamil

MOA: Inhibit slow, voltage-gated (L-type) **Ca^{2+} channels** resulting in ↓ Ca^{2+} influx. This causes relaxation of **arterial** smooth muscle and ↓ PVR.

Clinical Uses: **hypertension**, **angina**, Raynaud's phenomenon

Side Effects: headache, dizziness, peripheral edema, flushing, nausea

MOA: Nonpeptide angiotensin II receptor (AT_1 subtype) antagonist which inhibits the vasoconstrictor and aldosterone-secreting effects of angiotensin II (ATII).

Clinical Use: **hypertension**

Side Effects: headache, hypotension

MOA: Metabolized by smooth muscle cells to nitric oxide (**NO**) which activates guanylate cyclase and increases **cGMP**. This increase in cGMP results in the dephosphorylation of myosin light chains and the subsequent relaxation of smooth muscle.

Clinical Uses: **angina pectoris**, **myocardial infarction**, congestive heart failure

Side Effects: **headache**, **reflex tachycardia**, **postural hypotension**, **Monday disease**

MOA: Metabolized by red blood cells and smooth muscle cells to **nitric oxide** (NO, EDRF) which leads to the formation of **cGMP**. The ↑ cGMP leads to ↓ Ca^{2+} ions in **arteriolar** and **venous** vessels, causing vasodilation.

Clinical Uses: hypertensive emergencies, congestive heart failure

Side Effects: hypotension, arrhythmias, cyanide adn thiocyanate toxicity

MOA: Activates ATP-sensitive K^+ channels causing hyperpolarization of arteriolar smooth muscle cells. This results in arteriolar vasodilation.

Clinical Use: hypertensive emergencies

Side Effects: edema, tachycardia, hypoglycemia

MOA: Bind to **open Na^+ channels** preventing Na^+ influx thus decreasing the slopes of phase 0 and phase 4 (↑ QRS interval). Also inhibits K^+ currents, resulting in an ↑ repolarization time and action potential duration (↑ QT interval).

Clinical Uses: ventricular and supraventricular arrhythmias.

Side Effects: diarrhea, nausea and vomiting. Disopyramide exhibits strong anticholinergic effects.

MOA: Inhibit cAMP phosphodiesterase (PDE III) in cardiac and smooth muscle. This increase in cAMP results in a (+) **inotropic** effect and **vasodilation** (↓ preload and afterload).

Clinical Use: congestive heart failure

Side Effects: arrhythmias, hypotension, dizziness

MOA: Inhibits the **Na^+-K^+ ATPase** in myocardial cell membranes thereby increasing exchange of intracellular Na^+ for extracellular Ca^{2+} by the Na^+-Ca^{2+} exchanger. This ultimately results in a positive inotropic effect.

Clinical Uses: congestive heart failure, supraventricular arrhythmias

Side Effects: dysrhythmias, GI effects, Overdose is treated with digoxin antibodies

Class IB Drugs

Lidocaine
Tocainide
Mexiletine

Class IC Drugs

Flecainide
Propafenone
Moricizine

Class III Drugs

Amiodarone
Bretylium

Adenosine

Acetazolamide

Mannitol

Loop Diuretics

Furosemide
Bumetanide
Torsemide
Ethacrynic acid

Thiazide Diuretics

Hydrochlorothiazide
Chlorthalidone
Indapamide
Metolazone

Spironolactone

MOA: A class III antiarrhythmic which blocks K^+ channels resulting in a prolonged refractory period and action potential duration.

Clinical Uses: ventricular arrhythmias

Side Effects: neurotoxicity, photosensitivity

Notes: Amiodarone exhibits Class I, II, III and IV antiarrhythmic activity and is used infrequently due to its side effects.

Other: Bretylium

Page 124

MOA: A class IC agent which blocks Na^+ channels thus decreasing the phase 0 slope. No net effect on the action potential duration.

Clinical Uses: ventricular and supraventricular arrhythmias

Side Effects: **pro-arrhythmogenic**

Page 121

MOA: Block **activated** and **inactivated** Na^+ channels but exerts greater effects on inactivated channels. This blockade decreases the phase 0 slope. Also shortens the action potential duration.

Clinical Uses: ventricular arrhythmias

Side Effects: CNS effects. Tocainide may cause pulmonary fibrosis.

Page 120

MOA: Increases plasma osmolality thus drawing fluid from tissue to plasma. Also acts at the proximal tubule and loop of Henle to promote duiresis.

Clinical Uses: edema, cerebral edema, elevated intracranial pressure, glaucoma

Side Effects: headache, nausea, vomiting

Page 131

MOA: Inhibits carbonic anhydrase in the **proximal convoluted tubules**. This results in decreased reabsorption of Na^+ and HCO_3^- in the proximal convoluted tubules; however, some of the Na^+ is reabsorbed in the loop of Henle.

Clinical Uses: glaucoma, altitude sickness

Side Effects: drowsiness, paresthesias, metabolic acidosis

Page 131

MOA: Binds to G-protein coupled adenosine receptors resulting in activation of acetylcholine sensitive K^+ channels in the SA and AV nodes. This increase in conductance results in shortened action potential duration, hyperpolarization and decreased automaticity.

Clinical Use: DOC for acute termination of **supraventricular arrhythmias**

Side Effects: flushing, headache, dyspnea

Page 126

MOA: **Aldosterone antagonist** at mineralocorticoid receptors in the late distal tubule and collecting ducts leading to decreased synthesis of Na^+ channels and the Na^+-K^+-ATPase. This activity causes an increase in Na^+ clearance and a decrease in K^+ and H^+ excretion in the distal nephron

Clinical Uses: edematous states, hypertension, primary hyperaldosteronism

Side Effects: hyperkalemia, metabolic acidosis, endocrine effects

Page 134

MOA: Sulfonamide derivatives which inhibit the **Na^+-Cl^- symporter** on the luminal side of the epithelial cells in the early **distal convoluted tubules** (DCT) resulting in decreased reabsorption of NaCl. This decrease in Na^+ reabsorption promotes Na^+-Ca^{2+} exchange which leads to hypercalcemia and H_2O excretion.

Clinical Uses: **hypertension** , **edema**

Side Effects: hyponatremia, hypokalemic metabolic alkalosis

Page 133

MOA: Inhibit the **Na^+-K^+-$2Cl^-$ symporter** in the **thick ascending limb** of the loop of Henle. Delivery of these electrolytes to distal regions of the nephron results in secretion of K^+ and H^+.

Clinical Uses: edema, pulmonary edema, hypertension, hypercalcemia

Side Effects: orthostatic hypotension, hypokalemic metabolic alkalosis, hypersensitivity (furosemide, bumetanide, torsemide only)

Page 132

Amiloride

Triamterene

Antidiuretics

Vasopressin (ADH)
Desmopressin acetate

Ticlopidine

Dipyramidole

Heparin

Warfarin

Streptokinase

Tissue plasminogen activator (t-PA)

HMG-CoA Reductase Inhibitors

Lovastatin
Simvastatin
Pravastatin
Fluvastatin

MOA: Inhibits ADP-induced binding of fibrinogen to the platelet membrane at the glycoprotein IIb/IIIa complex.

Clinical Use: **stroke**

Side Effects: **GI effects**

Page 139

MOA: Activate $\mathbf{V_2}$ receptors on the renal tubule cells to increase the number of water channels in the kidney collecting tubules increasing the reabsorption of water and the formation of a concentrated urine.

Clinical Uses: central diabetes insipidus

Side Effects: headache, nausea, abdominal cramps, hyponatremia

Page 135

MOA: Blocks Na^+ channels in the late distal convoluted tubule and collecting ducts. This activity causes an increase in Na^+ clearance and a decrease in K^+ and H^+ excretion in the distal nephron.

Clinical Uses: **edematous states**, **hypertension** (mild to severe)

Side Effects: **hyperkalemia**, metabolic acidosis, headache

Others: Triamterene

Page 134

MOA: A coumarin derivative which inhibits the synthesis of **vitamin K** and thus prevents vitamin K-mediated **γ-carboxylation** of procoagulant factors **II** (prothrombin), **VII**, **IX**, **X**, as well as, anticoagulant factors **C** and **S**.

Clinical Uses: deep vein thrombosis, pulmonary thromboembolism

Side Effects: hemorrhage, skin rash, GI effects. Treatment of overdose: Vitamin K, fresh frozen plasma

Other: Dicumarol

Page 140

MOA: Enhances the proteolytic actions of **antithrombin III** which inactivates factors **IIa** (thrombin), **IXa**, **Xa**, **XIa** and **XIIa**.

Clinical Uses: anticoagulant (DOC during pregnancy), deep vein thrombosis, pulmonary thromboembolism

Side Effects: bleeding, thrombocytopenia, osteoporosis. Treatment of overdose: protamine

Page 140

MOA: Not fully elucidated but may increase adenosine levels resulting in coronary vasodilation and inhibition of platelet aggregation and activation.

Clinical Uses: **thromboemboli**

Side Effects: **angina**, **CV effects**, **GI effects**, **headache**

Page 139

MOA: **Reversibly** and **competitively inhibit HMG-CoA reductase**. This results in an increase of LDL receptors in the liver and a subsequent increase in LDL catabolism.

Clinical Uses: Type IIa, IIb hyperlipidemias

Side Effects: GI effects, myalgia, myositis, increased liver enzymes

Page 146

MOA: **Directly** converts only fibrin-bound plasminogen to plasmin.

Clinical Uses: acute myocardial infarction, acute pulmonary thromboembolism

Side Effects: increased incidence of stroke and cerebral hemorrhages than with other thrombolytics

Other: Urokinase converts both fibrin-bound and free plasminogen to plasmin.

Page 141

MOA: An **indirect** thrombolytic which combines with plasminogen to form an **activator complex** which converts free and fibrin-bound plasminogen to plasmin.

Clinical Uses: acute myocardial infarction

Side Effects: **systemic bleeding**, **antigenicity**

Other: Eminase is an anisoylated form of streptokinase

Page 141

Natural Penicillins

Penicillin G
Penicillin V
Penicillin V procaine
Penicillin G benzathine

Antistaphylococcal Penicillins

Methicillin
Nafcillin
Oxacillin
Dicloxacillin
Cloxacillin

Aminopenicillins

Ampicillin
Amoxicillin

Antipseudomonal Penicillins

Mezlocillin
Piperacillin
Azlocillin
Carbenicillin
Ticarcillin

1st Generation Cephalosporins

Cephalothin
Cephapirin
Cephradine
Cephalexin
Cefazolin
Cefadroxil

2nd Generation Cephalosporins

Cefamandole
Cefaclor
Cefoxitin
Cefotetan
Cefonicid
Cefprozil
Cefuroxime
Cefpodoxime proxetil

3rd Generation Cephalosporins

Ceftriaxone
Ceftazidime
Cefotaxime
Ceftizoxime
Moxalactam
Cefixime
Cefoperazone

Imipenem/ Cilastatin

Aztreonam

MOA: Attach to penicillin binding proteins and inhibit cell wall synthesis by **blocking transpeptidation** of **peptidoglycan**. Activate/ disinhibit intracellular cytotoxic "autolysins."

Spectrum: gram(-) bacteria

Clinical Uses: upper respiratory infections (*Strep. pyogenes, Strep. pneumoniae* and *H. flu*), urinary tract infection (Group-D *Enterococci*), bacterial meningitis (*L. monocytogenes*), invasive *Salmonella* infections, acute gastroenteritis

Side Effects: hypersensitivity reactions, nausea, vomiting and diarrhea, skin rashes

Page 157

MOA: Attach to penicillin binding proteins and inhibit cell wall synthesis by **blocking transpeptidation** of **peptidoglycan**. Activate/ disinhibit intracellular cytotoxic "autolysins."

Spectrum: narrow; *Staphylococcus*

Clinical Uses: **penicillinase producing *Staphylococci*** (DOC), some activity against *Streptococcus*

Side Effects: nephrotoxicity (methicillin)

Note: Methicillin and dicloxacillin are the most resistant to β–lactamases.

Page 156

MOA: Attach to penicillin binding proteins and inhibit cell wall synthesis by **blocking transpeptidation** of **peptidoglycan**. Activate/ disinhibit intracellular cytotoxic "autolysins."

Spectrum: gram(+), gram(-), spirochetes, many anaerobes.

Clinical Uses: pneumonia (*Strep. pneumoniae*), infections due to *Strep. pyogenes*, anaerobic infections, meningococcal infections, syphilis, diphtheria, anthrax, gas gangrene

Side Effects: hypersensitivity reactions, (+) Coombs' reaction

Page 155

MOA: Cell wall synthesis inhibitors with limited CNS penetration.

Spectrum: increased gram(-), decreased gram(+) coverage, some anaerobes.

Clinical Uses: UTI, respiratory infections, bone and soft tissue infections, bacterial meningitis (cefuroxime). **H**. *influenza*, **E***nterobacter aerogenes*, **N***eisseria*, **P***roteus mirabilis* (Indole-positive), **E**. *coli*, **K***lebsiella pneumonia*

Side Effects: Alcohol intolerance (disulfiram-like reaction) , bleeding, superinfection caused by gram(+) bacteria and fungi

Page 160

MOA: Cell wall synthesis inhibitors that do not Do not penetrate the CNS and thus can not be used to treat meningitis

Spectrum: excellent gram(+), poor gram(-), poor anaerobic coverage

Clinical Uses: surgical prophylaxis (DOC), minor *Staphylococcus* infections, UTI, **P***roteus mirabilis* (Indole-negative), **E**. *coli*, **K***lebsiella pneumoniae*, **S***taph. aureus*, **S***treptococcus* and *pneumococcus*

Side Effects: hypersensitivity reactions

Page 159

MOA: Attach to penicillin binding proteins and inhibit cell wall synthesis by **blocking transpeptidation** of **peptidoglycan**. Activate/ disinhibit intracellular cytotoxic "autolysins."

Spectrum: gram(-) bacilli

Clinical Uses: Serious *Pseudomonas* infections: in combination with aminoglycosides

Side Effects: decreased platelet agglutination, eosinophilia

Page 157

MOA: Cell wall synthesis inhibitor which is resistant to β-lactamases.

Spectrum: gram(-) aerobic rods including *P. aeruginosa* and *Serratia*.

Side Effect: superinfections with *Streptococci* and *Enterococci*

Page 162

MOA: Imipenem is a cell wall synthesis inhibitor. Cilastatin inhibits dehydropeptidase and thus prevents the cleavage of imipenem.

Spectrum: **broadest spectrum** β-lactam antibiotic currently available. Active against aerobic and anaerobic gram(+) and gram(-) organisms.

Clinical Uses: Covers *P. Aeruginosa* and *B. fragilis*, but not MRSA

Side Effects: high doses may cause seizures

Page 162

MOA: Cell wall synthesis inhibitors with good CNS penetration.

Spectrum: broad gram(-), moderate anaerobic and some aerobic activity.

Clinical Uses: **P**. *aeruginosa*, **H**. *flu*, **E***nterobacter aerogenes*, **N***eisseria*, **P***roteus mirabilis* (Indole-positive), **E**. *coli*, **K***lebsiella pneumonia*, **S**erratia

Side Effects: diarrhea, superinfection caused by gram(+) bacteria and fungi

Note: Ceftriaxone is DOC for gonorrhea and meningitis

Page 161

Vancomycin

Cycloserine

β-Lactamase Inhibitors

Clavulanic acid
Sulbactam
Tazobactam

Streptomycin

Other Aminoglycosides

Gentamicin
Tobramycin
Amikacin
Netilmicin

Tetracyclines

Tetracycline
Doxycycline
Minocycline
Demeclocycline
Oxytetracycline

Chloramphenicol

Macrolides

Erythromycin
Clarithromycin
Azithromycin

Lincosamides

Clindamycin
Lincomycin

MOA: Irreversibly bind to and **inactivate** β-**lactamases** preventing them from destroying β-lactam antibiotics. Contain a β-lactam ring, but have little antibacterial affect when given alone.

Clinical Uses: protect hydrolyzable penicillins and extend the spectrum of certain β-lactam agents.

Page 164

MOA: Structural analog of D-alanine which **antagonizes D-alanine** in bacterial cell-wall synthesis. Bactericidal and penetrates the CNS well

Spectrum: gram(+), gram(-), but primarily mycobacteria

Clinical Uses: tuberculosis

Side Effects: CNS effects, seizures

Page 164

MOA: Bactericidal cell wall inhibitor that binds to the **D-alanyl D-alanine** terminus of gram(+) cell wall precursors preventing **transpeptidation.**

Spectrum: gram(+) organisms: MRSA, MRSE, *Enterococcus*

Clinical Uses: pseudomembranous colitis (*C. difficile*), serious gram(+) infections resistant to β-lactam antibiotics, prophylaxis in patients with prosthetic heart valves undergoing dental procedures.

Side Effects: hearing loss, nephrotoxicity, red man syndrome

Page 163

MOA: Bacteriostatic agents which bind to the **30S** ribosomal subunit and block binding of **aminoacyl-tRNA** to the mRNA ribosomal complex.

Spectrum: broad; aerobic and anaerobic gram(+) and gram(-) bacteria.

Clinical Uses: Rocky Mountain Spotted Fever, Q-Fever, lymphogranuloma venereum, psittacosis, pneumonia, Lyme disease

Side Effects: GI irritation, tooth and bone discoloration

Page 168

MOA: **Aminoglycoside** which inhibits protein synthesis by binding irreversibly to the **30S** ribosomal subunit. Bactericidal.

Clinical Uses: pneumonia, urinary tract infections

Side Effects: ototoxicity, nephrotoxicity, neuromuscular blockade

Others: Neomycin and kanamycin

Page 167

MOA: An **aminoglycoside** which inhibits protein synthesis by binding irreversibly to the **30S** ribosomal subunit. Bactericidal.

Spectrum: aerobic gram(-) bacilli, some gram(+) and mycobacteria.

Clinical Uses: tuberculosis, bubonic plague

Side Effects: ototoxicity, nephrotoxicity, neuromuscular blockade

Page 167

MOA: Bacteriostatic agents which bind to the **50S** ribosomal subunit and inhibit protein synthesis by interfering translocation.

Spectrum: few clinical uses; aerobic gram(+) cocci, anaerobes

Clinical Uses: anaerobic infections

Side Effects: pseudomembranous colitis, diarrhea, skin rashes, pseudo tumor cerebri, vestibular problems

Page 172

MOA: Bacteriostatic inhibitor of protein synthesis which binds reversibly to the 23S rRNA of the **50S** ribosomal subunit and interferes with translocation. Poor CNS penetration.

Spectrum: aerobic gram(+) cocci and bacilli.

Clinical Uses: pneumonia, Legionnaires' disease, Pertussis, Diphtheria

Side Effects: nausea, vomiting, diarrhea, cholestatic hepatitis

Page 171

MOA: Bacteriostatic agent which binds **reversibly** to the **50S** ribosomal subunit and inhibits protein synthesis by interfering with chain elongation.

Spectrum: broad; aerobic and anaerobic gram(+) and gram(-) bacteria.

Clinical Uses: Typhoid fever, bacterial meningitis, rickettsial infections, psittacosis

Side Effects: nausea, vomiting, diarrhea, anemia, Gray Baby Syndrome

Page 169

Fluoroquinolones

Ciprofloxacin
Ofloxacin
Norfloxacin

Rifampin

Sulfonamides

Sulfisoxazole
Sulfamethoxazole
Sulfadiazine
Sulfamethizole
Sulfasalazine
Sulfadoxine
Sulfacetamide
Silver sulfadiazine
Mafenide

Trimethoprim

Trimethoprim/ Sulfamethoxazole

Isoniazid

Amphotericin B

Azole Antifungals

Ketoconazole
Fluconazole
Itraconazole
Miconazole
Clotrimazole

Flucytosine

MOA: Bacteriostatic agents which are competitive antagonists of **dihydropteroate synthase**, the enzyme responsible for incorporating PABA into dihydropteroic acid, the precursor to **folic acid**.

Spectrum: gram(+), gram(-)

Clinical Uses: toxoplasmosis, ulcerative colitis, enteritis, granulomatous colitis, urinary tract infections

Side Effects: hypersensitivity reactions, photosensitivity, GI effects, kernicterus

Page 178

MOA: **Inhibits DNA-dependent RNA polymerase** by blocking the β-subunit and suppressing chain initiation in RNA synthesis.

Spectrum: gram(+) and gram(-) bacteria.

Clinical Uses: tuberculosis, meningitis, prophylaxis, leprosy

Side Effects: generally well tolerated

Page 175

MOA: Bactericidal agents which prevent the replication of bacterial DNA by inhibiting **DNA gyrase**.

Spectrum: broad; aerobic gram(+), gram(-) bacteria, but **not** anaerobes.

Clinical Uses: urinary tract infections, sexually transmitted diseases, prostatitis, respiratory infections

Side Effects: generally well tolerated

Page 174

MOA: The mechanism is unknown, but thought to involve the **inhibition of mycolic acids synthesis**. Mycolic acids are necessary for the cell wall

Clinical Uses: tuberculosis

Side Effects: peripheral neuritis, hepatotoxicity

Others: pyrazinamide and ethambutol are also used to treat tuberculosis

Page 182

MOA: Synergistically active antimicrobial agent which blocks two sequential steps in the obligate enzymatic reaction in bacteria preventing the formation of nucleotides.

Spectrum: broad; gram(+) and gram(-) bacteria.

Clinical Uses: urinary tract infections, pneumonia, gonorrhea, bacterial prostatitis, bronchitis, otitis media

Side Effects: dermatologic effects, GI effects

Page 179

MOA: Bacteriostatic agent which inhibits **dihydrofolate reductase**

Spectrum: similar to sulfa drugs, gram(+), gram(-).

Clinical Uses: acute urinary tract infections, bacterial prostatitis

Side Effects: folate deficiency

Page 179

MOA: A narrow spectrum pyrimidine **antimetabolite** which is converted to 5-fluorouracil, an inhibitor of DNA and RNA synthesis.

Clinical Uses: cryptococcal infections, candidiasis

Side Effects: bone marrow suppression, hepatitis, GI effects

Page 189

MOA: Blocks ergosterol synthesis by inhibiting the cytochrome P_{450} enzymes. This causes depletion of ergosterol, resulting in disruption of the permeability of the cell membrane.

Clinical Uses: blastomycosis, oropharyngeal candidiasis, coccidioidomycosis, histoplasmosis

Side Effects: GI effects, endocrine effects (ketoconazole only)

Note: Miconazole and clotrimazole are used topically

Page 187

MOA: A polyene antifungal which binds ergosterol and punches holes in cell membranes. This increases fungal cell membrane permeability which results in cell death via osmotic disruption.

Clinical Uses: aspergillosis, blastomycosis, systemic candidiasis, coccidioidomycosis, cryptococcosis, histoplasmosis

Side Effects: acute febrile reactions, nephrotoxicity

Other: nystatin is used for topical applications

Page 186

Griseofulvin

Acyclovir

Foscarnet

Zidovudine

Amantadine
Rimantadine

Ribavirin

Chloroquine

Quinine

Pyrimethamine/
Sulfadoxine

MOA: Inhibits viral replication by blocking the pyrophosphate binding site of viral DNA polymerase.

Clinical Uses: CMV retinitis in AIDS patients, treatment of HIV patients with acyclovir-resistant herpes virus

Side Effects: nephrotoxicity, GI effects, electrolyte imbalances

MOA: A **guanine** analog which is converted to acyclovir monophosphate (by the herpes simplex virus encoded enzyme **thymidine kinase**) then converted to the diphosphate and triphosphate forms by cellular enzymes.

Clinical Uses: Herpes virus types I and II, varicella-zoster virus

Side Effects: nephrotoxicity, neurotoxicity at high doses

Other: Ganciclovir is used for CMV infections

MOA: Inhibits mitosis of cells, by disrupting spindle formation. Binds to tubulin involved in mitotic division and arrests cells in metaphase. May also bind to other proteins such as keratin.

Clinical Uses: dermatophytic infections, *Tinea* infections

Side Effects: CNS effects, GI effects

MOA: A **guanosine** analog whose mechanism of action is not fully defined but is related to a reduction of intracellular guanosine triphosphate pools and inhibition of viral RNA and protein synthesis.

Clinical Uses: Respiratory syncytial virus, Lassa fever, Influenza A and B virus

Side Effects: anemia

MOA: Inhibits uncoating of the **Influenza A** virus after it enters the cell by blocking the viral M2 membrane protein. The M2 protein forms a pump, which moves protons into the endosome and lowers its pH. The low pH facilitates viral uncoating.

Clinical Uses: Influenza type A virus, Parkinson's disease

Side Effects: CNS effects, GI effects

MOA: A structural analog of **thymidine** which is phosphorylated by cellular enzymes into its triphosphate. Zidovudine triphosphate is incorporated into viral DNA by reverse transcriptase and inhibits viral DNA synthesis.

Clinical Uses: HIV

Side Effects: anemia, neutropenia, neurotoxicity

Others: Didanosine and zalcitabine are also used to treat HIV.

MOA: **Pyrimethamine** inhibits **dihydrofolate reductase** which inhibits the synthesis of tetrahydrofolate and leads to inhibition of DNA synthesis. **Sulfadoxine** competitively inhibits dihydropteroate synthase.

Clinical Uses: toxoplasmosis, malaria due to P. *falciparum*

Side Effects: GI effects, bone marrow suppression, hypersensitivity reactions

MOA: The *MOA* is unknown but may involve inhibition of plasmodium hemoglobin polymerase or an increase in the pH of plasmodia vacuoles.

Clinical Uses: malaria due to chloroquine- or multidrug resistant *P. falciparum*, nocturnal leg cramps, babesiosis

Side Effects: cinchonism, blackwater fever

Other: mefloquine

MOA: The mechanism in unknown, however, may involve DNA intercalation, inhibition of plasmodium hemoglobin polymerase or an increase in the pH of plasmodia vacuoles.

Clinical Uses: malaria, extra-intestinal amebiasis

Side Effects: stomach upset, headache, visual disturbances, CV effects

Metronidazole	Stibogluconate	Suramin
Pentamidine	Pyrantel pamoate	Diethylcarbamazine
Ivermectin	Mebendazole	Praziquantel

MOA: The mechanism is unclear but may involve inhibition of enzymes required for energy metabolism.

Clinical Uses: African sleeping sickness without CNS involvement, onchocerciasis

Side Effects: GI effects, CNS effects

Others: Melarsoprol is used to treat African sleeping sickness with CNS involvement; nifurtimox is used to treat American trypanosomiasis

Page 203

MOA: Pentavalent antimony compound whose *MOA* is unclear but is thought to inhibit glycolysis.

Clinical Uses: Cutaneous, mucocutaneous, and visceral leishmaniasis

Side Effects: GI effects, cardiac arrhythmias

Page 202

MOA: An electron acceptor that causes the formation of chemically reactive species which interact with DNA and proteins.

Clinical Uses: luminal and extraluminal amebiasis used in combination with diloxanide furoate, giardiasis, *Trichomonas vaginali*

Side Effects: GI effects, CNS effects, metallic taste

Others: diloxanide furoate is used alone for asymptomatic amebiasis or in combination with metronidazole for luminal and extraluminal amebiasis.

Page 201

MOA: Not well understood but is thought to work by decreasing the muscular activity of the organisms and/or by increasing the susceptibility of microfilaria to phagocytosis.

Clinical Uses: filariasis, Ascariasis, Loiasis

Side Effects: Mazzotti reaction

Page 206

MOA: Depolarizing neuromuscular blocking agent which results in paralysis of the worm.

Clinical Uses: ascariasis, *Necator americanus, Enterobius vermicularis*

Page 206

MOA: Not well understood. Appears to interfere with nuclear metabolism and inhibit the synthesis of DNA, RNA, proteins and phospholipids.

Clinical Uses: Pneumonia due to *Pneumocystis carinii*, African sleeping sickness

Side Effects: hypotension, pancreatic β-cell dysfunction

Page 203

MOA: **Increases calcium permeability** leading to calcium efflux. This causes initial contraction, spasm and eventual paralysis of the worms.

Clinical uses: Schistosomiasis, *Clonorchis sinensis, Paragonimus westermani, T. saginata, T. solium, D. latum* and *H. nana*, cysticercosis

Side Effects: CNS effects, fever, GI effects

Page 208

MOA: Binds to tubulin and inhibits **microtubule** polymerization.

Clinical Uses: Pinworm infections caused by *E. vermicularis*, Whipworm infections caused by *T. trichiura, Necator americanus*

Side Effects: abdominal pain, diarrhea

Others: Thiabendazole is used to treat *S. stercoralis*, cutaneous larva migrans, visceral larva migrans

Page 207

MOA: Increases GABA mediated neurotransmission in nematodes resulting in paralysis of the parasites.

Clinical Uses: River blindness

Side Effects: Mazzotti reaction

Page 206

6-Mercaptopurine	Methotrexate	Cytarabine
5-Fluorouracil	Hydroxyurea	Mechlorethamine
Cyclophosphamide	Melphalan	Lomustine Carmustine

MOA: **Pyrimidine analog** which is activated to the monophosphate nucleotide (AraCMP) which can then form AraCDP and **AraCTP** the latter of which **inhibits DNA synthesis** by preventing DNA chain elongation.

Cell-cycle specific for **S-phase**

Clinical Uses: AML (DOC), ALL, CML, Non-Hodgkin's lymphoma

Side Effects: bone marrow suppression, stomatitis

Page 213

MOA: A **folic acid antagonist** which prevents the conversion of dihydrofolate to tetrahydrofolate (THF) by inhibiting dihydrofolate reductase (**DHFR**). THF is required for the synthesis of thymidylate, DNA, RNA and some amino acids (Ser, Met).

Cell cycle specific for **S-phase**

Clinical Uses: psoriasis, rheumatoid arthritis, breast carcinoma, lung cancer, ALL

Side Effects: **Leucovorin** is used to treat overdose

Page 212

MOA: A purine antimetabolite which is converted by hypoxanthine-guanine phosphoryl transferase (**HGPRT**) to the active form 6-thioinosinic acid which inhibits key enzymes in the **purine synthetic pathway**. This results in inhibition of DNA synthesis.

Cell cycle specific for **S-phase**

Clinical Uses: **ALL**, **AML**

Side Effects: bone marrow suppression

Page 212

MOA: Bifunctional **alkylating agent** which forms an ethylenimmonium that cross links strands of DNA and RNA.

Cell cycle **non-specific**

Clinical Use: **Hodgkin's disease** (component of MOPP)

Page 214

MOA: Urea analog which **prevents DNA synthesis** by inhibiting **ribonucleotide reductase**, the enzyme which converts ribonucleotides to deoxyribonucleotides.

Cell cycle specific for **S-phase**

Clinical Use: **CML**

Page 213

MOA: Ribosylated or phosphorylated to 5-F-UMP. 5-F-UMP can inhibit RNA synthesis. It also prevents DNA synthesis by inhibiting thymidylate synthetase

Cell cycle specific for **S-phase**

Clinical Uses: **Breast carcinomas, GI carcinomas**

Page 213

MOA: Inhibit DNA, RNA and protein synthesis via bifunctional alkylation and protein modification (carbamoylation of lysine residues).

Cell cycle **non-specific**. Crosses BBB

Clinical Uses: **brain tumors**

Page 215

MOA: **Phenylalanine** derivative of nitrogen mustard. Forms an ethylenimmonium ion that cross links strands of DNA and RNA.

Cell cycle non-specific

Clinical Uses: ovarian carcinoma, multiple myeloma

Page 214

MOA: **Prodrug** which is metbolized to a **phosphoramide mustard** (active metabolite) and **acrolein** (toxic metabolite). The **phosphoramide mustard** metabolite cross-links DNA and RNA.

Cell cycle non-specific

Clinical Uses: ovarian, breast carcinoma, Hodgkin's and Non-Hodgkin's lymphoma

Side Effects: hemorrhagic cystitis at high doses (due to acrolein)

Page 214

Streptozocin	Cisplatin	Busulfan
Dacarbazine	Dactinomycin	Doxorubicin Daunorubicin
Bleomycin	Vinblastine	Vincristine

MOA: An alkylsulfonate type bifunctional alkylating agent which alkylates and cross-links strands of DNA.

Cell cycle **non-specific**

Clinical Use: DOC for **CML**

Page 216

MOA: Platinum coordination complex which is hydrolyzed to form an activated electrophile that alkylates DNA.

Cell cycle **non-specific**

Clinical Uses: testicular carcinoma (component of VBC), bladder carcinoma

Side Effects: nephrotoxicity, ototoxicity

Other: Carboplatin is used for ovarian carcinoma and exhibits less toxicity.

Page 216

MOA: Alkylating agent which inhibits DNA synthesis by cross linking strands of DNA. Diabetogenic agent in experimental animals due to high affinity for and toxicity to pancreatic β cells.

Cell cycle **non-specific**.

Clinical Uses: pancreatic carcinoma (insulinoma)

Page 215

MOA: Antitumor activity may result from any of several mechanisms including DNA intercalation, single-stranded DNA breaks and membrane disruption.

Cell cycle specific: predominantly **S-phase** specific but at low doses cells may proceed through S-phase and die in G2.

Clinical Uses: AML, ALL

Page 217

MOA: Antibiotic which binds double-stranded DNA and intercalates between adjacent G-C base pairs. This inhibits **DNA-dependent RNA polymerase**. Also causes single-stranded DNA breaks.

Cell cycle non-specific

Clinical Uses:: Wilm's tumor (component of VAC), rhabdomyosarcoma (VAC)

Page 217

MOA: Hepatically activated alkylating agent which is thought to inhibit DNA and RNA synthesis via formation of carbonium ions.

Cell cycle **non-specific**

Clinical Use: Hodgkin's lymphoma: component of ABVD

Page 217

MOA: A **spindle poison** which binds **tubulin** and prevents assembly of **microtubules**. This inhibits formation of the mitotic spindle and blocks cells in mitosis.

Cell-cycle phase specific for **M phase**

Clinical Uses: Hodgkin's Disease (component of MOPP), rhabdomyosarcoma (component of VAC)

Side Effects: neurotoxicity

Page 219

MOA: A **spindle poison** which binds **tubulin** and prevents assembly of microtubules. This inhibits formation of the mitotic spindle and blocks cells in mitosis.

Cell-cycle phase specific for **M phase**

Clinical Uses: testicular carcinoma (component of VBC and VBE), Hodgkin's Disease (component of ABVD)

Side Effects: bone marrow suppression

Page 219

MOA: Combines with iron to form a complex that reacts with oxygen producing free radicals which cause strand scission and **DNA fragmentation**.

Cell cycle specific for **G2 phase**

Clinical Uses: testicular carcinoma (component of VBC or VBE), Hodgkin's disease (component of ABVD)

Side Effects: pulmonary toxicity

Page 218

Bromocriptine

Levothyroxine sodium
(T4)

Liothyronine sodium
(T3)

Propylthiouracil
(PTU)

Methimazole

^{131}I

Glucocorticoids

Cortisol
Cortisone
Corticosterone
Prednisolone
Prednisone
Methylprednisolone
Triamcinolone
Dexamethasone
Betamethasone

Glucocorticoid
Antagonists

Aminoglutethimide
Metyrapone
O.p'DDD
RU486

Aldosterone

Estrogens

Estradiol
Estrone
Ethinyl estradiol
Mestranol

Tamoxifen

MAO: Inhibit thyroid peroxidase thereby preventing iodination of tyrosyl residues of thyroglobulin and coupling of iodotyrosine residues. PTU also inhibits the peripheral deiodination of T4 to T3.

Clinical Uses: Graves' disease, radiation adjuvant and conversion of a hyperthyroid patient to euthyroid prior to surgical treatment.

Side Effects: transient leukopenia, fever, skin rash, itching, joint pain, hypothyroidism and agranulocytosis

Page 234

Clinical Uses: hypothyroidism, hormone replacement therapy, prevention of cretinism in hypothyroid newborns and treatment after thyroid cancer

Side Effects: palpitations, arrhythmias and thyrotoxicosis

Page 233

MAO: An ergot-derived dopamine agonist which decreases pituitary prolactin secretion.

Clinical Uses: prolactinoma, amenorrhea, galactorrhea, infertility, acromegaly and parkinsonism

Side Effects: nausea, lightheadedness, vasospasm and CNS effects

Page 226

MOA: Prevents the synthesis (aminoglutethimide, metyrapone, O.p'DDD) of glucocorticoids or inhibit the glucocorticoid and progesterone receptors (RU486).

Clinical Uses: Aminoglutethimide for breast cancer and Cushing;s syndrome; metyrapone for diagnosis of adrenal function; O.p'DDD for adrenocortical carcinoma; RU486 is an abortifacient.

Side Effects: lethargy, edema, hirsuitism

Page 242

MOA: Among glucocorticoids and analogs available, there is variation in their anti-inflammatory and mineralocorticoid acitivities.

Clinical Uses: Cortisol, cortisone and corticosterone are used for **replacement therapy**; prednisone is part of the MOPP **chemotherapy** regimen; dexamethasone is used in the diagnosis of Cushing's disease.

Side Effects: adrenal suppression, salt retention, immunosuppression, hyperglycemia, osteoporosis

Page 241

MAO: Specifically taken up by the thyroid gland, incorporated into thyroglobulin and concentrated in colloid. Cytotoxic effects eventually destroy the thyroid gland

Clinical Uses: hyperthyroidism, Graves' disease refractory to other therapies, toxic nodular goiter

Side Effects: hypothyroidism, delayed onset of therapeutic effects

Page 236

MOA: A **nonsteroidal antiestrogen** which competitively inhibits estrogen at the estrogen receptor.

Clinical Use: breast cancer

Side Effects: hot flashes, ovarian enlargement.

Page 247

MOA: Bind the estrogen receptor and form a complex which stimulates transcription of target genes. Exogenous administration inhibits FSH secretion and prevents ovulation.

Clinical Uses: oral contraceptives, postmenopausal hormone therapy, hypogonadism in girls.

Side Effects: hypertension, breast tenderness, endometrial hyperplasia, breakthrough bleeding.

Page 247

MOA: An endogenous mineralocorticoid which increases Na^+ and water retention.

Others: Fludrocortisone exhibits weaker mineralocorticoid activity and is used to treat **Addison's disease**.

Page 243

Progestins

Medroxyprogesterone
Norethindrone
Norethindrone acetate

Mifepristone

Androgens

Testosterone
Methyltestosterone
Fluoxymesterone

Antiandrogens

Finasteride
Spironolactone
Cyproterone
Flutamide

Calcium Salts

Calcium carbonate
Calcium chloride
Calcium gluceptate
Calcium gluconate

Vitamin D Forms

Bisphosphonates

Etidronate
Pamidronate

Calcitonin

MAO: Bind the androgen receptor and stimulate transcription from genes containing androgen responsive elements..

Clinical Use: **hormone replacement therapy**, anemia, breast cancer, osteoporosis

Side Effects: masculinizing effects in women, alteration in serum lipid profiles, hepatocellular carcinoma

MOA: A **competitive inhibitor** of progestins at progesterone receptors in the presence of progestin. In the absence of progestin, mifepristone acts as a **partial agonist**. Mifepristone is also a competitive inhibitor of glucocorticoids at the glucocorticoid receptor.

Clinical Use: abortifacient, postcoital contraception

Others: Danazol

MAO: bind to progestin receptors and stimulate transcription of target genes.

Clinical Use: contraception, postmenopausal hormone therapy

Side Effects: weight gain, edema, depression, thrombophlebitis

MAO: increase Ca^{2+} and PO_4^{2-} absorption from the intestine, decrease renal excretion of Ca^{2+} and increase renal excretion of PO_4^{2-}

*Clinical Use:*Nutritional rickets, metabolic rickets, osteomalacia, hypoparathyroidism, osteoporosis, chronic renal failure, vitamin D deficient states and chronic forms of tetany

Side Effects: vascular calcification, nephrocalcinosis, soft tissue calcification, growth arrest in children

Clinical Uses: hypocalcemic tetany and dietary supplement

MAO: Either inhibit the synthesis of dihydortestosterone (fiansteride) or act as antagonists at androgen receptors (spironolactone, cyproterone, flutamide).

Clinical Use: benign prostatic hyperplasia, hirsutism

MAO: interact with receptors on osteoclasts producing a decrease in the ruffled membrane surface area resulting in a decrease in resorptive activity. Reduces Ca^{2+} and PO_4^{2-} reabsorption in the kidney..

Clinical Use: Paget's disease of bone

Side Effects: allergic reactions, flushing, redness, or tingling of the face, ears, hands and feet and GI effects

MAO: adsorbed to bone, where it is taken up by osteoclasts and inhibits their activity. This slows the formation and dissolution of hydroxyapatite crystals (anti-resorptive effect).

Clinical Use: Paget's disease of bone, heterotopic ossification (myositis ossificans), malignancy-associated hypercalcemia and osteoporosis

Side Effects: bone pain in patients with Paget's disease usually around the pagetic lesion, osteomalacia, bone fractures and diarrhea

Indomethacin

Ibuprofen

Aspirin

Probenecid

Colchicine

Acetaminophen

Second Generation H_1-Blockers

Terfenadine
Loratadine
Astemizole

First Generation H_1-Blockers

Diphenhydramine
Dimenhydrinate
Chlorpheniramine
Meclizine

Allopurinol

MOA: **Irreversibly** inhibits cyclooxygenase decreasing the production of prostaglandins and thromboxane

Clinical Uses: myocardial infarction, antiplatelet, analgesia, antipyretic, anti-inflammatory

Side Effects: bleeding complications, gastric intolerance, hypersensitivity reactions, renal toxicity, hepatotoxicity, **Reye's Syndrome**

Page 272

MOA: **Reversibly** inhibit cyclooxygenase decreasing the production of prostaglandins and thromboxane

Clinical Uses: analgesia, rheumatoid arthritis, osteoarthritis

Side Effects: GI disturbances

Other: Naproxen

Page 273

MOA: **Reversibly** inhibits cyclooxygenase decreasing the production of prostaglandins and thromboxane.

Clinical Uses: acute gout, ankylosing spondylitis, Barter's syndrome, rheumatoid arthritis, osteoarthritis, closure of PDA

Side Effects: CNS effects, GI effects, Hypersensitivity reactions, renal toxicity

Other: Sulindac

Page 274

MOA: Inhibits prostaglandin synthesis, primarily in the CNS, through an unclear mechanism. A minor route of acetaminophen metabolism is via the P_{450} system which produces toxic species.

Clinical Uses: **analgesia**, antipyretic: especially children with febrile viral illnesses.

Side Effects: allergic reactions, Overdose: nausea, vomiting, anorexia, abdominal cramps and ultimately, fatal hepatic necrosis

Page 275

MOA: **Inhibits microtubule formation** in leukocytes causing a decrease in motility, phagocytosis and release of chemotactic factors.

Clinical Uses: acute and chronic gout

Side Effects: diarrhea, nausea, vomiting, abdominal pain, bone marrow depression and alopecia with long term use

Page 278

MOA: **Inhibits tubular reabsorption** of uric acid in the proximal convoluted tubule thereby increasing its excretion

Clinical Uses: **chronic gout**, adjuvant in antibiotic therapy.

Side Effects: **acute gouty attacks**

Others: Sulfinpyrazone

Page 279

MOA: Allopurinol and its metabolite, alloxanthine (oxypurinol), **inhibit xanthine oxidase (XO)**, the enzyme which catalyzes the formation of uric acid from hypoxanthine

Clinical Uses: **chronic gout**, hyperuricemia secondary to blood dyscrasias or antineoplastic therapy, renal calculi, hyperuricemia of Lesch-Nyhan syndrome

Side Effects: hypersensitivity reactions, acute gouty attacks, GI upset, inhibits P_{450} system

Page 279

MOA: **Reversible**, competitive inhibitors of histamine at H_1-receptors.

Clinical Uses: **allergies**, motion sickness, sedation, vestibular disturbances (Menière's disease, vertigo), drug-induced extrapyramidal effects: *diphenhydramine*.

Side Effects: **sedation**, anticholinergic effects, GI disturbances, loss of appetite

Page 282

MOA: **Reversible**, competitive inhibitors of histamine at H_1-receptors. Do not cross the blood-brain barrier therefore are **non-sedating**.

Clinical Uses: **allergies**

Side Effects: arrhythmias: ventricular tachycardia (torsades de pointes): terfenadine or astemizole

Page 282

Cyclosporine

Tacrolimus

Azathioprine

Muromonab CD3 (OKT-3)

Rh_0(D) Immune Globulin

Granulocyte colony stimulating factor (G-CSF)
and
Granulocyte-macrophage colony stimulating factor (GM-CSF)

Levamisole

Aldesleukin

Sumatriptan

MOA: **Pro-drug** activated to **mercaptopurine**, an **antimetabolite** which inhibits purine synthesis preventing T cell proliferation.

Clinical Uses: organ transplant rejection, rheumatoid arthritis

Side Effects: bone marrow suppression, leukopenia, infection, megaloblastic anemia, nausea, vomiting

Page 286

MOA: **Inhibits T cell activation** by binding the FK506 binding protein. This complex decreases **calcineurin** activity ultimately preventing production of IL-2, IL-3 and IFN-γ.

Clinical Uses: **organ transplantation**

Side Effects: **nephrotoxicity**, hepatotoxicity, neurotoxicity, hypertension, hyperglycemia, vomiting, diarrhea

Page 286

MOA: **Blocks T cell activation** by binding cyclophilin and decreasing the activity of **calcineurin**. This ultimately prevents production of IL-2, IL-3 and IFN-γ.

Clinical Uses: **organ transplantation**, graft-vs-host disease subsequent to bone marrow transplantation.

Side Effects: **nephrotoxicity**, hepatotoxicity, neurotoxicity, hypertension, hyperglycemia, hirsutism, gingival hyperplasia

Page 286

MOA: Recombinant proteins which stimulate the proliferation and activation of **neutrophils** (G-CSF) or **macrophages/granulocytes** (GM-CSF).

Clinical Use: recovery from chemotherapy

Side Effects: excessive leukocytosis, fever, allergic reactions, capillary leak syndrome

Page 288

MOA: Prevents maternal antibody response to Rh_0(D)-positive cells which may enter Rh-negative mother's bloodstream.

Clinical Uses: **Rh-hemolytic disease** of newborn (erythroblastosis fetalis): prophylaxis. Administered to Rh_0(D)-negative mothers within 72 hours after the birth of a Rh_0(D)-positive baby.

Side Effects: pain and erythema at injection site

Page 287

MOA: Murine monoclonal antibody directed against the **CD3** molecule of the T-cell antigen receptor complex. This interaction initially causes cytokine release (first-dose) but ultimately blocks the actions of **T-cells**.

Clinical Uses: Acute renal transplant rejection, acute rejection of cardiac or hepatic transplants

Side Effects: **Cytokine-release syndrome**due to the initial activation of lymphocytes. Observed as diarrhea, dizziness and fever, anaphylaxis, hypersensitivity

Page 287

MOA: **Serotonin agonist** which selectively stimulates **5-HT$_{1D}$** receptors and causes vasoconstriction of cerebral vessels.

Clinical Use: acute migraine headaches

Side Effects: dizziness, tingling, muscle weakness and neck pain

Page 289

MOA: Recombinant preparation of **IL-2** which promotes the proliferation and differentiation of lymphocytes into cytotoxic cells and natural killer cells

Clinical Use: **renal cell carcinoma**

Side Effects: capillary leak syndrome, renal failure, cardiac arrest, stroke, severe anemia

Page 288

MOA: Stimulates delayed hypersensitivity and T-cell mediated immunity

Clinical Uses: **colorectal cancer**, Hodgkin's disease, rheumatoid arthritis

Side Effects: blood dyscrasias, ataxia

Page 288

Ergotamine

Antacids

Calcium carbonate
Aluminum hydroxide
Magnesium hydroxide

Omeprazole

Bismuth, tetracycline and metronidazole

Misoprostol

Cisapride

Metoclopramide

Odansetron

Granisetron

Prochlorperazine

MOA: A **prodrug** which is activated at an acidic pH to a sulfenamide derivative that binds **irreversibly** to the **H^+-K^+ ATPase** proton pump on the luminal surface of stomach parietal cells. This results in decreased H^+ secretion.

Clinical Uses: **gastroesophageal reflux**, hypersecretory conditions, duodenal ulcer

Side Effects: nausea, diarrhea, abdominal colic

Page 292

MOA: React chemically to buffer stomach acid with little effect on acid secretion.

Clinical Uses: hyperacidity, duodenal/gastric ulcer, gastroesophageal reflux

Side Effects metabolic acidosis (calcium carbonate). constipation (aluminum hydroxide), diarrhea (magnesium hydroxide)

Page 292

MOA: An ergot alkaloid which stimulates **$5\text{-}HT_{1D}$** and α-adrenergic receptors providing relief of acute headaches by causing vasoconstriction of cerebral vessels.

Clinical Use: **acute** migraine attacks, cluster headaches

Side Effects: nausea, vomiting, diarrhea, vasospasm, muscle weakness in the extremities

Other: Methylsergide is another ergot alkaloid with agonist activity at 5-HT receptors.

Page 289

MOA: Enhances esophageal sphincter tone and esophageal clearance by ↑ the release of acetylcholine in the **myenteric plexus** (prokinetic activity).

Clinical Uses: **gastroesophageal reflux**, gastroparesis, chronic constipation, colonic hypomotility

Side Effects: abdominal cramping, constipation, diarrhea

Page 294

MOA: A PGE_1 analog which inhibits gastric acid secretion. Also stimulates the secretion of bicarbonate and mucus which can prevent ulcer development or progression.

Clinical Uses: duodenal/gastric ulcers

Side Effects: diarrhea

Page 293

MOA: Treatment regimen to eradicate *Helicobacter pylori*, a putative etiologic agent in peptic ulcer disease and gastric carcinoma, from the GI tract.

Clinical Uses: peptic ulcer disease, gastroesophageal reflux (*bismuth*), diarrhea(*bismuth*)

Side Effects: nausea, diarrhea, dizziness

Page 293

MOA: An antipsychotic agent that blocks **D_2** receptors in the medullary chemoreceptor trigger zone as well as the vagus nerve in the GI tract.

Clinical Use: antiemetic

Side Effects: drowsiness, hypotension, extrapyramidal effects

Page 295

MOA: Selectively and **competitively inhibits serotonin** at **$5\text{-}HT_3$** receptors in the periphery (vagal nerve terminals) and CNS (area postrema). It is not yet established which of these 2 effects is responsible for antiemesis.

Clinical Use: **antiemetic**

Side Effects: headache, constipation, diarrhea, dizziness

Page 295

MOA: **Antagonist** at **D_2** and **$5\text{-}HT_3$** receptors in gastric smooth muscle resulting in acceleration of GI emptying and intestinal transit time (prokinetic activity). **Antagonist** at **D_2** receptors in the chemoreceptor trigger zone (antiemetic effect).

Clinical Uses: diagnostic procedures, gastroparesis, gastroesophageal reflux, antiemetic

Side Effects: extrapyramidal side effects, diarrhea, drowsiness, dizziness

Page 294

Bulk Forming Laxatives

Dietary fiber
Methylcellulose
Psyllium

Saline Laxatives

Magnesium hydroxide
Magnesium citrate

Lactulose

Stimulant Laxatives

Phenolphthalein
Bisacodyl
Senna
Casarca sagrada

Docusate sodium

Polaxamers

Benzonatate

Guafenesin

Carbon monoxide

Nitrogen dioxide

MOA: Synthetic disaccharide which is not absorbed and acts as an **osmotic laxative** to attract water into the intestinal lumen.

Clinical Uses: constipation, chronic hepatic encephalopathy

Side Effects: flatulence, abdominal cramps, nausea, vomiting, diarrhea

Others: glycerin, polyethylene glycol are other osmotic diureticsis

Page 297

MOA: Hypertonic solution of non-absorbable salts that retain water within the colonic lumen by osmotic forces leading to distention and increased peristaltic activity.

Clinical Uses: constipation, colonic lavage, elimination of parasites, poisoning

Side Effects: dehydration, electrolyte imbalance

Page 307

MOA: Undigestible plant, fruit and vegetable parts which form gels within the large intestine causing water retention and distention leading to an increase in GI peristaltic activity.

Clinical Use: constipation

Side Effects: flatulence

Page 306

MOA: A **local anesthetic** which suppresses stretch or cough receptors of vagal afferents located in respiratory passages, lungs and pleura. Also may inhibit transmission of the cough reflex to the medulla.

Clinical Uses: antitussive

Side Effects: constipation, dizziness, drowsiness, skin rash

Page 299

MOA: Anionic surfactants which emulsify and soften the stool facilitating the passage of feces. Increase net water and electrolyte secretion into the intestine.

Clinical Use: constipation

Side Effects: diarrhea, nausea, abdominal cramps, rash

Page 298

MOA: Reduces the net absorption of fluid and electrolytes and induces GI motility by stimulating Auerbach's plexus.

Clinical Uses: constipation, evacuation of the bowel prior to surgery or diagnostic exams

Side Effects: fluid and electrolyte deficiencies, abdominal cramps, pink coloration of urine and feces: *phenolphthalein*

Page 298

MOA: Brown, irritating gas which accesses the **lower respiratory tract** and causes irritation of lungs, eyes, nose and throat and pulmonary edema. At high concentrations acute pulmonary edema may be fatal.

Effects: exposure to high levels of NO_2 leads to **Silo-Fillers disease** which is characterized by cough and dyspnea presenting ≤ 30 hrs after exposure.

Page 302

MOA: A colorless, odorless and non-irritating gas which causes **tissue hypoxia** by competing with oxygen for hemoglobin binding (forms carboxy-Hb). Its affinity for hemoglobin is 200 times greater than that of oxygen.

Effects include headaches, decreased visual acuity, tachycardia and tachypnea, coma, respiratory failure, convulsions and death. **Treatment** includes removal of source and administration of pure oxygen gas.

Page 302

MOA: Acts as an **expectorant** to increase the volume and decrease the viscosity of tracheal and bronchial secretions.

Clinical Use: antitussive

Side Effects: rare

Page 299

Bipyridyls

Lead (Pb)

Arsenic

Mercury (Hg)

Vitamin B1 (thiamine)

Vitamin B3 (niacin, nicotinic acid)

Vitamin B12 (cobalamin)

Folic acid

Vitamin C (ascorbic acid)

Exposure: skin, lungs, GI

Acute effects: GI distress (vomiting, rice water stools), garlic breath, capillary transudation and hypotension.

Chronic effects: skin discoloration, malaise, fatigue and neurological symptoms

Page 304

Most common cause of heavy metal poisoning. Exposure by ingestion (70%) and by inhalation. A common means of exposure in children is by ingestion of lead-containing paint (pica).

Acute effects: abdominal colic and CNS alterations.

Chronic effects: GI distress, weight loss, peripheral neuropathy (including **wrist-drop** and foot-drop), lead lines on long bones in X-ray, anemia (microcytic, hypochromic), and infertility. Childhood encephalopathy: behavioral effects, ataxia, stupor, coma.

Page 304

Includes **paraquat**. Results in the formation of O_2 radicals and is only toxic if ingested.

Effects: GI irritation which initially presents as hematemesis and or blood in the stools; progressive pulmonary impairment and death.

Page 303

Deficiency: **Pellagra**: **dermatitis, diarrhea** and **dementia** (3 D's); glossitis, degeneration of posterior and lateral columns, death.

Clinical Uses: **pellagra**, **hyperlipidemia**, especially type IIb

Toxicology: flushing, pruritus, cramps, nausea, vomiting, hepatotoxicity, arrhythmias

Page 308

Deficiency: **Dry beri-beri**: peripheral neuropathy with muscle atrophy; **wet beri-beri**: characterized by high cardiac output failure.

Commonly observed in chronic alcoholics as **Wernicke syndrome** (dementia, ataxia, and ophthalmoplegia) and **Korsakoff's psychosis**.

Clinical Use: thiamine deficiency

Page 308

Elemental mercury: *Acute effects* include bronchitis, pneumonitis, tremor, excitability. *Chronic effects* include neurasthenic symptoms, tremor, personality changes.

Inorganic mercury: *Acute effects* include GI ulceration, bleeding and necrosis. Renal failure. *Chronic effects* include renal tubular toxicity and neurological alterations.

Organic mercury: *Chronic effects* include visual field and hearing changes, ataxic gait. Also, impaired intelligence and speech abnormalities

Page 304

Deficiency: **Scurvy**: subperiosteal, skin, subungual, and joint hemorrhages due to inadequate collagenous support of capillaries. Observed as tooth loss, gingivitis, inability to limit infections, poor wound healing, arrested skeletal development (children).

Clinical Uses: scurvy, supplementation during pregnancy

Page 309

Deficiency: Megaloblastic anemia and growth failure.

Folic acid deficiency can develop within months.

Clinical Uses: Megaloblastic anemia, **pregnant** or lactating women

Page 309

Deficiency: Hematologic: megaloblastic anemia, CNS: degeneration of the posterior columns of the spinal cord.

Vitamin B12 deficiency takes years to develop because body stores are used up slowly.

Clinical Use: **Megaloblastic anemia**

Page 308

Insulin Preparations

Ultrashort Acting:
- Zinc insulin ("regular insulin")
- Prompt insulin zinc (semilente)

Short Acting:
- Isophane insulin suspension (NPH)
- Insulin zinc suspension (lente)

Long Acting:
- Protamine zinc insulin (PZI)
- Extended zinc insulin (ultralente)

Oral Hypoglycemics

Sulfonylureas:
- Tolbutamide
- Acetohexamide
- Tolazamide
- Chlorpropamide
- Glyburide
- Glipizide

Metformin

Ethanol

Disulfiram

Amphetamines

- Dextroamphetamine
- Methamphetamine
- Methylphenidate

Cocaine

Marijuana

Niclosamide

MAO: Thought to decrease hepatic glucose production and improve insulin sensitivity by increasing peripheral glucose uptake and utilization. Does not stimulate the β cells of the pancreas to secrete insulin.

Clinical Use: type II diabetics (NIDDM) refractory to dietary modifications alone

Side Effects: anorexia, diarrhea, nausea, vomiting, flatulence, and lactic acidosis

Page 269

MAO: Stimulate secretion of insulin by β-cells of the pancreas by blocking K^+ channels causing depolarization. This triggers insulin release from the β-cells of the pancreas. In addition, the sulfonylureas decrease glucagon levels and increase the binding of insulin to its receptors.

Clinical Use: type II diabetics (NIDDM) refractory to dietary modifications alone

Side Effects: hypoglycemia, nausea, vomiting, cutaneous reactions and hematologic effects

Page 268

Clinical Use: type I diabetics (IDDM)

Side Effects: insulin shock, antigenic response, weight gain, local sensitivity at injection site.

Page 267

MOA: Stimulates presynaptic dopamine release. Effects include: euphoria, increased attention, insomnia, decreased appetite and increased motor activity.

Clinical Uses: attention deficit hyperactivity disorder (ADHD), narcolepsy, obesity

Overdose is observed as anxiety, aggressiveness, delusions, headache, hallucinations, cardiac arrhythmias and circulatory collapse.

Page 80

MOA: An **aldehyde dehydrogenase inhibitor** which causes the accumulation of acetaldehyde when ethanol is consumed

Clinical Use: **alcoholism**

Side Effects: flushing, nausea, hypotension and tachycardia due to an accumulation of acetaldehyde

Page 78

MOA: A CNS depressant which works through GABA receptors to enhance GABA mediated synaptic neurotransmission

Clinical Uses: methanol overdose, ethylene glycol overdose

Side Effects: acute effects include sedation, disinhibition, euphoria and ataxia. Chronic effects include tolerance and dependence, ↓ liver function, GI irritation, Wernicke-Korsakoff syndrome, Fetal alcohol syndrome.

Page 78

MOA: Inhibits oxidative phosphorylation in the mitochondria of cestodes.

Clinical Uses: DOC for most cestode infections, including *T. saginata, T. solium, D. latum and H. nana.* It is only effective against these intestinal tapeworms; it is ineffective against cysticercosis (praziquantel is used) and in treating *E. granulosus* (mebendazole is used).

Side Effects: GI effects

Page 208

MOA: The active component is **∂-9THC** which acts on its own receptors. Effects include euphoria, sedation and altered judgement and time sense. Peripheral effects include increased heart rate, blood pressure, hunger, **reddening of conjunctiva**, dry mouth and bronchodilation.

Clinical Uses: **Dronabinol**, a pharmaceutical preparation of ∂-9THC, is used in AIDS-related anorexia and as an antiemetic agent in chemotherapy.

Page 82

MOA: Blocks the dopamine transporter (↑ dopaminergic stimulation) and prevents norepinephrine and serotonin reuptake. Effects include increased alertness, arousal, euphoria, increased heart rate and blood pressure.

Clinical use: local anesthetic

Overdose is observed as excitation, psychosis (formication, "cocaine bugs"), convulsions, respiratory depression and coma.

Page 81

Resins

Cholestyramine
Colestipol

Niacin

Gemfibrozil

Paclitaxel

Etoposide

Leuprolide

H_2-Blockers

Cimetidine
Ranitidine
Famotidine
Nizatidine

Cromolyn Sulfate

MOA: Decreases serum triglycerides by decreasing hepatic secretion of VLDL and increasing lipoprotein lipase activity in capillary endothelial cells.

Clinical Uses: **Type IIb**, III, **IV** and **V** hyperlipidemias

Side Effects: stomach pain, gas, rash, gallstones

Other: Clofibrate is similar to gemfibrozil but used infrequently due to its toxicities.

Page 147

MOA: Decreases production of VLDL resulting in ↓LDL. Increases HDL via an unknown mechanism.

Clinical Uses: **Type IIa**, **IIb**, **III**, **IV** and **V** hyperlipidemias, niacin deficiency, **Pellagra**

Side Effects: GI effects, intense cutaneous flush, pruritus,

Page 146

MOA: Promote the excretion of bile salts by forming an insoluble complex in the small intestine. This increases the conversion of cholesterol to bile acids and increases the number of LDL receptors in the liver which removes LDL from the plasma.

Clinical Uses: **Type IIa**, **IIb** hyperlipidemias,

Side Effects: **constipation**, steatorrhea, **decreased absorption** of fat soluble vitamins and certain drugs

Page 146

MOA: Long acting **synthetic GnRH analog** which are used to inhibit the release of FSH and LH from the anterior pituitary when administered in a continuous fashion.

Clinical Uses: Prostatic carcinoma, endometriosis

Page 220

MOA: Stabilizes the **DNA topoisomerase II**-DNA complex causing double strand DNA breaks during DNA replication.

Cell cycle specific for **S** and **G2** phases

Clinical Uses: Testicular carcinoma (component of VBE

Page 219

MOA: Binds to tubulin promoting the **formation** and preventing the dissolution of microtubules.

Cell-cycle phase specific for **M phase**

Clinical Use: Ovarian carcinoma

Page 219

MOA: Inhibits the release of histamine from mast cells.

Clinical Use: **asthma** prophylaxis

Side Effects: bronchospasm, cough or wheezing

Page 283

MOA: Competitively inhibits histamine at H_2-receptors

Clinical Uses: duodenal and gastric ulcers, Zollinger-Ellison syndrome, gastroesophageal reflux disease

Side Effects: sedation, headache, dizziness, GI distress, muscle pain, endocrine effects, inhibits P_{450} enzymes

Note: Ranitidine, famotidine and nizatidine have less CNS, endocrine effects than cimetidine and do not inhibit the P_{450} system

Page 283